PROGRESS IN CLINICAL AND BIOLOGICAL RESEARCH

Series Editors

RECENT TITLES

Please contact the publisher for information about previous titles in this series.

EORTC Genitourinary Group Monograph 5

PROGRESS AND CONTROVERSIES IN ONCOLOGICAL UROLOGY II

European Organization for Research on the Treatment of Cancer
Genitourinary Group Monograph Series

SERIES EDITORS

Louis Denis
Department of Urology
A.Z. Middelheim
Antwerp, Belgium

Fritz H. Schröder
Department of Urology
Erasmus University Rotterdam
Rotterdam, The Netherlands

Monograph 1: **Progress and Controversies in Oncological Urology,**
Karl H. Kurth, Frans M.J. Debruyne, Fritz H. Schroeder,
Ted A.W. Splinter, and Theo D.J. Wagener, *Editors*

Monograph 2: Published in two volumes: **Part A: Therapeutic Principles in
Metastatic Prostatic Cancer. Part B: Superficial Bladder Tumors,**
Fritz H. Schroeder and Brian Richards, *Editors*

Monograph 3: **Developments in Bladder Cancer,** Louis Denis, Tadao Niijima,
George Prout, Jr., and Fritz H. Schröder, *Editors*

Monograph 4: **Management of Advanced Cancer of Prostate and Bladder,**
Philip H. Smith and Michele Pavone-Macaluso, *Editors*

Monograph 5: **Progress and Controversies in Oncological Urology II,**
Fritz H. Schröder, Jan G.M. Klijn, Karl H. Kurth, Herbert M. Pinedo,
A.W. Splinter, and Herman J. de Voogt, *Editors*

EORTC Genitourinary Group Monograph 5

PROGRESS AND CONTROVERSIES IN ONCOLOGICAL UROLOGY II

Proceedings of an International Symposium Held in Amsterdam, March 19–21, 1987

Editors

Fritz H. Schröder
Department of Urology
Erasmus University Hospital
3000 DR Rotterdam
The Netherlands

Jan G.M. Klijn
Department of Internal Medicine
Rotterdam Radiotherapeutic Institute
3075 EA Rotterdam
The Netherlands

Karl H. Kurth
Department of Urology
Erasmus University Hospital
3000 DR Rotterdam
The Netherlands

Herbert M. Pinedo
Department of Internal Medicine
Free University Hospital
1007 MB Amsterdam
The Netherlands

Ted A.W. Splinter
Department of Oncology
Erasmus University Hospital
3000 DR Rotterdam
The Netherlands

Herman J. de Voogt
Department of Urology
Free University Hospital
1007 MB Amsterdam
The Netherlands

ALAN R. LISS, INC. • NEW YORK

Address all Inquiries to the Publisher
Alan R. Liss, Inc., 41 East 11th Street, New York, NY 10003

Copyright © 1988 Alan R. Liss, Inc.

Printed in the United States of America

Library of Congress Cataloging in Publication Data

Congress on Progress and Controversies in Oncological
    Urology II (1987 : Amsterdam, Netherlands)
    Progress and controversies in oncological urology II.

    (Progress in clinical and biological research ;
v. 269) (EORTC Genitourinary Group monograph ; 5)
    Includes bibliographies and index.
        1. Genitourinary organs—Cancer—Congresses.
2. Prostate—Cancer—Congresses. I. Schröder, F. H.
II. Title. III. Series. IV. Series: Genitourinary
Group monograph series ; monograph 5. [DNLM: 1. Uro-
genital Neoplasms—congresses.   Wl PR668E v.269 /
WJ 160 C749p 1987]
RC280.G4C59 1987   616.99'46   88-680
ISBN 0-8451-5119-3

Contents

Contributors

N.K. Aaronson, The Netherlands Cancer Institute, Department of Social Medicine, 1066 CX Amsterdam, The Netherlands [261]

Nina Aass, Department of Medical Oncology and Radiotherapy, The Norwegian Radiumhospital, Oslo, Norway [481]

Ryoetsu Abe, Department of Urology, Akita University School of Medicine, Akita 010, Japan [551]

R. Ackermann, Department of Urology, University of Düsseldorf, D-4000 Düsseldorf, Federal Republic of Germany [313]

Hideyuki Akaza, Department of Urology, Faculty of Medicine, The University of Tokyo, Tokyo 113, Japan [243,539]

H.W. Bauer, Department of Urology and Outpatient Clinic, Freie Universität Berlin, Federal Republic of Germany [33]

Marluce Bibbo, Section of Cytopathology, The University of Chicago, Chicago, IL 60637 [11]

Jan H.M. Blom, Department of Urology, Erasmus University Hospital, Rotterdam, The Netherlands [209,509,533,601]

E.A. Boedefeld, Studienzentrale, Medizin Univ. Klinik, 53 Bonn 1, Federal Republic of Germany [407]

C.G.G. Boeken Kruger, Department of Urology, Zuiderziekenhuis, Rotterdam, The Netherlands [579]

Claude Bollack, Service de Chirurgie Urologique, Hospices Civils, Strasbourg Cedex, France [233]

Aldo Bono, Department of Urology, Osp. Di Cicolo e Fundazione E.S. Macchi, Varese, Italy [199]

C. Bouffioux, Department of Urology, University of Liege, Liege, Belgium [525]

E. Boven, Free University Hospital, Amsterdam, The Netherlands [461]

R. Bussar-Maatz, Urologische Klinik, Urban Krankenhaus, 1 Berlin 61, Federal Republic of Germany [407]

Gerald W. Chodak, Section of Urology, Department of Surgery, The University of Chicago, Chicago, IL 60637 [11,87]

E.H. Cooper, Unit for Cancer Research, University of Leeds, Leeds LS2 9NL, England [43]

F. Calais da Silva, Hopital Desterro, Venda Nova, 2700 Amadora, Portugal [261]

The numbers in brackets are the opening page numbers of the contributors' articles.

C.J. Davis, Jr., Armed Forces Institute of Pathology, Washington, DC 20306 **[329]**

F.M.J. Debruyne, Department of Urology, University Hospital, Nijmegen, The Netherlands **[511]**

W.H. de Jong, Dutch National Institute of Public Health and Environmental Hygiene, Bilthoven, The Netherlands **[511]**

Jean B. deKernion, Department of Surgery, Division of Urology, UCLA School of Medicine, Los Angeles, CA 90024 **[347]**

L. Denis, Department of Urology, University Hospital Middelheim, Antwerp, Belgium **[579]**

M. de Pauw, EORTC Data Center, Brussels, Belgium **[381,461,525,579]**

Herman J. de Voogt, Department of Urology, Free University Hospital, Amsterdam, The Netherlands **[69,97,109,121,139,261,579]**

E.G.E. de Vries, Department of Internal Medicine, University Hospital, Groningen, The Netherlands **[429]**

John P. Donohue, Department of Urology, Indiana University, University Hospital A112, Indianapolis, IN 46223 **[451]**

C. Estrada Arras, Department of Clinica de Noroeste, Juares y Yucatan, Hermosillo, Sonora, Mexico **[199]**

William R. Fair, Urology Service, Memorial Sloan-Kettering Cancer Center, New York, NY 10021 **[289]**

Sophie D. Fosså, Department of Medical Oncology and Radiotherapy, The Norwegian Radiumhospital, Oslo, Norway **[481]**

M.P.H. Franssen, Department of Urology, University Hospital, Nijmegen, The Netherlands **[511]**

Hubert G.W. Frohmüller, Department of Urology, University of Würzburg Medical School, D-8700 Würzburg, Federal Republic of Germany **[21]**

Hermann Frommhold, Department of Urology and Radiotherapy, University of Innsbruck, A-6020 Innsbruck, Austria **[591]**

A.D.H. Geboers, Department of Urology, University Hospital, Nijmegen, The Netherlands **[511]**

Richard P. Golding, Departments of Urology and Radiology, Free University Hospital, Amsterdam, The Netherlands **[69]**

R.R. Hall, Department of Urology, Freeman Hospital, Newcastle Upon Tyne, United Kingdom **[569]**

A. Harris, Newcastle General Hospital, Newcastle, United Kingdom **[461]**

Franz Hering, Division of Urology, Department of Surgery, University of Basel, CH-4031 Basel, Switzerland **[227]**

A. Horwich, Institute of Cancer Research and The Royal Marsden Hospital, Sutton, Surrey, SM2 5PT, United Kingdom **[471]**

D. Jacqmin, Service de Chirurgie, Hospices Civils de Strasbourg, Strasbourg Cedex, France **[579]**

Gerhard Jakse, Department of Urology and Radiotherapy, University of Innsbruck, A-6020 Innsbruck, Austria **[591]**

David R. Jones, Department of Urology, Gwent Urological Centre, St. Woolos Hospital, Newport, Gwent NP9 4SZ; and Academic Department of Radiology, University Hospital of Wales, Cardiff, United Kingdom **[57]**

W.G. Jones, University Department of Radiotherapy, Cookridge Hospital, Leeds LS16 6QB, Great Britain [159,243,381,461,579]

Roland Kath, Innere Klinik und Poliklinik (Tumorforschung), West German Tumour Center, Universitaetsklinikum, D-4300 Essen 1, Federal Republic of Germany [439]

Tetsuro Kato, Department of Urology, Akita University School of Medicine, Akita 010, Japan [551]

S.B. Kaye, Gartnavel Hospital, Glasgow, United Kingdom [381,461]

Paul Keller, Section of Urology, Department of Surgery, The University of Chicago and the Pritzker School of Medicine, Chicago, IL 60637 [87]

K. Kleinschmidt, Urologische Klinik, Urban Krankenhaus, 1 Berlin 61, Federal Republic of Germany [407]

Jan G.M. Klijn, Department of Internal Medicine, Rotterdam Radiotherapeutic Institute, 3075 EA Rotterdam, The Netherlands [327,345,357,379]

T. Kotake, University Department of Radiotherapy, Cookridge Hospital, Leeds LS16 6QB, United Kingdom [243]

Karl H. Kurth, Department of Urology, Erasmus University Hospital, 3000 DR Rotterdam, The Netherlands [157,175,193,525]

Donald L. Lamm, Department of Urology, WVU Medical Center, Morgantown, WV 26506 [497]

Masatsugu Moriyama, Department of Urology, Akita University School of Medicine, Akita 010, Japan [551]

F.K. Mostofi, Armed Forces Institute of Pathology, Washington, DC 20306 [209,329]

N.H. Mulder, Department of Internal Medicine, University Hospital, Groningen, The Netherlands [429]

P.O.M. Mulder, Department of Internal Medicine, University Hospital, Groningen, The Netherlands [429]

Gerald P. Murphy, Department of Urology, State University of New York at Buffalo, School of Medicine and Urologic Cooperative Oncology Group, Buffalo, NY 14214 [131,187]

Donald W.W. Newling, Department of Urology, Princess Royal Hospital, Hull, United Kingdom [43,199,579]

Norbert Niederle, Innere Klinik und Poliklinik (Tumorforschung), West German Tumour Center, Universitaetsklinikum, D-4300 Essen 1, Federal Republic of Germany [439]

Kenichiro Okada, Department of Urology, Faculty of Medicine, Kyoto University, Kyoto 606, Japan [211]

Robert F. Ozols, Medicine Branch, Clinical Oncology Program, Division of Cancer Treatment, National Cancer Institute, Bethesda, MD 20892 [419]

David F. Paulson, Division of Urology, Duke University Medical Center, Durham, NC 27710 [211,359]

M.J. Peckham, British Postgraduate Medical Federation, London WC1N 3EJ, United Kingdom [471]

W. Brian Peeling, Department of Urology, Gwent Urological Centre, St. Woolos Hospital, Newport NP9 4SZ, United Kingdom [57]

Martin I. Resnick, Division of Urology, Case Western Reserve University School of Medicine, Cleveland, OH 44106 [111]

Brian Richards, Department of Urology, York District Hospital, York, England **[177, 233]**

Alastair W.S. Ritchie, Department of Surgery, Division of Urology, UCLA School of Medicine, Los Angeles, CA 90024 **[347]**

Ernest E. Roberts, Academic Department of Radiology, University Hospital of Wales, Cardiff, United Kingdom **[57]**

Melville R.G. Robinson, Department of Urology, The General Infirmary, Pontefract, West Yorkshire, WF8 1PL, England **[43,147]**

E.J. Ruitenberg, Dutch National Institute of Public Health and Environmental Hygiene, Bilthoven, The Netherlands **[511]**

Georg Rutishauser, Urologische Klinik, Abteilung fuer Chirurgie der Universitaet, Kantonspital Basel, CH-4031 Basel, Switzerland **[211, 227]**

Peter G. Ryan, Department of Urology, Gwent Urological Centre, St. Woolos Hospital, Newport NP9 4SZ, United Kingdom **[57]**

Kazunari Sato, Department of Urology, Akita University School of Medicine, Akita 010, Japan **[551]**

Max E. Scheulen, Innere Klinik und Poliklinik (Tumorforschung), West German Tumour Center, Universitaetsklinikum, D-4300 Essen 1, Federal Republic of Germany **[439]**

Carl G. Schmidt, Innere Klinik und Poliklinik (Tumorforschung), West German Tumour Center, Universitaetsklinikum, D-4300 Essen 1, Federal Repubic of Germany **[439]**

Harry W. Schoenberg, Section of Urology, Department of Surgery, The University of Chicago and the Pritzker School of Medicine, Chicago, IL 60637 **[11,87]**

H. Schraffordt Koops, Department of Surgical Oncology, University Hospital, Groningen, The Netherlands **[429]**

L.M.H. Schreinemachers, Department of Urology, Groot Ziekengasthuis, Den Bosch, The Netherlands **[511]**

Fritz H. Schröder, Department of Urology, Erasmus University Hospital, 300 DR Rotterdam, The Netherlands **[xxi,19,31,55,67,71,579]**

Siegfried Seeber, Innere Klinik und Poliklinik (Tumorforschung), West German Tumour Center, Universitaetsklinikum, D-4300 Essen 1, Federal Republic of Germany **[439]**

I.A. Sesterhenn, Armed Forces Institute of Pathology, Washington, DC 20306 **[329]**

C. Th. Smit Sibinga, Regional Red Cross Blood Bank Groningen-Drenthe, Groningen, The Netherlands **[429]**

Jill K. Siddall, Unit for Cancer Research, University of Leeds, Leeds LS2 9NL, England **[43]**

D. Th. Sleijfer, University Hospital, Groningen, The Netherlands **[381,429,461]**

Franklin L. Smith, Section of Urology, Department of Surgery, The University of Chicago, Chicago, IL 60637 **[11]**

P.J. Spaander, Department of Pathology, Red Cross Hospital, The Hague, The Netherlands **[209,381]**

Ted A.W. Splinter, Department of Oncology, Erasmus University Hospital, 3000 DR Rotterdam, The Netherlands [393,405,417,427,437,459,461,469,479, 493,579]

P.A. Steerenberg, Dutch National Institute of Public Health and Environmental Hygiene, Bilthoven, The Netherlands [511]

Gerrit Stoter, Free University Hospital, Amsterdam, The Netherlands [381,461,549,567,577,579,589,599]

Stefan Suciu, EORTC Data Center, 1000 Brussels, Belgium [275]

Richard J. Sylvester, EORTC Data Center, 1000 Brussels, Belgium [275,381,461,525]

W.W. ten Bokkel Huinink, Netherlands Cancer Institute, Amsterdam, The Netherlands [381,461]

F.J.W. ten Kate, University Hospital Dijkzigt, Rotterdam, The Netherlands [579]

Jaap Valk, Departments of Urology and Radiology, Free University Hospital, Amsterdam, The Netherlands [69]

A.J. van der Eb, Department of Medical Biochemistry, University of Leiden, Sylvius Laboratories, 2300 RA Leiden, The Netherlands [1]

A.P.M. van der Meijden, Department of Urology, University Hospital, Nijmegen, The Netherlands [511]

Erik P. van der Weijer, Department of Urology, Free University Hospital, Amsterdam, The Netherlands [69]

M.J.W. van Leeuwen, IKO Cancer Center, Nijmegen, The Netherlands [511]

A.T. van Oosterom, Department of Oncology, Hospital of Antwerp, Antwerp, Belgium; and University Hospital, Leiden, The Netherlands [243,381,461]

H. van Ormondt, Department of Medical Biochemistry, University of Leiden, Sylvius Laboratories, 2300 RA Leiden, The Netherlands [1]

Thea E.G. van Zanten, Department of Radiology, Free University Hospital, Amsterdam, The Netherlands [69]

C.P.J. Vendrik, University Hospital, Utrecht, The Netherlands [381]

Ursula B. Wandl, Innere Klinik und Poliklinik (Tumorforschung), West German Tumour Center, Universitaetsklinikum, D-4300 Essen 1, Federal Republic of Germany [439]

Hiroki Watanabe, Department of Urology, Kyoto Prefectural University of Medicine, Kyoto, Japan 602 [99]

L. Weissbach, Urologische Klinik, Urban Krankenhaus, 1 Berlin 61, Federal Republic of Germany [407]

John N. Wettlaufer, Division of Urology, Department of Surgery, University of Colorado Health Sciences Center, Denver, CO 80262 [395]

Willet F. Whitmore, Jr., Memorial Sloan-Kettering Cancer Center, New York, NY 10021 [123]

P.H.B. Willemse, Department of Internal Medicine, University Hospital Groningen, The Netherlands [429]

Manfred Wirth, Department of Urology, University of Würzburg Medical School, D-8700 Würzburg, Federal Republic of Germany [21]

Hidetoshi Yamanaka, Department of Urology, Gunma University, Gunma, Japan [275]

Osamu Yoshida, Department of Urology, Faculty of Medicine, Kyoto University, Kyoto City, Japan [211]

Preface

This volume is the fifth EORTC-Genitourinary Group Monograph to be published within three years and the second complete report resulting from a congress on the issue "Progress and Controversies in Oncological Urology II." The volume was conceived for professionals involved in planning and carrying out clinical research in oncological urology. It can serve as a reference book, but progress in this field is rapid, so its value will be limited to a number of years. The editors hope that the issue will serve as a guideline for rational management of urological malignancies by giving an update of most controversial issues in this field.

In this volume a first attempt is made to reach international consensus on a number of features of prostatic carcinoma. The process of achieving consensus was as follows. A group of internationally recognized experts was brought together as a working party to deal with each one of the eight issues for consensus. A chairman and co-chairmen were nominated. The chairman prepared a position paper and rotated it to the members of his working party prior to the meeting. The position paper was commented upon and returned to the chairman, who then considered all comments and revised the paper accordingly. During the meeting in Amsterdam in March 1987, the audience was split into groups of 30–40 participants in consensus seminars. During those seminars the revised position paper was discussed in detail and again revised by the chairman and/or his co-chairmen according to comments and discussion. These papers are finally included in this issue.

Clinical research in oncology represents a very powerful tool for further progress. However, knowledge and consensus concerning basic facts like minimal requirements for clinical studies, the role of prognostic factors and response criteria, and a trial technology adapted to the needs of each individual tumor are prerequisites if one wants to obtain proper and meaningful results that withstand international comparison. The editors hope that with this book a small step in this direction can be made.

The congress on "Progress and Controversies in Oncological Urology II" was sponsored by Hoechst A.G., Federal Republic of Germany; Imperial Chemical Industries (I.C.I.), U.K.; and Schering Corporation, U.S.A.

F.H. Schröder

EORTC Genitourinary Group Monograph 5: Progress and Controversies in Oncological Urology II, pages 1-9

DOMINANT AND RECESSIVE ONCOGENES IN CARCINOGENESIS

H. van Ormondt and A.J. van der Eb

Department of Medical Biochemistry, University of Leiden, Sylvius Laboratories, P.O.Box 9503, 2300 RA Leiden, The Netherlands

INTRODUCTION

When a normal cell becomes cancerous it does so because something goes awry in the intricate system of controls that govern its proliferation. The most obvious way one could envisage this to occur was through the loss of one or more regulatory functions. However, when it became possible to study oncogenesis at the molecular level, the first experimental data pointed in another direction: cancer was found to be caused by mutations or DNA rearrangements that change normal genes into dominant oncogenes rather than abolish regulatory genes. But the most recent evidence suggests that both models contribute to our understanding of how malignancies arise.

Dominant oncogenes

The first known examples of dominant oncogenes were the oncogenes of tumor viruses. In the case of RNA tumor (retro-)viruses, these oncogenes were later found to be of animal cellular origin, having accidentally found their way into the viral genomes by some illegitimate recombination event. More than 20 different oncogenes have been discovered in retroviruses which all proved to be derived from the animal hosts.

Activation by mutation

In 1979 Weinberg and his colleagues discovered that DNA isolated from human bladder carcinoma cells was capable of transforming the murine cell line NIH 3T3 into oncogenic cells. From this they deduced that the tumor cells contained a gene that had acquired oncogenic properties, presumably due to mutation. Subsequent characterization showed it to be identical to the H-ras gene, a human homolog of the oncogene of the Harvey rat sarcoma virus (a retrovirus). Further experiments revealed that between 15-20% of the human tumor DNAs had transforming activity in NIH 3T3 cells, and that in most cases a ras gene was responsible. The difference between the normal ras protooncogenes and their transforming counterparts in all cases was a point mutation resulting in a single amino-acid substitution, at positions 12, 13 or 61 of the ras protein. This change, apparently, was sufficient to alter the protein's functional properties. With this discovery it was proved for the first time that the old theory claiming that cancer is a result of somatic mutation, was indeed correct.

Activation by enhanced expression

In the years following Weinberg's discovery, a number of other oncogenes (see Table 1) were found to be

TABLE 1. Examples of oncogenes involved in human neoplasia

gene	(putative) function in normal cell
ras (H-, K-, N-)	GTPase; possible role in transfer of growth factor signals
myc (c-, N-, L-)	transcription activator (?); role in initiation of cell proliferation by growth factors
erb-B	EGF receptor; protein kinase
abl	protein kinase
sis (?)	PDGF (platelet-derived growth factor)

implicated in various human malignancies. It became clear that the mode of activation just described for the ras genes, i.e. mutation, is not the only pathway by which a proto-oncogene is converted into an active oncogene.

In a number of instances, rearrangement of proto-oncogenes is the cause of activation. This is best illustrated for the case of myc, which is one of the most prominent oncogenes, and is activated by DNA arrangements

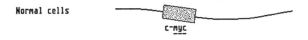

Normal cells

c-myc

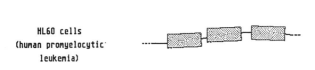

HL60 cells
(human promyelocytic
leukemia)

amplification of c-myc (20-30x) ⟶ elevated c-myc expression

Activated second oncogene: N-ras

Fig.1. The human cell line HL60 which is derived from a promyelocytic leukemia contains 20-30 copies of the myc proto-oncogene. As a result, these cells exhibit an elevated expression of this gene.

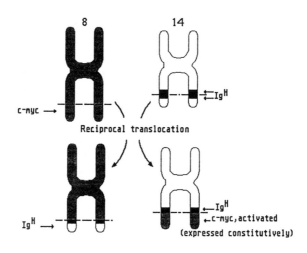

8   14

c-myc ⟶   Ig^H

Reciprocal translocation

Ig^H ⟶   ←Ig^H
                          ←c-myc, activated
                          (expressed constitutively)

Fig.2. In Burkitt's lymphoma cells a reciprocal translocation has taken place between chromosomes 8 and 14. As a result, the myc gene alights in a region where active transcription (of Ig heavy chain RNAs) takes place. This causes the myc gene to be overexpressed.

resulting in deregulated or enhanced expression. E.g., in
the human leukemic cell line HL-60 the myc gene is amplified 20-30x, which in its turn leads to an elevated myc
protein level (Fig.1). In some tumors, gene amplification
is a recurrent phenomenon (e.g. in small-cell lung carcinoma or in neuroblastoma), but it can also occur as an
occasional abnormality in numerous other cancers. Wherever
it has been found, myc gene amplification appears to
correlate with tumor progression and hence must be a late
event. How amplification arises, is as yet unknown.

Activation of myc can also be caused by chromosomal
translocations, as is the case in Burkitt lymphoma cells.
In these cells the most frequent translocation involves
chromosomes 8 and 14, as a result of which the myc gene
moves from its original location on chromosome 8 to a
region on chromsome 14 where the immunoglobulin heavy
chain genes are situated. One assumes that by this move
the myc gene is freed from its normal regulatory constraints, and, having alit in a transcriptionally active
region (Burkitt lymphoma consists of partially differentiated B-lymphoid cells which produce immunoglobulins) may
be expressed constitutively (Fig.2). This mode of expression, as recent information has borne out, will force the
cells to remain in the proliferative state, and block the
way to differentiation. Only if myc expression is ar-
rested, cells will stop dividing or may initiate terminal
differentiation.

Chimaeric oncoprotein

Chromosomal translocation may have yet another
result also leading to oncogene activation, as is exempli-
fied by the Philadelpha translocation. Here, a reciprocal
translocation between chromosomes 9 and 22 results in the
transfer of the abl protooncogene from chromosome 9 to a
specific gene on chromosome 22. As a consequence, a new
hybrid gene is formed starting in the bcr gene of chromosome 22 and continuing in abl. The resulting chimaeric
protein has altered enzymatic properties. So in this case,
the chromosomal translocation affects biochemical function, and not the regulation of expression.

More than one oncogene in cancer cells

In the past few years evidence has accumulated
indicating that activation of just one oncogene is not
sufficient to convert the cell to a cancerous state, but
that for this transition more steps are required. Similar
observations were done in our own laboratory, when it was
established that oncogenic transformation of primary

rodent cells by adenovirus DNA required the introduction of both the E1A and E1B transcription units into the target cells.

The human leukemic cell line HL-60 of which we mentioned above that it harbours an amplified myc gene, was found to have a mutated ras gene, as well. Burkitt lymphoma cells, in addition to the chromosomal transposition, have also incurred a mutation in a member of the ras gene family.

Direct proof that at least two oncogenes are required for oncogenesis came from experiments with cultured cells exposed to myc and ras genes, as shown in Table II. The 3T3 cell line requires the transfection of only one oncogene

TABLE 11. Transfection of cultured cells with ras and myc

Cells + oncogenes	Oncogenic transformation
3T3 cells + T24 ras	+
REF cells + T24 ras	-
REF cells + T24 ras + myc	+

to become oncogenic, whereas the primary (diploid) rat embryo fibroblasts need two, the ras gene and the myc gene, the myc gene apparently being required to immortalize the cells. In the 3T3 cell line this immortalization had already occurred spontaneously (apparently not as a result of myc activation).

Functions of protooncogenes.

In order to understand how oncogenes cause cancer, it is necessary to understand their function in the normal cell. All available information indicates that the proto-oncogenes are involved in the regulation of cell proliferation (and possibly cell differentiation). If a cell is to divide, it will do so under the influence of growth factors in the surrounding medium which bind to specific receptors on the cell surface and by doing so activate their receptors. These activated membrane proteins then transmit a growth-stimulating signal into the cell, which will eventually reach the nucleus by way of a number of intermediary steps. The result is the onset of expression of a number of genes, among which the proto-oncogenes myc and fos. The myc and fos gene products are proteins that

exert their functions in the nucleus. A few hours after
their induction, one observes the onset of DNA replication
followed by cell division. It should be noted, however,
that at least two growth factors are required for efficient progression through the cell cycle. It then turned
out that several of the intermediate stages in the signal
transduction pathway were, in fact, regulated by products
of protooncogenes: the oncogene sis encodes a subunit of
the platelet-derived growth factor (PDGF), erb-B the EGF
receptor, ras genes are assumed to code for membrane-asso-
ciated signal transfer proteins, while myc and fos are at
the end of the command chain in the nucleus. From the
above it is evident that changes in the structure or in
the expression level of the proto-oncogenes may cause the
deregulation of cell growth, which is one of the changes
characteristic of cancer cells.
Alternative pathways.
        In the preceding sections we have attempted to
describe the picture that has emerged in the years following Weinberg's original discovery: dominant oncogenes
arise from the mutational activation of cellular genes and
at least two such steps (often involving myc and ras) are
required for oncogenic transformation. However, this
picture apparently is an oversimplification which does not
fully explain a number of observations:
1. not more than 20% of tumors contain activated ras
   genes;
2. a similar proportion contains activated myc;
3. only a few examples with both activated ras and myc
   have become known.
        Some arguments can be made that should at least
partially meet the above problems. First, there certainly
must be more oncogenes than the ones identified to date.
And, secondly, as far as the activated ras genes are
concerned, several are known already that are so weakly
transforming in the customary NIH 3T3 cell assay that they
failed to be detected. To circumvent the latter problem,
Dr. Bos in our laboratory devised a methodology that
allows detection of all possible mutations at codons 12,
13 and 61 of the H-, K- and N-ras genes. The method which
makes use of hybridization of synthetic oligonucleotide
probes to in vitro amplified portions of the various ras
genes, is very sensitive and much faster than the original
laborious biological assay. In cooperation with Dr.
Vogelstein (Johns Hopkins, Baltimore) he screened a larger
number of colon cancers, and found 40% of them to contain

an activated K-<u>ras</u> gene.

A third way to explain the inconsistencies of the dominant oncogene theory would be, that there are alternative pathways to cancer which do not involve dominant oncogenes.

"Recessive oncogenes" and "Tumor suppressor" genes.

In fact, evidence is accumulating that not only dominant but also recessive mutations play a role in oncogenesis. Today, there are two major lines of evidence for this contention.

First, examples are known of tumors that are characterized by homozygosity of a specific chromosomal aberration. This situation is found in individuals with a hereditary predisposition for development of specific types of neoplasia, such as the hereditary form of retinoblastoma and Wilm's tumor. The normal cells of such patients already are heterozygous for this specific aberration. Thus, the risk that the patient will incur a similar mutation in the unaffected allel is fairly high. In the case of retinoblastoma, homozygosity (or hemizygosity) of the mutation, which has been mapped to chromosome 13q, will only lead to cancer when it occurs in a retina cell. The same patients may at a later age develop osteosarcoma characterized by the same chromosomal abnormality. The chromosomal locus for this disease has been cloned and, apparently, involves only one gene whose function is lost in the affected cells. In the latter case, and in Wilm's tumor, where the lesion has been mapped to chromosome 11p, the genes in question differ from e.g. <u>myc</u> and <u>ras</u> in that they must be inactivated in order for the tumor to develop. Their function in normal cells is still unknown, but they probably have a role in the control of differentiation of specific cells or tissues.

Secondly, fusion of tumor cells with normal diploid cells may cause suppression of the oncogenic phenotype (Fig.3). For instance, a gene present in normal human cells suppress the oncogenic activity of the mutated H-<u>ras</u> gene of bladder carcinoma (EJ) cells. From this, it should be inferred that the tumor cells were already defective for the tumor suppressor gene in question, which in this case seemed to be located also on chromosome 11. A further conclusion to be drawn from such experiments is that dominant oncogenes may only be able to exert their full activity when a tumor suppressor gene first is inactivated. Evidence has recently been presented that a high proportion of human bladder carcinomas is characterized

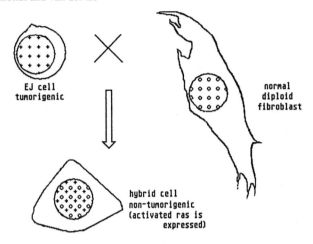

Fig.3. Fusion or normal rat fibroblasts with oncogenic human bladder tumor cells (harboring an activated H-ras gene) results in a hybrid in which the oncogenic activity of that gene is suppressed, presumably by a suppressor gene present in the normal cells.

also by homozygosity of a particular deletion of chromosome 11p. This suggests that bladder carcinoma also belongs to the group of tumors in which homozygosity of a specific gene mutation is an essential prerequisite for the tumor to develop.

CONCLUSION

The question whether the two (dominant and recessive) categories of oncogenes or cancer-related genes each are responsible for distinct pathways or carcinogenesis, or, on the other hand, cooperate in this process, remains to be resolved. However, the cell fusion experiments described in the previous paragraph suggests that they may work simultaneously, or even in collusion. The coming years hopefully will provide an answer to this important question.

REFERENCES

The reader is referred to the following review articles:
1. J.M. Bishop (1985) Cell 42, 23-38.
2. J.M. Bishop (1987) Science 235, 305-311.
3. M.D. Cole (1986) Ann.Rev.Genet. 20, 361-384.
4. T. Hunter (1984) Sci.Amer., Aug. 60-69.
5. R. Müller (1986) Trends Biochem. Sci. 11, 129-132.
6. L. Ratner, S.F. Josephs and F. Wong-Staal (1985)
   Ann.Rev.Microbiol. 39, 419-449.
7. H.E. Varmus (1984) Annu. Rev. Genet. 18, 553-612.
8. R.A. Weinberg (1985) Science 230, 770-776.

For a dissenting view:
9. P.H. Duesberg (1987) Cancer Res. 47, 1199-1220.

EORTC Genitourinary Group Monograph 5: Progress
and Controversies in Oncological Urology II, pages 11-18
© 1988 Alan R. Liss, Inc.

THE ROLE OF TRANSRECTAL ASPIRATION BIOPSY IN THE DIAGNOSIS OF CARCINOMA OF THE PROSTATE

Gerald W Chodak, Franklin L Smith, Marluce Bibbo
and Harry W Schoenberg

Section of Urology, Department of Surgery and Section
of Cytopathology, The University of Chicago, Chicago
Illinois 60637

INTRODUCTION

A fundamental problem with carcinoma of the prostate is that early detection is not easily accomplished. As a result, in the past 20 years, the mortality rate from this disease has continued to rise (American Cancer Society, 1983). In a recent survey, over 40% of patients had extracapsular spread of tumor at the time of diagnosis (Murphy et al., 1982).

One way to reduce the mortality rate from this disease is to detect a higher percentage of tumors that are still localized to the prostate. This may require a biopsy method that can detect smaller tumors.

The most common biopsy methods include transrectal and transperineal core punch biopsies (Murphy et al., 1982), which have false negative rates of 10% - 28% (Zincke et al., 1973, Bissada et al., 1977, Straus, 1968, Seka and Lindquist, 1963, Berletson, 1966). An alternative method is transrectal aspiration biopsy which employs a fine needle that can be safely passed through the rectum. Prompted by the current controversy over the role of aspiration biopsy, we have analyzed our data to determine the factors that impact on the reliability of this procedure.

MATERIALS AND METHODS

Transrectal aspiration biopsy was performed either

alone or in conjunction with a transperineal core biopsy as previously described (Chodak et al., 1984). At least three aspirates were made for each patient. These biopsies were performed on any male who had an abnormal digital rectal examination. The aspiration biopsy was performed without anesthesia or antibiotics, however, the transperineal biopsy was performed under spinal or general anesthesia. All of the aspiration biopsies were performed by either of two urologists, whereas the core biopsy was performed by the private physician for that case. Prostate cancer was confirmed either by a core biopsy, a radical prostatectomy, a pelvic lymph node dissection, the presence of metastases or at autopsy. If prostate cancer was diagnosed, patients were staged by chest X-ray, acid and alkaline phosphatase, and transrectal ultrasonography.

The criteria for malignant cytology included a loss of normal nuclear polarity, the presence of nucleoli and nuclear pleomorphism, a variation in cell size and shape,the presence of chromatin clumping, and the presence of acinar structures. Carcinoma was diagnosed by cytology providing that the slide showed a predominance of malignant cells. Many samples contained a small number of malignant appearing or highly atypical cells and these were interpreted as suspicious for cancer. Whenever possible, repeat biopsies were performed in these cases.

RESULTS

In order to gain experience with transrectal aspiration biopsy, we initially conducted a trial comparing this method to transperineal core biopsy. We found that the aspiration biopsy method was suspicious or diagnostic for prostate cancer in 98% (47/48) of the samples compared to a sensitivity of only 81% (38/47) for the transperineal core biopsy method.

Based on these results, the aspiration biopsy method was adopted as the initial procedure to evaluate all prostate abnormalities that warranted a biopsy. A total of 230 cases have been reviewed and the diagnosis on the cytology report has been recorded. The diagnosis was adenocarcinoma in 70 cases (30%), no evidence of cancer in 112 (49%), and in 48 (21%), the sample was suspicious for cancer or atypical cells were present. Because we believe that the latter category is abnormal, repeat biopsies have been recommended to this group. Thus far, a repeat biopsy has been performed in 28 cases in which the initial cytology showed highly atypical or slightly atypical cells. We found malignant cells in 73% of 22 patients whose initial biopsy showed highly atypical cells and 14% continued to show highly atypical cells (Table 1).

TABLE 1:   REBIOPSY RESULTS FOR PATIENTS
            WITH HIGHLY ATYPICAL CYTOLOGY

FINAL DIAGNOSIS	NO. (%)
Adenocarcinoma	16 (73%)
Highly atypical cytology	3 (14%)
Slight atypia	2 (9%)
Benign	1 (4%)
TOTAL	22

Only one patient had a completely benign repeat sample. A repeat biopsy was also performed on six patients with slight atypia and only one showed adenocarcinoma. The remaining five again showed slight atypia (N=3) or were benign (N=2). No complications have been observed for patients who only had an aspiration biopsy.

These results have enabled us to treat patients based solely on the cytology interpretation. Usually, each case of cancer is reviewed with the cytopathologist in order to reconfirm the diagnosis. If the malignant cells obtained by the aspiration biopsy are well-differentiated, we usually perform a core biopsy before proceeding with a radical prostatectomy because well-differentiated cells can be confused with atypical hyperplasia. The outcome for 53 patients who were diagnosed with prostate cancer only by aspiration biopsy is shown in Table 2. Twelve patients had a core biopsy performed prior to radical surgery.

TABLE 2:   TREATMENT OF PATIENTS BASED ON ASPIRATION
BIOPSY SHOWING MALIGNANT CELLS

TREATMENT	NO. PATIENTS
Core biopsy followed by surgery	12
Radical prostatectomy	9
Radiation therapy	12
Hormone therapy	13
I125 seed implants	2
Pelvic lymph node dissection	1
No treatment	4
Total	53

Four patients have not been treated because a core
biopsy was negative (N=2) or the patient refused (N=2).
In one patient, the radical prostatectomy specimen did not
confirm the diagnosis. This cytology has been re-reviewed
by two independent cytopathologists, and they confirmed
the diagnosis of moderately-differentiated adenocarcinoma.

DISCUSSION

Although prostate cancer can be suspected by the
digital rectal examination, confirmation by biopsy is an
absolute necessity. In one study, smooth or elevated
nodules or stony hardness were benign more often than they
were malignant (Jewett, 1956).

The most commonly used biopsy methods involve
removing a core of tumor by a punch biopsy procedure. The
disadvantages of these methods are that anesthesia is
required, there is a variable false negative rate,
infections may occur, and other complications, such as
bleeding or urinary retention may result.

The alternative procedure is transrectal aspiration
biopsy which was first described by Ferguson (Ferguson,
1930), and modified by Franzen and co-workers (Franzen   et
al., 1962). The advantages of aspiration biopsy are that
no anesthesia is required, it can be performed in the
office, the sensitivity is high, the complication rate is
low, and the cost is lower than most core biopsies.

For the past three years, we have used this method to

evaluate lesions detected by the digital examination. In a comparative study, we found that the sensitivity of the aspiration method was much higher than the sensitivity of the core procedure. The results reported in the literature, however, vary considerably.

In reviewing our data, several factors have been identified which might explain the poor results obtained by some investigators. In one report, the sensitivity with the aspiration method was only 73% (Lin et al., 1979). In that study, however, atypia was not considered abnormal. In contrast, we found that cancer was present in 73% of the patients with highly atypical cells on the aspiration. As a result, any patient with an atypical cytology should undergo a repeat procedure or have close follow-up observation.

Another important factor is the learning curve associated with this procedure. In our experience, the first 10 - 15 samples were of lesser quality than subsequent samples. To insure quality control, only two physicians performed the aspiration biopsy. Other studies in which many more physicians perform the biopsy will not have the same sensitivity. Nevertheless, for physicians who are interested in using this procedure, regular use of the aspiration method should result in excellent accuracy.

If an equivocal aspiration biopsy sample is obtained or if the cytology is negative but the lesion is very suspicious, performing a repeat aspiration is far easier than repeating the core biopsy. In the United States, many urologists employ general or spinal anesthesia to perform a transperineal core biospy. Repeating this method is much more costly and more of an inconvenience to the patient than is the aspiration biopsy. Although a transrectal core biopsy does not require the same amount of anesthesia, antibiotics must be administered and this method still has a significantly higher complication rate than the other procedures (Davison et al., 1971, Fawcett et al., 1975, Ruebust et al., 1979). Furthermore, the transrectal core biopsy does not always result in a high sensitivity. Both Ostroff (Ostroff et al., 1975) and Bissada (Bissada et al., 1977) reported a sensitivity of only 81%. Therefore, transrectal aspiration biopsy appears to be the ideal method to use because it is convenient and it has a low complication rate.

Two other explanations for our high sensitivity may
relate to our technique. We routinely take at least three
aspirates in order to assure an adequate sample, and test
different regions of the lesion. The accuracy associated
with each method will also depend on the size of the
lesion to be examined. Our interest in the aspiration
method developed because we were conducting a screening
program for prostate cancer and many of the patients had
only a slightly abnormal examination. In many of these
cases, we had little confidence that the core biopsy could
accurately sample the lesion. The aspiration biopsy
offered the advantage that the needle could be inserted
directly into the suspicious area that was adjacent to the
finger in the rectum. One reason to recommend greater use
of this procedure is that it may be possible to detect a
higher percentage of potentially curable tumors.

Although the aspiration biopsy method has many clear
advantages over the core procedures, it also has a few
potential disadvantages. First, the success is dependent
on the quality of the cytopathologist. As more experience
is gained, however, physicians will be able to gain
confidence in the interpretation. Until sufficient
expertise is available, samples can be referred to more
experienced cytopathologists. Also, because of the
learning curve, we recommend initially performing both the
aspiration biopsy and core biopsy in order to avoid
missing a tumor.

The last concern involves treating patients based
only on the cytology report. In the largest series,
Esposti (Esposti et al., 1975) found no false positive
cases using the aspiration method. We have found a single
case in which no tumor was found on the radical
prostatectomy specimen. Two explanations are that the
tumor was not completely resected or the lesion was small
and it was not found on routine histologic sectioning. To
avoid any potential problems, we recommend performing a
core biopsy if only well-differentiated cells are
aspirated.

In summary, transrectal aspiration biopsy is an
excellent method to use to examine lesions in the
prostate. The advantages of this method over other biopsy
methods support greater use of this procedure. We believe

that it should be used as the initial method to evaluate all prostate lesions detected by the digital examination. Furthermore, the procedure is sufficiently reliable to permit patients to be treated based solely on the result from the cytology. Attention to certain technical details should result in a high sensitivity with this procedure.

REFERENCES

American Cancer Society (1983). Cancer facts and figures.
Bertelsen S (1966). Transrectal needle biopsy of the prostate. Acta Chir Scand 357:266.
Bissada NK, Rountree GA and Sulieman JS (1977). Factors affecting accuracy and morbidity in transrectal biopsy of the prostate. Surg, Gyn & Obs 145:869.
Chodak GW, Bibbo M, Straus FH II and Wied GL (1984). Transrectal aspiration biopsy versus transperineal core biopsy for the diagnosis of carcinoma of the prostate. J Urol 132:480.
Davison P, Malament M (1971). Urinary contamination as a result of transrectal biopsy of the prostate. J Urol 105:545.
Esposti PL, Elman A and Norlen H (1975). Complications of transrectal aspiration biopsy of the prostate. Scand J Urol Nephrol 9:208.
Fawcett DP, Eykyn S, Bultitude MI (1975). Urinary tract infection following transrectal biopsy of the prostate. Br J Urol 47:679.
Ferguson RS (1939). Diagnosis and treatment of early carcinoma of the prostate. J Urol 42:774.
Franzen S, Giertz G and Zajicek J (1960). Cytological diagnosis of prostatic tumors by transrectal aspiration biopsy: A preliminary report. Br J Urol 32:193.
Hoskins JH and Mehlinger GT (1966). Needle biopsy of the prostate. Am Fam Physician GP 34:88.
Jewett HJ (1984). Prostatic Cancer: A personal view of the problem. J Urol 131:845.
Kaufman JJ, Ljung BM, Walther P and Waisman J (1982). Aspiration biopsy of prostate. Urol XIX:587.
Lin BPC, Davies WEL and Harmata PA (1979). Prostatic aspiration cytology. Pathology 11:607.
Murphy GP, Natarajan N, Pontes JE, Schmitz RI, Smart CR, Schmidt JD and Mettlin C (1982). The National Survey of Prostate Cancer in the United States by the American College of Surgeons. J Urol 82:928.

Ostroff EB, Almario J and Kramer H (1975). Transrectal
    needle method for biopsy of the prostate: Review of 90
    cases. Am Surg, pp 659.

Ruebush TK, McConville JH, Calia FM (1979). A double blind
    study of trimethoprim-sulfamethoxazole prophylaxis in
    patients having transrectal needle biopsy of the
    prostate. J Urol 122:492.

Sika JV and Lindquist HD (1963). Relationship of needle
    biopsy diagnosis of prostate to clinical signs of
    prostatic cancer; an evaluation of 300 cases. J Urol
    89:737.

Straus II FS (1968). Surgical pathology of prostatic
    needle biopsies. The Bulletin of Pathology, pp 236.

Zincke H, Campbell JT, Utz DC, Farrow GM, Anderson MJ
    (1973). Confidence in the negative transrectal needle
    biopsy. Surg. Gyn & Obs 136:78.

EORTC Genitourinary Group Monograph 5: Progress
and Controversies in Oncological Urology II, pages 19-20
© 1988 Alan R. Liss, Inc.

Discussion: The Role of Transrectal Aspiration Biopsy in
the Diagnosis of Carcinoma of the Prostate

Fritz H. Schroder, Rotterdam, The Netherlands

Schröder: Dr. Chodak, before you started fine needle aspiration biopsies, did the core biopsy delay your radical
prostatectomy in any way?

Chodak: I believe that some people feel that delay after
core biopsy is warranted because there may be inflammation
in the area due to the multiple core procedures. Indeed,
after fine needle aspiration biopsy one could decide to
proceed to radical prostatectomy more immediately.

Mostofi: I should just like to make the point that aspiration cytology is reliable only in the hands of the trained
cytologists. Those pathologists that usually do only histopathology are not capable to reliably read cytological
slides. This requires training. Training can best be obtained in Sweden. Fortunately, there are also three loca-
tions in the United States that can provide such training,
one in New York, one in Washington and one in Chicago.

Paulson: I should like you to lay aside that comment about
having to delay radical prostatectomy after a core biopsy.
Our experience with more than 500 radical prostatectomies
indicates that you do not have to delay the procedure after
core biopsy. Inflammation and scarring are reasonable concerns but from a clinical standpoint you do not have to wait
and delay the procedure.

Chodak: I would acknowledge that that is the case. But
certainly some people feel that a previous aspiration biopsy
facilitates a radical prostatectomy. I do know that Walsh
feels that way.

Schröder: I am wondering about your comment that only the
Gleason score predicts accurately the incidence of lymph
node involvement. Any other grading system, if properly
applied, should do the same thing. There should also be some

correlation between grading obtained on cytological specimens and lymph node involvement. Do you have any data on
that?

Chodak: Our data would indicate that the correlation is
quite inaccurate, mainly because most of the specimens are
moderately differentiated. My comment regards the individual
patient. In most cases grading does not help you to decide
what to do. In spite of that, we would not want to proceed
and do a core biopsy first, just to know the Gleason sum and
to have a better predictor of lymph node involvement. For
cytology specimens eventually the correlation will be the
same as has been shown in the literature, but I do not think
it will help in decision making as far as lymph node
involvement is concerned.

Debruyne: Dr. Chodak, you said that aspiration cytology can
be used as a means of follow-up control of radiotherapy. My
question is, how reliable is this method, since we all know
that radiotherapy itself can alter the morphological
appearance of the cells.

Chodak: I would like to get back to Dr. Mostofi's comments,
which indicated that you need a trained cytopathologist to
interpretate the specimens. The reason why we got involved
is that often after radiotherapy you feel a normal appearing
area where the previous nodule was located. Then, if you do
an aspiration biopsy of that area, you may find vital
looking malignant cells. By means of rectal palpation we may
think that a patient is fine, the aspiration cytology in
this situation may help to identify the patient that still
has residual tumors. We do have well-trained cytopathologists and they are able to make that distinction.

Jacobi: Thank you for this clear statement. If there are no
more questions we should procede to the next presentation.

EORTC Genitourinary Group Monograph 5: Progress
and Controversies in Oncological Urology II, pages 21–29
© 1988 Alan R. Liss, Inc.

TRANSRECTAL ASPIRATION BIOPSY AND PUNCH BIOPSY IN THE
DIAGNOSIS OF PROSTATE CARCINOMA - A COMPARATIVE STUDY
AND LITERATURE REVIEW

Hubert G.W. Frohmüller and Manfred Wirth

Department of Urology
University of Würzburg Medical School
Josef Schneider-Strasse 2, D-8700 Würzburg
Fed. Rep. of Germany

INTRODUCTION

Digital rectal examination of the prostate gland is
currently the most sensitive method of detecting prostatic
carcinoma at an early stage. The specificity of physical
examination, however, is only 50 per cent. Since the diagnosis of prostatic cancer requires a cytological or morphological analysis, a biopsy is necessary in every patient
suspect of having a carcinoma of the prostate. The traditional methods are the perineal and the transrectal punch
biopsy, of which the latter is followed by a higher incidence of complications (Maier et al, 1984; Meyer et al,
1987; Schmiedt, 1972). Whereas these two procedures require
local anesthesia, transrectal fine needle aspiration biopsy, as described by Franzén and associates in 1960, is a
minor procedure with hardly any complications or contraindications. By the latter method a cytological diagnosis
is obtained as compared to the morphological diagnosis
procured by the other two modes. In the Scandinavian countries as well as in other parts of Europe the diagnosis of
prostate cancer is based to a large degree on the results
of transrectal aspiration biopsy (Faul et al, 1980).

MATERIAL AND METHODS

At the Department of Urology of Würzburg University
simultaneous transrectal aspiration biopsy and transperineal punch biopsy have been routinely utilized as an out-
patient procedure for the diagnosis of prostatic cancer

since 1971. Biopsy is performed when rectal digital examination revealed a lesion suspicious of prostate cancer. Perineal punch biopsy of both lobes of the prostate was done under local anesthesia using the Vim-Silverman needle (Silverman, 1938) until July 1972, thereafter the TruCut needle has been utilized (Mellinger and Blackard, 1968). Simultaneous transrectal aspiration biopsy from both lobes of the prostate has been carried out using the original instrument described by Franzén in 1960. During the past 16 years 33 members of the permanent staff and the residents of our institution have been involved in performing these biopsies at various periods of time. Cytological analysis of the aspiration biopsy specimen was performed by one pathologist/cytologist, whereas several members of the pathological department were involved in the examination of the histological specimens obtained by perineal punch biopsy. The data of all 1609 transrectal aspiration biopsies and perineal punch biopsies simultaneously performed during the years 1971 to 1986 were evaluated for this retrospective study.

RESULTS

The results of both transrectal aspiration biopsy and perineal punch biopsy are summarized in table 1. Prostate cancer was diagnosed in 33.2 per cent of the cases. Other malignancies, namely 5 urothelial carcinomas and 2 leiomyosarcomas, were detected in 0.4 per cent. Suspected cancer and unsatisfactory preparations were noticed in 6.1 per cent. In these cases the biopsy procedures were repeated. Non-malignant tissue or cells were diagnosed in 60.3 per cent of the cases.

TABLE 1. Cytological and Histological Diagnosis by Simultaneous Transrectal Aspiration Biopsy and Perineal Punch Biopsy

Diagnosis	No. of biopsies	%
Prostatic carcinoma	534	33.2
Other malignancies	7	0.4
Suspected cancer and unsatisfactory preparations	98	6.1
Non malignant	970	60.3
Total	1609	100.0

Perineal punch biopsy by itself (table 2) led to the diagnosis of prostatic cancer in 32.1 per cent of the cases. Other malignancies were detected by this method in all 7 patients with these diseases. Unsatisfactory preparations and suspected cancer were found in 6.8 per cent, and non-malignant tissue was obtained in 60.7 per cent.

TABLE 2. Histological Diagnosis by Perineal Punch Biopsy

Diagnosis	No. of biopsies	%
Prostatic carcinoma	517	32.1
Other malignancies	7	0.4
Suspected cancer and un-satisfactory preparations	109	6.8
Non malignant	976	60.7
Total	1609	100.0

The results obtained by transrectal aspiration biopsy alone are presented in table 3. Prostatic cancer was detected by this method in only 308 out of 1609 cases, i.e. 19.2 per cent. Other malignancies, namely 4 urothelial carcinomas and 1 leiomyosarcoma, were found in 5 of 7 cases. Suspected cancer and unsatisfactory preparations were seen in 25.6 per cent, and non malignant cells were diagnosed in 54.9 per cent of the cases.

TABLE 3. Cytological Diagnosis by Transrectal Aspiration Biopsy

Diagnosis	No. of biopsies	%
Prostatic carcinoma	308	19.2
Other malignancies	5	0.3
Suspected cancer and un-satisfactory preparations	412	25.6
Non malignant	884	54.9
Total	1609	100.0

A comparison of positive results obtained by transrectal aspiration biopsy on one hand and perineal punch biopsy on the other hand is presented in table 4. In 55.1 per cent of the cases prostatic cancer was detected by the combined procedure of transrectal aspiration biopsy and perineal punch biopsy. By perineal punch biopsy alone prostate cancer was found in 41.7 per cent. Aspiration biopsy by itself, when punch biopsy was negative, was positive in only 3.2 per cent. There was no case of false positive cytology. These data demonstrate that in our hands transperineal punch biopsy was superior to transrectal aspiration biopsy.

TABLE 4. Prostatic Cancer Diagnosed by Simultaneous Transrectal Aspiration Biopsy and Perineal Punch Biopsy

Diagnoses based on:	No. of biopsies	%
Both methods	294	55.1
Punch biopsy only	223	41.7
Aspiration biopsy only	17	3.2
Total	534	100.0

Complications following simultaneous transrectal aspiration biopsy and perineal punch biopsy (table 5) were seen in a total of 101 out of 1609 patients, i.e. in 6.3 per cent of the cases. Fever occurred in 3.2 per cent, hematuria in 2.9 per cent, 2 patients developed an epididymitis and another one noticed hematospermia. Since aspiration biopsy and punch biopsy were performed during the same session, the individual complication rate for each procedure could not be estimated. Because of the well known low incidence of complications associated with fine needle aspiration it can be safely assumed that the majority of the complications observed were caused by the punch procedure.

TABLE 5. Complications After 1609 Simultaneous Transrectal Aspiration Biopsies and Perineal Punch Biopsies

	n	%
Fever	51	3.2
Hematuria	47	2.9
Epididymitis	2	0.1
Hematospermia	1	0.1
Total	101	6.3

DISCUSSION

Needle aspiration biopsy was first utilized by Ferguson (1930) almost 60 years ago. Since its reintroduction by Franzén et al in 1960, the advantages and disadvantages of aspiration biopsy in comparison with punch biopsy in the diagnosis of prostate cancer have kindled a continuous discussion. While some authors prefer aspiration biopsy (Chodak et al, 1986; Faul, 1974; Hosking et al, 1983; Schmiedt, 1972), others find the punch biopsy to be superior (Chodak et al, 1984). Ackermann and Müller (1977) as well as Epstein (1976) demonstrated that the simultaneous utilization of both methods offers an additional factor of reliability. Since transrectal punch biopsy is troubled by a considerably higher incidence of complications (Maier et al, 1984; Meyer et al, 1987; Schmiedt, 1972), perineal punch biopsy is regarded as the method of choice, when a morphological diagnosis is desired.

The proportion of positive biopsies for the aspiration as well as the punch procedure varies in the literature, depending mainly on the indication for performing the procedures. In this series of 1609 cases the biopsies were performed after rectal examination had revealed a lesion suspicious of prostate cancer. Utilizing both methods, namely perineal punch biopsy and transrectal aspiration biopsy, 33.2 per cent of the patients were diagnosed as harbouring a prostatic carcinoma. These results are comparable to those reported by Melograna et al (1982), Droese et al (1976) and Kaulen and Davidts (1972) with a range from 31.6 to 38.7 per cent. Ekman et al (1967), Epstein (1976), Chodak et al (1984) and Carter et al (1986) found a higher incidence of prostatic carcinoma ranging from 33.9 to 60.5 per cent using one or both of these diagnostic procedures. This higher incidence can be explained by the assumption that only highly suspicious lesions were considered an indication for performing a biopsy. However, if this be the case, it is conceivable that a certain number of early cancer cases will escape detection.

The occurrence of the relatively small number of prostatic cancers detected by transrectal aspiration biopsy in this study calls for an explanation. In the literature the accuracy of transrectal aspiration biopsy in detecting prostatic cancer differs considerably. It was found to be as low as 46 per cent, whereas authors like Faul (1974), Chodak et al (1984) as well as Ljung et al (1986) reported transrectal aspiration biopsy to be superior to perineal punch biopsy. Bandtlow (1972) as well as Reuter et al (1971) reported a positive aspiration biopsy in 14.4 to 16 per cent. Comparable results to the herein reported series of 19.2 per cent are related by Droese et al (1976) and Melograna et al (1982). Esposti (1966), Ekman et al (1967), Epstein et al (1976), Maier et al (1984), Chodak et al (1984) and Carter et al (1986) reported a higher incidence in the diagnosis of prostatic carcinoma by transrectal aspiration biopsy ranging from 35.6 to 55.2 per cent.

The discrepancies in these different series could be in part due to the fact that some authors classified suspicious findings as positive, as well as to the circumstance that the number of aspirations done per patient varies greatly from one study to another.

Other reasons for failure in the cytological diagnosis could be artefacts in the fixation material, misinterpretations by the cytologist, and limited experience in performing the technique of transrectal aspiration biopsy. Since in our series the 1609 biopsies were carried out by all members of the teaching staff, as well as the residents, a limited technical skill during the learning phase of this procedure must be taken for granted. DeKernion (1983), among others, called attention to the fact that aspiration biopsy is more difficult to learn than perineal punch biopsy.

By combining transrectal aspiration biopsy with perineal punch biopsy, prostatic cancer was detected in only 3.2 per cent additionally by the aspiration technique (table 4). The advantage of performing both, transrectal aspiration biopsy and perineal punch biopsy simultaneously, has been established in all corresponding series reported in the literature (Ackermann and Müller, 1977; Chodak et al, 1984; Chodak et al, 1986; Droese et al, 1976; Ekman et al, 1967; Epstein, 1976; Esposti, 1966; Heinau et al, 1972; Kaulen and Davidts, 1972; Maier et al, 1984; Melograna et al, 1982).

The rate of complications following simultaneous perineal punch biopsy and transrectal aspiration biopsy amounted to 6.3 per cent in our series. In the literature, the complication rate after transrectal aspiration biopsy only has been reported to range from 0 to 2 per cent (Chodak et al, 1986; Faul, 1974; Jocham et al, 1983; Reuter and Schuck, 1971).

The complication rate following perineal punch biopsy is considerably higher, ranging from 3.5 to 19.5 per cent (Andersson et al, 1967; Fortunoff, 1962; Wendel and Evans, 1967). The complication rate of transrectal aspiration biopsy and perineal punch biopsy, performed at the same session, was reported by Maier et al (1984) to be 4.4 per cent and by Andersson et al (1967) to be 20 per cent.

Finally, contrary to the opinion of Chodak et al (1986) we have never found it necessary to delay radical prostatectomy in patients in whom a perineal core biopsy had been performed.

SUMMARY

It can be concluded from the data presented here, that perineal punch biopsy is able to supply more reliable results than fine needle aspiration biopsy in the diagnosis of prostate cancer. The advantage of aspiration biopsy, however, is its low incidence of complications.

Since the application of both methods, namely transrectal aspiration biopsy and perineal punch biopsy, offers an additional factor of reliability, it appears worth-while to utilize both procedures in the diagnosis of carcinoma of the prostate.

REFERENCES

Ackermann R, Müller H-A (1977). Retrospective analysis of 645 simultaneous perineal punch biopsies and transrectal aspiration biopsies for diagnosis of prostatic carcinoma. Eur Urol 3:29-34.

Andersson L, Jönsson G, Brunk U (1967). Puncture biopsy of the prostate in the diagnosis of prostatic cancer. Scand J Urol Nephrol 1:227-234.

Bandtlow K (1972). Ergebnisse und Treffsicherheit der transrektalen Saugbiopsie nach Franzén. Z Urol 5:383-387.

Carter HB, Riehle RA, jr, Koizumi JH, Amberson J, Vaughan ED (1986). Fine needle aspiration of the abnormal prostate: A cytohistological correlation. J Urol 135:294-298.

Chodak GW, Bibbo M, Straus FS II, Wied GL (1984). Transrectal aspiration biopsy versus transperineal core biopsy for the diagnosis of carcinoma of the prostate. J Urol 132:480-482.

Chodak GW, Steinberg GD, Bibbo M, Wied G, Straus FS II, Vogelzang NJ, Schoenberg HW (1986). The role of transrectal aspiration biopsy in the diagnosis of prostatic cancer. J Urol 135:299-302.

DeKernion JB (1983). Aspiration biopsy of the prostate: The urologists viewpoint. Seminars Urol 1:166-171.

Droese M, Soost H-J, Voeth C (1976). Zytodiagnostik des Prostatakarzinoms nach transrektaler Saugbiopsie. Urologe A 15: 13-17.

Ekman H, Hedberg K, Persson PS (1967). Cytological versus histological examination of needle biopsy specimens in the diagnosis of prostatic cancer. Brit J Urol 39:544-548.

Epstein NA (1976). Prostatic biopsy: A morphologic correlation of aspiration cytology with needle biopsy histology. Cancer 38:2078-2087.

Esposti PL (1966). Cytologic diagnosis of prostatic tumors with the aid of transrectal aspiration biopsy: A critical review of 1110 cases and a report of morphologic and cytochemical studies. Acta Cytol 10:182-186.

Faul P, Göttinger H, Jocham D, Schmiedt E (1980). Kritische Betrachtungen zum derzeitigen diagnostischen Stellenwert der Prostata-Zytologie. Verh Dtsch Ges Urol 32:53-56.

Faul P (1974). Die klinische Bedeutung der Prostata-Zytologie und ihre diagnostischen Möglichkeiten. Münch Med Wschr 116: 15-18.

Ferguson RS (1930). Prostatic neoplasms. Their diagnosis by needle punction and aspiration. Amer J Surg 9:507.

Fortunoff S (1962). Needle biopsy of the prostate: A review of 346 biopsies. J Urol 87:159-163.

Franzén S, Giertz G, Zajicek J (1960). Cytological diagnosis of prostatic tumors by transrectal aspiration biopsy: a preliminary report. Brit J Urol 32:193-196.

Heinau H, Knuth O, Löhe E, Fiedler U, Kirstaedter HS (1972). Vergleichende Untersuchungen der Saug- und Stanzbiopsie der Prostata. Verh Dtsch Ges Urol 24:256-260.

Hosking DH, Paraskevas M, Hellsten R, Ramsey EW (1983). Cytological diagnosis of prostatic carcinoma by transrectal fine needle aspiration. J Urol 129:998-1000.

Jocham D, Schmiedt E, Göttinger H, Faul P, Schmeller N, Laible V (1983). Die Prostatazytologie - 12 Jahre Erfahrung mit der transrektalen Feinnadelbiopsie. Urologe A 22:120-126.

Kaulen H, Davidts HH (1972). Diagnostische Möglichkeiten und Nachteile der transrektalen Aspirationsbiopsie mit cytologischer Beurteilung beim Prostata-Carcinom. Verh Dtsch Ges Urol 24:268-271.

Ljung B-M, Cherrie R, Kaufman JJ (1986). Fine needle aspiration biopsy of the prostate gland: a study of 103 cases with histological followup. J Urol 135:955-958.

Maier U, Czerwenka K, Neuhold N (1984). The accuracy of transrectal aspiration biopsy of the prostate: an analysis of 452 cases. Prostate 5:147-151.

Mellinger GT, Blackard CE (1968). A new instrument for needle biopsy of the prostate. J Urol 99:228-231.

Melograna F, Oertel YC, Kwart AM (1982). Prospective controlled assessment of fine-needle prostatic aspiration. Urology 19:47-51.

Meyer WH, Huland H, Becker H (1987). Transrektale Prostatastanzbiopsie: Beeinflussung der fieberhaften Komplikationsrate durch Antibiotika. Akt Urol 18:22-24.

Reuter HJ, Schuck W (1971). Die Nadelbiopsie der Prostata zur zytologischen Karzinomdiagnostik: Erfahrungen an 1500 Fällen. Z Urol 11:857-862.

Schmiedt E (1972). Prostatabiopsie und -cytologie aus klinischer Sicht. Verh Dtsch Ges Urol 24:260-263.

Silverman J (1938). A new biopsy needle. Am J Surg 40:671-672.

Wendel RJ, Evans AT (1967). Complications of punch biopsy of the prostate gland. J Urol 97:122-126.

EORTC Genitourinary Group Monograph 5: Progress
and Controversies in Oncological Urology II, pages 31-32
© 1988 Alan R. Liss, Inc.

Discussion: Transrectal Aspiration Biopsy and Punch Biopsy
in the Diagnosis of Prostate Carcinoma - A Comparative
Study and Literature Review

Fritz H. Schroder, Rotterdam, The Netherlands

Jacobi: Some controversial standpoints are expressed in this
presentation as compared to the previous speaker. Is there
any discussion?

Fosså: Some of the different results you report may in fact
be due to a different patient population. The proportion of
positive biopsies should be different if one uses fine
needle aspiration cytology in patients with clinically mani-
fest carcinoma or if it is used as a pure screening procedure.

Frohmüller: No, this is not the case. We will do a biopsy
only if we have a clinical suspicion of carcinoma. I must,
however, admit that even the slightest irregularity in the
surface of the prostate will be reason for us to a biopsy,
but this does not mean that aspiration cytology is done as a
screening procedure in our hands.

Collste: At our institution aspiration biopsy is a specia-
list procedure. Actually, the urologist involved does not
even do the biopsy, the procedure is entirely in the hands
of the cytopathologist. I think that we are much closer to
Dr. Chodak's figures of accuracy, actually it should be
close to a 100 per cent. So I advise against a lot of people
within a department doing the procedure.

Frohmüller: Thank you for these comments. I have previously
discussed this problem with Dr. Chodak. I realize that in
the United Stated in some areas the biopsy is done by the
cytopathologist. In Germany, as far as I know, it is always
done by a urologist and I think this will stay so. The main
difference between Dr. Chodak's and our series is that in
our institution all the biopsies have been done by various
members of our staff and by the urology residents. On the
other hand, all slides have been reviewed by one cytopathologist of whom I believe that he is excellent. We certainly

cannot blame our poor results on our cytopathologist.

Scardino: Dr. Frohmüller, can you tell me what you do when you have a positive cytology and a negative core biopsy? Does your pathologist identify that immediately, does he react by cutting more sections? Would you then repeat the biopsy? We find in our experience that either one of the biopsies is positive at first and essentially the results obtained with those techniques are quite similar.

Frohmüller: Fortunately, the number of positive cytological and negative histological diagnoses was very small. If this ever would happen, we would do a second poor biopsy. We have never done a radical prostatectomy on aspiration cytology evidence only. We always wish to have a morphological diagnosis confirmed by a perineal punction biopsy.

Schröder: I wonder how those who would only do an aspiration biopsy would recognize a false positive result?

Frohmüller: One would recognize it later on when doing the radical prostatectomy.

Chodak: I would like to draw attention to what I think is an important feature in these series. When we do a biopsy we review the specimen together with the cytopathologist. The criteria for malignancy is that a predominant number of cells is malignant. You could still see areas of normal cells, but still, this patient does not have a normal biopsy. If one reads only the pathology report, one may become convinced that we are dealing with a normal biopsy. However, if one reviews the case together with the pathologist, one would go back and repeat the biopsy and come to definite diagnosis. That, I believe, is the reason why we have a high sensitivity.

Frohmüller: I must admit that our relationship with our pathologist is not as close. If the pathologist says there is no cancer, we believe that. If he says there is cancer, we also believe that. When we, however, felt on clinical grounds that there was suspicion in face of a negative biopsy, we would go back and re-biopsy the patient.

EORTC Genitourinary Group Monograph 5: Progress
and Controversies in Oncological Urology II, pages 33–42
© 1988 Alan R. Liss, Inc.

ACID PHOSPHATASE, ALKALINE PHOSPHATASE AND PROSTATE-
SPECIFIC ANTIGEN - USEFULNESS IN THE DIAGNOSIS OF
METASTATIC DISEASE AND FOLLOW-UP

H.W. Bauer
Department of Urology and Outpatient Clinic,
Freie Universität Berlin, Klinikum Steglitz

INTRODUCTION

The search for a prostate tumor-associated marker that
is sufficiently reliable for diagnosing and therapeutic
monitoring of the disease has not yet been successful.

Nevertheless, biochemical markers such as acid phosphatase, alkaline phosphatase and the prostate-specific
antigen can be helpful in the management of prostatic
cancer patients. However, it is extremely important for
the clinicians to understand the biology and limitations
of the individual tumor marker. As long as we are not informed about the biology of the tumor markers to a greater
extent, the results following from this consequently cannot be more reliable than the clinical parameters on the
basis of which their value is measured. This knowledge is
the only way in which markers will be ordered in a cost-
effective way and errors in the interpretation will be
kept at a minimum.

Acid Phosphatase

Acid phosphatases are enzymes that are capable of hy-
drolyzing phosphate esters at a pH below 7, and are classified as orthophosphoric monoester hydrolases. The observation that elevation of acid phosphatase in serum is
associated with metastatic carcinoma of the prostate is
now 50 years old (Gutman AB, Gutman EB, 1938).

Subsequent studies established a relationship between serum acid phosphatase levels and disease progression and response (Robinson et al., 1939; Huggins C, Hodges CV, 1941; Sullivan et al., 1942). Acid phosphatases are produced in bone, leukocytes, erythrocytes, platelets, kidneys, liver and various tissues other than the prostate. For this reason it is not an adequate marker for prostate cancer in the sense of specificity.

There was an increase in the specificity by differentiation of the tartrate sensitive fraction of the total acid phosphatase (Fishman and Lerner, 1953). But due to the susceptibility of enzyme activity to changes in temperature, pH and the influence of hemolytic processes the increase of the specificity was too low for the procedure to reach broad acceptance. In addition to this, the tartrate sensitive fraction consists of different isoenzymes, i.e. the isoenzymes 2, 3 and 4, but only the isoenzyme 2 is a prostate-specific isoenzyme the values of which are increased in sera of patients with prostatic cancer (Lam et al., 1982).

A large number of reports have been published concerning the clinical significance of the total acid phosphatase and the tartrate sensitive fraction in prostatic cancer patients (Table 1).

Acid Phosphatase – enzymatic
Sensitivity for diagnosing prostatic cancer with metastases (Stage D)

author	year	n	sensitivity
FOTI et al.	1977	25	60%
LEE et al.	1980	14	36%
PONTES et al.	1981	10	60%
JACOBI et al.	1981	18	53%
WIRTH et al.	1981	12	39%
FLÜCHTER et al.	1982	19	68%
VIHKO et al.	1982	18	47%
ROMAS et al.	1982	18	65%
BAUER et al.	1982	110	65%
LAM et al.	1984	24	30%
ANDERSSON	1985	96	75%
LEWENHAUPT et al.	1985	26	75%
VIHKO et al.	1985	110	36%

Table 1

Acid phosphatase
Follow-up in patients with prostatic cancer
Stage D
Sensitivity enzym:

author	year	n	sensitivity
Resp.			
BAUER	1983	72	67%
ZWEIG	1985	19	79%
Nonresp.			
BISHOP et al.	1985	56	64%
MERRICK et al.	1985	22	48%
SOHNS et al.	1986	46	50%

Table 2

Summarizing the results of parallel determination, it seems that the tartrate sensitive acid phosphatase activity is slightly more sensitive than the total acid phosphatase activity in diagnosing stage D prostatic cancer patients.

The recognition of responders and nonresponders to hormonal treatment in prostatic cancer patients by the total acid phosphatase or the tartrate sensitive fraction is very similar and shows results between 50 and 70% (Table 2).

The bone marrow acid phosphatase measured by colorimetric assays is of no additional value as compared to the imaging technique in staging prostatic cancer (Romas et al., 1950; Bauer, 1983).

Prostatic Acid Phosphatase

Since enzymatic methods lack the specificity to measure any single isoenzyme, their immunological characteristics have to be investigated. In 1964 Schuhman and coworkers were able to detect the serum acid phosphatase, the isoenzyme 2 (PAP), by gel diffusion techniques.

PAP has been identified as a glycoprotein with a molecular weight of 100,000 daltons; its subunits have been identified, the site of possible enzymatic reactions have been located, and amino acid analysis has been performed (Choe et al. 1982).

Since then, a large number of assays have become available. Some investigators also combine the immunologic and enzymatic approach employing a specific antibody to isolate the enzyme in order to provide a functional assay (IEA) (Hackenberg, Bauer, 1983). The usefulness of the immunochemical PAP determination in the diagnosis of metastatic disease has been evaluated in many centers (Table 3). The advantages of the immunoassays, i.e. sensitivity, specificity and reproducibility over colorimetric assays are now accepted.

The overall sensitivity of metastatic prostate cancer disease is about 80 - 85% at a specificity of about 90%. The main problem for all immunoenzymatic assays now commercially available is that there is no defined standard for PAP. For that reason, the results are not comparable at the moment.

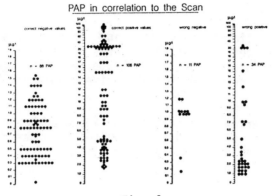

Fig. 1

Figure 1 shows a correlation of 112 patients in prostatic cancer stage C and D monitored over a period of 2 years with bone scans and PAP. The 239 comparable examinations showed only 11 false-negative results and 34 false-positive results for PAP. The reason for the false-positive PAP results would be that PAP also detects metastases in other organ systems and refers not only to the skeleton system. It is undisputable that the scans were the more sensitive indicators of progressive disease in the bone system.

Sensitivity PAP

Sensitivity for diagnosing prostatic cancer with metastases (Stage D)

author	year	n	sensitivity	method
FOTI et al.	1977	25	92%	RiA
LEE et al.	1980	14	79%	iEA
CHOE et al.	1980	23	78%	iEA
PONTES et al.	1981	10	80%	RiA
JACOBI et al.	1981	18	87%	EiA
WIRTH et al.	1981	12	83%	RiA
FLÜCHTER et al.	1982	19	94%	RiA
VIHKO et al.	1982	18	89%	RiA
GRIFFITH et al.	1982	25	84%	EiA
			76%	RiA
ROMAS et al.	1982	18	94%	iEA
BAUER et al.	1982	61	92%	EiA
BAUER et al.	1982	51	95%	iEA
LAM et al.	1984	24	85%	EiA
MAATMAN et al.	1984	10	50%	RiA
ANDERSSON	1985	96	78%	RiA
			96%	ELiSA
LEWENHAUPT et al.	1985	26	78%	RiA
			96%	ELiSA
VIHKO et al.	1985	110	70%	RiA
ZWEIG et al.	1985	34	83-91%	RiA
CHU et al.	1986	116	73%	RiA

Table 3

PAP
Follow-up in patients with prostatic cancer Stage D

author	year	n	sensitivity
Resp.			
KONTURRI et al.	1985	5	100%
ZWEIG et al.	1985	19	84-89%
Nonresp.			
RUBEY et al.	1985	15	74%
ZWEIG et al.	1985	10	60-70%

Table 4

However, in patients responding to therapy, changes in serum acid phosphatase or alkaline phosphatase frequently occur before any improvement in the bone scan appears.

The usefulness for PAP determination in monitoring prostate cancer patients is shown in Table 4. The positive predictive value for elevated PAP results regarding a nonresponding patient is lower than the negative predictive value of an unchanged PAP value for a responding person.

PAP might be a prognostic parameter for patients under systemic treatment such as hormonal management or chemotherapy.

Figure 2 shows the follow-up of 100 prostatic cancer patients who underwent castration by orchiectomy or endocrine therapy. Half of them had normal PAP values 3 months later and had a much better prognosis than those with constant high PAP levels.

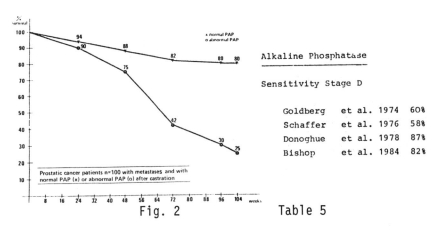

Fig. 2

Table 5

Alkaline Phosphatase

Sensitivity Stage D

Goldberg	et al.	1974	60%
Schaffer	et al.	1976	58%
Donoghue	et al.	1978	87%
Bishop	et al.	1984	82%

Alkaline Phosphatase

The alkaline phosphatases are a series of enzymes that hydrolyse phosphatase esters at a pH greater than 7. Four isoenzymes are known: bone, liver, intestinal tract and from the placenta, also called Regan isoenzyme. In the adult, the majority of serum alkaline phosphatase is of liver or gastrointestinal mucosal origin, only 10% are from the skeleton system. The alkaline isoenzyme from the bone is a parameter for the activity of the osteoblasts. Increased values may stand for bone metastases, morbus Paget, osteoporosis or the healing of bone fractures as well as live bone scans. It is therefore not surprising that the results of elevated alkaline phosphatase and bone scans are very comparable in prostatic cancer patients. Clinical sensitivity for the total alkaline phosphatase in prostatic cancer patients stage D_2 is shown in Table 5. The highly specific bone isoenzyme cannot be used routinely since a commercial test is not yet available. And even if it were, this isoenzyme reflects only the skeleton system and not the prostate cancer disease. Therefore, the biological features of PAP and PSA alone should already make them more helpful in diagnosing and monitoring prostatic cancer patients.

Prostate-Specific Antigen

The prostate-specific antigen and the prostate-specific acid phosphatase are well-defined glycoproteins and enzymes (Wang et al., 1979). PSA has recently been reported to exhibit a mild activity of protease. A profound inhibitory effect of Zn on the enzymatic activity has been observed in addition (Chu and Murphy, 1986).

The PSA concentration in malignant prostate tissue is not different from that in normal or benign hyperplastic prostate. The antigen is primarily found in seminal plasma. In the prostate tissue the antigen is localized in the ductal elements of the gland.
The same localization was found for PAP.
There is no immunological cross-reactivity between PAP and PSA. It is evident that PAP and PSA are expressed independently by tumor cells.
The pattern of immunostaining for PSA in prostate cancer is similar to that of PAP.
Both antigens had a cytoplasmic localization in tumor cells.
Several investigators showed that there was a correlation between the loss of the immunohistologically identified expression of PAP and PSA and the loss of differentiation; but this point is still controversial, since other authors did not find the same results (Nadji et al. 1981).

It is ndisputable that both antigens, PAP and PSA, should always be explored, for it could be possible that only one antigen is expressed.

Although no quantitative difference was found in serum PSA levels between BPH and stage A and B of prostate cancer patients, patients with stage C or D exhibit significantly elevated PSA levels (Kuriyama et al., 1982; Bauer, 1975; Wang et al., 1986).

Like most other tumor markers, PSA is of high clinical value in monitoring the course of disease, especially the response to treatment.

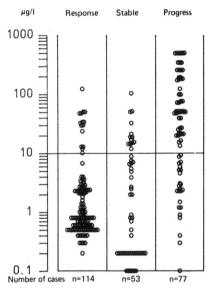

Fig. 3:
PSA in Prostatic Cancer
[p<0.001 Response/Progress]

Pretreatment serum PSA, quantified on patients with stage D_2 prostate cancer who were unresponsive to prior hormonal therapy and were randomized to chemotherapy has revealed that PSA is of prognostic value in patients' survival irrespective of the treatment regimen. The lower the pretreatment PSA, the longer the survival (Killian et al. 1985).

Figure 3 shows PSA levels in prostatic cancer patients used to distinguish between tumor response and progressive disease. The criteria for response and progression were according to the NPCP.

Proposal for Therapy Monitoring and Follow-Up of Prostate cancer patients

use both: PSA and PAP

1. A positive treatment response will be indicated by decreasing levels of both PSA and PAP to their normal background.
   There might be a difference between endocrine treatment and chemotherapy.

2. A partial treatment response will be indicated by the failure of either PAP or PSA, or both do not return to their normal background.

3. An impending recurrence is usually indicated by a rise in serial serum PSA or PAP, or both.

SUMMARY

PSA and PAP are effective immunohistologic markers for prostatic cancer metastases.

PSA seems to be more sensitive than PAP for diagnosing metastatic prostatic cancer.

Simultaneous determination of PSA and PAP yields an additive clinical value in diagnosing and follow-up of prostatic cancer.

The prognostic reliability for disease progression (recurrence and treatment response) seems to be PSA > PAP > AcidP > Alkal. P.

REFERENCES

Bauer HW (1983). Phosphatasen: Relevanz der einzelnen Analyse-Verfahren. In Faul P, Altwein J (eds): 'Aktuelle Diagnostik und Therapie des Prostatakarzinoms," Informed Verlag, pp 75-83.
Bauer HW (1985). Vergleich von prostataspezifisch saurer Phosphatase (PAP) und prostataspezifischem Antigen (PSA) in der Diagnostik und Verlaufskontrolle des Pro-

statakarzinoms. Lab Med 9: 149.

Braun JS, Habig H, Griesemann D (1974). Die diagnostische Bedeutung der sauren Phosphatase im Serum beim Prostatacarcinom. Urologe A 13: 236.

Choe BK, Pontes JE, Morrison MK, Rose NR (1978). Prostatic acid phosphatase II. A double-antibody radioimmunoassay. Arch Androl 1: 227.

Chu TM, Murphy GP (1986). What's new in tumor markers for prostate cancer. Urology 27: 487.

Cook WB, Fishman WH, Clard BG (1962). Serum acid phosphatase of prostatic origin in the diagnosis of prostatic carcinoma. Clinical evaluation of 2408 tests by Fishman-Lerner method. J Urol 88: 281.

Cooper JF, Foti A (1974). A radioimmunoassay for prostatic acid phosphatase. I. Methodology and range of normal male serum values. Invest Urol 12: 98.

Fishman WH, Dast RM, Bonner CD, Leadbetter WF, Lerner F, Homburger F (1953). A new method for estimating serum acid phosphatase of prostatic origin applied to the clinical investigation of cancer of the prostate. J Clin Invest 32: 1034.

Fishman WH, Lerner FA (1953). A method for estimating serum acid phosphatase of prostatic origin. J Biol Chem 200: 89.

Gutman AB, Gutman EB (1938). An "acid" phosphatase occurring in the serum of patients with metastasizing carcinoma of the prostate gland. J Clin Invest 17: 473-478.

Hackenberg H, Hennrich N, Bauer HW (1983). Ein neuer Festphasen-Immunoassay für saure Prostata-Phosphatase. In Keller H (ed.): "Methodik und Diagnostische Bedeutung der Sauren Prostataphosphatase", GIT-Verlag, pp 17-28.

Hofstädter F (1986). Tumoren des männlichen Urogenitalsystems. Verh Dtsch Ges Path 70: 172-183.

Huggins C, Hodges CV (1941). The effect of castration, of estrogen and of androgen injection on serum phosphatases in metastatic carcinoma of the prostate. Cancer Res 1: 293-297.

Jacobi GH, Prellwitz W (unpublished data).

Killian CS, Yang N, Emrich LJ et al. (1985). Prognostic importance of prostate-specific antigen for monitoring patients with stages B_2 to D_1 prostate cancer. Cancer Res 45: 886-891.

Kuriyama M, Wang MC, Lee CC et al. (1982). Multiple marker evaluation in human prostate cancer with the use of tissue-specific antigens. J Natl Cancer Inst 68: 99-105.

Lam KW , Li CY, Yam LT, Smith RS, Hacker B (1982). Comparison of prostatic and nonprostatic acid phosphatase. Annals of the NY Academy of Sciences 390: 1-15.

Mathes G, Richmont SG, Sprunt (1956). Use of L-tartrate in determining prostatic serum acid phosphatase. Report of 514 cases. J Urol 75: 143.

Murphy GP, Reynoso G, Kenny GM, Gaeta JF (1969). Comparison of total and prostatic fraction serum acid phosphatase levels in patients with differentiated and undifferentiated prostatic carcinoma. Cancer 23: 1309.

Nadji M, Tabei S, Castro A et al. (1981). Prostate specific antigen, an immunohistologic marker for prostatic neoplasms. Cancer 48: 1229-1232

Nobles ER, Ker WS, Dutoit ChH (1957). Serum prostatic acid phosphatase levels in patients with carcinoma of the prostate. JAMA 164: 2020.

Robinson JN, Gutman EB (1939). Clinical significance of increased serum "acid" phosphatase in patients with bone metastases secondary to prostatic carcinoma. J Urol 42: 602-618.

Romas N, Veenema RJ, Konrad CH, Tomashefsky M (1980). Bone marrow acid phosphatase in prostatic cancer: an assessment by immunoassay and biochemical methods. J Urol 123: 392-395.

Romas NA, Hsu KC, Tomashefsky P, Tannenbaum M (1978). Counterimmunoelectrophoresis for detection of human prostatic acid phosphatase. Urology 12: 79.

Solms A, Weinstock N, Hennich G (1986). Die saure Phosphatase beim Prostatakarzinom. Git Labor Medizin 146.

Sullivan TJ, Gutman EB, Gutman AB (1942). Theory and application of the serum "acid" phosphatase determination in metastasizing prostatic carcinoma: early effects of castration. J Urol 48: 426-458.

Vihko P, Soganti E, Järne O, Peltonen L, Vihko R (1978). Serum prostate specific acid phosphatase: development and validation of a specific radioimmunoassay. Clin Chem 24: 1915.

Wang MC, Valenzuela LA, Murphy GP, Chu TM (1979). Purification of a human prostate specific antigen. Invest Urol 17: 159.

Wang TY, Kawaguchi TP (1986). Preliminary evaluation of measurement of serum prostate-specific antigen level in detection of prostate cancer. An Clin Lab Sc 16: 461.

EORTC Genitourinary Group Monograph 5: Progress
and Controversies in Oncological Urology II, pages 43–53
© 1988 Alan R. Liss, Inc.

ACID PHOSPHATASE, ALKALINE PHOSPHATASE AND PROSTATE SPECIFIC
ANTIGEN : WHICH MARKERS SHOULD WE CHOOSE ?

E.H. Cooper, J.K. Siddall, D.W.W. Newling and
M.R.G. Robinson.
Unit for Cancer Research, University of Leeds,
Leeds LS2 9NL (E.H.C., J.K.S.), The Princess
Royal Hospital, Hull (D.W.W.N.) and Pontefract
General Infirmary, Pontefract (M.R.G.R.).

The biochemical monitoring of prostatic cancer has for
many years relied on the measurement of the serum enzymatic
activity of acid phosphatase, using various substrates and
inhibitors to restrict the activity of the prostatic
fraction.   In the 1970s prostatic acid phosphatase was
isolated and immunochemical assays devised for this antigen
(Foti et al., 1977).   These assays were soon generally
available as commercial kits and have been widely adopted
in parts of Europe and North America.   Population screening
was advocated prematurely before the sensitivity and specificity of the assays were critically evaluated.   This
eventually led to many publications about the limitations
of this test (see Pontes, 1983, for review).

Our view, based on experience of several PAP kits
produced by Behringwerke (Cooper et al., 1983), Merck
(Cooper et al., 1986) and Hybritech (Siddall et al., 1986a)
was the assay was more precise than enzymatic measurements
of the activity of serum acid phosphatase (prostatic
fraction).   Its clinical advantages were mainly associated
with those situations in which small changes in PAP levels
were important, for example in the monitoring of patients
not receiving any treatment, and the identification of the
risks of progression.

More recently another protein - prostate specific
antigen (PSA) - has been isolated and characterised and
shown to have the properties to make it a good tumour
marker.   The introduction of a commercial assay for PSA
by Hybritech, San Diego, California, has enabled many

urologists to gain first hand experience of this new test.
Finally in Japan, studies of antigens in seminal fluid have
identified γ-seminoprotein (γ-Sm)(Hara et al., 1966) which
subsequently has been found to be another biomarker for
prostatic cancer (Okabe et al., 1985).

This sequence of progress is somewhat confusing for
the clinician when having to decide which test to use. The
enzymatic measurement of serum acid phosphatase activity is
cheap, it is moderately accurate when in high range but
notoriously difficult to interpret with confidence when in
the normal or near normal range. This test, despite its
faults, fits into the routine of clinical chemistry practice
and is suitable for small batch running. To introduce new
tests, especially in countries such as the United Kingdom
where control is tight and the state pays most of these
costs, requires strong argument and conviction on the part
of those requesting the test that the results can help their
clinical judgement. We shall look at this evidence, but
first some background about PSA and γ-Sm, details about PAP
have been covered by Dr. Bauer.

Prostate specific antigen was isolated and characterised by Wang et al. in 1979. It is a glycoprotein, 7%
carbohydrate by weight, with a molecular weight of 34,000 d.
It is distinct from PAP and is synthesised in the acinar
cells of the normal prostate and is present in prostatic
fluid. Benign hyperplastic prostatic acini and primary
and metastatic prostatic cancer also synthesise this protein.
The antigen does not occur in any other tissue. PSA is
distinct from PAP and is synthesised independently of PAP.
PSA is now known to be a serine protease (Watt et al., 1986).

Gamma seminoprotein (γ-Sm) was isolated by Hara (1966)
and at first was used as an indicator of seminal stains in
forensic medicine. Later its serum levels were shown to
reflect the tumour burden of prostatic cancer (Okabe et al.,
1985; Kuriyama et al., 1986). γ-Sm and PSA show many
features in common. They are both glycoproteins, molecular
weight of γ-Sm is 23,000 d. In a comparative study of γ-Sm
and PSA we found there was a close similarity in the serum
levels of these two antigens. The overall correlation
coefficient of their levels was highly significant (r=0.68,
p<0.001). The distribution of levels for γ-Sm and PSA
were similar when the untreated patients were subdivided
into extent of disease and histological grade (Siddall et al.,

1986c). It is possible that γ-Sm is a part of the PSA molecule. At present tests for γ-Sm are only available in Japan. We shall not discuss γ-Sm any further, it appears to have all the properties we will describe for PSA and its use may grow especially in Japan.

During the evaluation of PSA as a marker for prostatic cancer studies were organised in several centres in the United States and in Leeds by Hybritech to compare PSA and PAP using their Tandem^R double monoclonal antibody radio-immunoassays. A meeting was held last summer in New York to consolidate the data available at that time (Lange et al., 1986). In this presentation we draw on the results from our multicentre studies in Yorkshire and those from the United States.

Normal Levels.

There are various ways of determining normal levels of an analyte in the serum. The simplest is to test healthy blood donors. This indicated 99% of 265 males <40 years old have a PSA <4 ng/ml. In 207 healthy males >40 years old 97% were still <4 ng/ml. Bearing the results of the PSA levels in BPH in mind it seems that a working level of 10 ng/ml be set as a discriminant in patients with no previous PSA levels for comparison, but as the patient's own normal level, when he is in remission, becomes apparent by sequential measurements, it becomes clear that the level will tend to fall to <4 ng/ml and often reach a low basal level of <2 ng/ml. In 27 patients who remained in remission for 2-3 years after endocrine manipulation the mean PSA was <2 ng/ml, and 95% of the observations were <5 ng/ml (Siddall et al.,1986a).

PSA and PAP in Patients at Presentation.

We have measured serum PSA and PAP levels in 274 patients with carcinoma of the prostate at the time of diagnosis before giving any treatment. They are divided into patients without skeletal metastases ($T_{0-4} N_x M_0$) shown in Table I and those with skeletal metastases ($T_{0-4} N_x M_1$) which are shown in Table II.

TABLE 1. Distribution (%) of Serum PSA in Prostatic Cancer at Diagnosis

	Number	PSA ng/ml			
		<4	4 - 10	10 - 100	>100
M_O	168	44% (72)	18% (31)	31% (53)	5.9% (10)
M_1	106	1.8% (2)	5.6% (6)	46% (49)	46% (49)

Number of patients in parenthesis

TABLE 2. Distribution (%) of Serum PAP in Prostatic Cancer at Diagnosis

	Number	PAP ng/ml			
		<2	2.1 - 10	10.1 - 100	>100
M_O	168	73% (124)	21% (35)	5.3% (9)	-
M_1	106	24% (26)	33% (35)	32% (34)	9% (10)

Number of patients in parenthesis

Of 168 patients with M_O disease 56% had PSA values above 4.0 ng/ml and 38% above 10 ng/ml, whilst PAP was raised (>2 ng/ml) in 44 (26%). By contrast in 106 patients with skeletal metastases 62% had PSA above 4 ng/ml and in 58% it was greater than 10 ng/ml.

In the non-metastatic patients there was a relationship between tumour stage and PSA levels so that in 60 patients with T_{1-O} tumour 25% had a PSA >4 ng/ml, in 46 with T_2 tumours 67% had a PSA >4 ng/ml and in 62 with T_3 or

T_4 tumours 78% had a PSA >4 ng/ml. We also observed there was a relationship between histological grade and PSA levels with the highest levels being in the least well differentiated tumours (Siddall et al., 1986).

The American studies reported by Lange et al. (1986) showed that the PSA levels in 553 patients with prostatic cancer at presentation when subdivided by stage were as follows:- Of 70 cases of stage A tumours 63% had values above 4 ng/ml and 30% above 10 ng/ml, in 90 cases of stage B tumours 71% had values above 4 ng/ml and 50% above 10 ng/ml. In 393 cases of stage C and D cancer 85% had values above 4 ng/ml and 75% above 10 ng/ml. The corresponding percentage elevation of PAP >4 ng/ml by stage were A 8%, B 22%, C 43% and D 63%.

Benign Prostatic Hyperplasia (BPH)

In Lange's survey the serum PSA levels in 352 cases of BPH showed that 80% had levels <4 ng/ml, 18% 4.1-10 ng/ml, and in 2% it was >10 ng/ml.

A practical point to emerge is the value of measuring PSA in patients with symptoms and signs of apparent BPH, a persistent high level could constitute a warning that the patient may have a carcinoma and further investigation should not be delayed.

Can PSA Be Used for Population Screening ?

Schwartz (1986) has calculated the likely impact of using the Hybritech PSA assay for population screening. He used the following parameters : 1) the prevalence of prostatic cancer in men >55 years is 10%, therefore screening 100,000 asymptomatic men >55 years should show 10,000 cases (stages A and B); 2) 99% of normal men have a PSA <4 ng/ml; 3) the data quoted by Lange on the distribution of PSA levels in prostatic cancer (see above). Then using a PSA >4 ng/ml as a positive test he estimates the test would detect 6,500 cancers but at the same thime there would be 18,000 false positives due to the prevalence of BPH. Thus there would be 24,500 positives that include 6,500 cancers but 3,500 cancers would be missed. This is

unacceptable. Raising the discriminant to >10 ng/ml then
4,100 cases would be detected plus 1,800 false positives
and 69% of the positives would have cancer but 5,900 cases
of cancer would not be detected. This suggests the detection rate would be too low to warrant such a screening
programme.

PSA, PAP and Prediction of Outcome

It is generally agreed that about 30% of patients with
localised prostatic cancer will progress in 5 years, and
50% of those with distant metastases will die within two
years. But to translate these general predictions into a
well informed estimate of what will happen to the individual
patient is usually impossible. The changing attitudes
about the management of apparently localised prostate
cancer has focused our attention on the predictive values
of PSA and PAP. In particular, we have been interested to
look at the value of the presentation level of PSA in
patients who are managed by a deferred treatment policy.
We have observed 52 patients who were watched without
treatment until they developed symptoms or evidence of
progression, none were staged surgically, they were assessed clinically and by scintigraphy and judged to be T_{0-3}
$N_x M_0$. The relationship between the PSA at presentation
and the incidence of progression is shown in Table 3.

TABLE 3. Relationship of the serum PSA levels at presentation to the occurrence of progression in 52 patients with
non-metastatic disease kept under surveillance without
treatment.

	PSA level at presentation	
	< 10 ng/ml	> 10 ng/ml
Progression 0.5 - 5 y * median 1.5 y	5[†]	12
No progression 1 - 5 y * median 3 y	32	3

* = duration of observation
[†] = 3 patients progressed >3 y after presentation.

In this small series a level >10 ng/ml carried a strongly raised probability that progression will occur within 2 years. Patients who developed progression after a 2 - 5 year interval did not have a raised PSA when they were first diagnosed.

The corresponding PAP levels showed that among those patients who progressed in 2 years 5/13 (38%) had a PAP >2 ng/ml at presentation. A single case had a raised PAP (4 ng/ml) but showed no progression up to two years. The PAP level had no predictive value for 3 patients who progressed 4 - 5 years after presentation.

In the recent large scale EORTC study of laboratory based prognostic factors in metastatic prostatic cancer in the clinical trial No. GU 30805 only haemoglobin level (p=<0.0001) and alkaline phosphatase levels (p=0.0231) had a prognostic significance, acid phosphatase levels were of no prognostic significance (p=0.9859).

In a cohort of 68 patients with metastatic disease followed up 2 - 3 years we found that the 15 who presented with a pre-treatment serum PSA <30 ng/ml had a significantly longer survival than the 53 with a PSA >30 ng/ml, median survival 60 months and 34 months respectively. This raises the question of whether in future trials of metastatic disease the PSA at the time of entry might be a stratification factor, albeit only used in the final analysis, but it will require a large series to define the real significance of PSA as a prognostic factor.

Monitoring Disease Progress and Response to Treatment

Any surgery of the prostate is associated with a rapid release of PSA and PAP into the circulation which usually declines to the base line level in a few days. In untreated disease (M_o) without signs of progression the PSA can remain unchanged for up to 4 years or show a very slow rise at a rate of approximately 2 ng/ml/year (Siddall et al. 1986a).

Patients presenting with a raised PSA generally show a fall to normal levels following orchiectomy, oestrogen therapy or LH-RH therapy. The rate of fall varies considerably, in some it occurs within 1-2 weeks, in other

patients it is over several months.   In patients with
localised disease and long term survivors in patients with
metastatic disease the PSA is frequently <3 ng/ml during
the time of clinical complete remission or stable metastatic
disease.

Killian et al. (1986) have made a comparative study of
PSA, PAP, total alkaline phosphatase (TAP) and bone alkaline
phosphatase (BAP) to predict progression at an early or
advanced stage of the disease.   In stage B2 to D1 (after
correction for effects of stage, initial therapy and
adjuvant therapy on the risk of progression) showed that
only PSA (p=0.0002) was a clinical important marker of
imminent progression, PAP was marginal (p=0.07), TAP and
BAP were not significant.   PSA levels were predictive of
an increased risk six months prior to progression. However,
in stage D2 markers were prognostically important; using a
discriminant level of twice the upper limit of normal for
each test the order of reliability of indicating progression
was PSA, BAP and PAP.   BAP was well correlated with the
extent of the bone tumour load.

Sequential measurements show that a rising PSA is
usually associated with or precedes progression.   Several
examples of the change of levels of PSA have been published
(Siddall et al., 1986 a & b; Hetherington et al., 1987;
Killian et al., 1985).

However, the exact lead time depends on the intervals
between sequential PSA measurements and the timing of other
investigations, especially scintigraphic bone scans to
evaluate the patient's status.   We have examined these
relationships in 54 patients who have undergone repeated
scintigraphic examinations at intervals that are standard
in the EORTC protocols.   In this study of 54 patients who
presented with a negative bone scan 20 developed skeletal
metastases, the serum PAP and PSA were rising at the time
the scan became positive in 5 and 9 of these patients
respectively.   Local progression occurred in a further 9
patients, the serum PSA was rising in all of them, and the
PAP in 8.   In 66 patients with previously documented
evidence of skeletal metastases bone scan evidence of
progression was seen in 36.   At the time of progression
serum PAP was rising in 20 (55%) and the PSA in 26 (72%).
In 4 patients neither marker was raised at the time of first
evidence of progression (Hetherington et al., 1987).

Finding a Cost Effective Biomarker

Undoubtedly the switch from an enzymatic assay of acid phosphatase to PSA involves increased cost, the kits currently available for PSA are radioimmunoassays which are unsuitable for small batch running:- ELISA kits have been announced. Many requests for acid phosphatase in general hospitals are part of a routine work up of older men admitted to medical wards. The occasional high level can alert the physician to a case of disseminated prostatic cancer. Most of these requests do not require PSA measurement, hence there is the problem of making the test generally available, it would only be cost effective if there was appropriate education about its value. Within the narrower confines of urology and oncology the PSA would seem to be the marker of choice. The information given by the PSA at presentation when taken into account with clinical and histological data is considerable, in isolation it can raise suspicions but generally it gives little firm information. Once treatment or observation has been initiated the frequency of measurement will determine the lead time when there is progression. Usually the rate of evolution of prostatic cancer makes a monitoring schedule of 4 times a year during the higher risk periods (first two years in M_O disease) and coincidental with routine visits for M_1 disease an adequate schedule. Repeat measurements are advised when there is suspicion of a rise.

Are There any Indications for Using PSA Today ?

Serial serum PSA tests are at present the most sensitive biomarker of progression in localised and metastatic cancer. There appear to be two clinical situations in which the measurement of PSA can be very helpful. The first is the monitoring of patients with regionally confined prostatic cancer who are being managed by deferred treatment. The second is the early identification of the onset of hormone resistance in patients with low volume disease, to enable alternative treatments to be started before there has been a down grading of the patient's performance status.

No doubt other indications will emerge especially when the range of effective treatment is increased.

Acknowledgement

    EHC and JKS are supported by the Yorkshire Cancer
Research Campaign.   This study is made on behalf of the
Yorkshire Urological Cancer Research Group.

REFERENCES

Cooper EH, Pidcock NB, Daponte D, Glashan RW, Rowe E,
    Robinson MRG (1983).   Monitoring of prostate cancer by
    an enzyme-linked immunosorbent assay of serum prostatic
    acid phosphatase. Eur Urol 9: 17-23.
Cooper EH, Newling DWW, Siddall JK (1986). Verlaufskontrolle
    des nicht metastasierenden Prostatakarzinoms mit Hilfe der
    Bestimmung der sauren Prostata-Phosphatase im Serum.   In:
    Neue Erkenntnisse zur klinischen Wertigkeit und Methodik
    der sauren Prostataphosphatase, Bauer HW und Froschle MC
    (eds), Darmstadt, Git, pp 43-46.
Foti A, Cooper J, Herschman H, Malvaez R (1977). Detection
    of prostatic cancer by solid-phase radioimmunoassay of
    serum prostatic acid phosphatase. N Engl J Med 297:1357
Hara M, Inone T, Koyangi Y, Goto J, Yamazaki H, Fukuyama T
    (1966). Preparation and immunoelectrophoretic assessment
    of antisera to human seminal plasma. Jpn J Legal Med 20:
    356-362.
Hetherington JW, Siddall JK, Cooper EH (1987). The contri-
    bution of bone scintigraphy prostatic acid phosphatase
    and prostatic specific antigen to the monitoring of
    prostate cancer. Eur Urol (in press).
Killian CS, Yang N, Emrich LJ (1985). Prognostic importance
    of prostatic specific antigen for monitoring patients with
    B2 to D1 prostate cancer. Cancer Res 45: 886-891.
Killian CS, Emrich LJ, Vargas FP, Constantine R, Wang MC,
    Chu TM (1986). Prognostic importance of prostate-specific
    antigen and other markers for monitoring of prostate
    cancer patients. In: Tumor Markers in Prostate Cancer,
    Princetown, NJ, Excerpta Medica, pp 24-36.
Kuriyama M, Takeuchi T, Shinoda I, Okano M, Nishiura T (1986).
    Clinical evaluation of seminoprotein in prostate cancer.
    The Prostate 8: 301-311.
Lange PH, Ercole CJ, Vessella RL (1986). Tumor markers in
    the follow up of initial therapy of prostate cancer. In:
    Tumor Markers in Prostate Cancer, Lange PH (ed), Prince-
    town, NJ, Excerpta Medica, pp 16-23.

Okabe T, Noda S, Sagawa K, Yokoyama M, Kamachi S (1985). Clinical evaluation of prostate specific antigens. (γ-Seminoprotein). Jpn J Urol 76: 165-173.

Pontes JE (1983). Biological markers in prostate cancer. J Urol 130: 1037-1047.

Schwartz MK (1986). Can prostate specific antigen be used in screening ? In: Tumor Markers in Prostate Cancer, Lange PH (ed), Princetown, NJ, Excerpta Medica, pp 47-51.

Siddall JK, Cooper EH, Newling DWW, Robinson MRG, Whelan P (1986a). An evaluation of the immunochemical measurement of prostatic acid phosphatase and prostatic specific antigen in carcinoma of the prostate. Eur Urol 12: 123-130.

Siddall JK, Hetherington JW, Cooper EH, Newling DWW, Robinson MRG, Richards B, Denis L (1986b). Biochemical monitoring of carcinoma of the prostate treated with an LH-RH analogue (Zoladex). Br J Urol 58: 678-682.

Siddall JK, Shetty SD, Cooper EH (1986c). Measurements of serum γ-seminoprotein and prostatic specific antigen evaluated for monitoring carcinoma of the prostate. Clin Chem 32: 2040-2043.

Wang MC, Valenzuela LA, Murphy GP, Chu TM (1979). Purification of a human prostate-specific antigen. Invest Urol 17: 159-163.

Watt KWK, Lee PS, Timkulu TM, Chan WP, Loor R (1986). Human prostate-specific antigen : Structural and functional similarity with serine proteases. Proc Natl Acad Sci USA 83: 3166-3170.

EORTC Genitourinary Group Monograph 5: Progress
and Controversies in Oncological Urology II, pages 55–56
© 1988 Alan R. Liss, Inc.

Discussion: Acid Phosphatase, Alkaline Phosphatase and
Prostate Specific Antigen: Which Markers Should We Choose?

Fritz H. Schroder, Rotterdam, The Netherlands

Dubernard: Is there any discussion?

Schmidtbauer: What is the ideal timing for determining the
markers as related to rectal examination?

Cooper: We have conducted a small experiment to this fact.
There is undoubtedly a small group of patients in whom a
vigorous rectal examination will result in a rise of PSA.
But usually these patients will have high levels before they
start. Very few patients who have otherwise normal levels,
will show any change after rectal examination. My view on
the subject is that in the group of patients where an elevated marker in the initial diagnostic phase is of greatest
importance, the group with localized disease, there is rarely any pressure for making a quick decision. The important
examination that should be relied on would be a repeat
examination without previous rectal palpation.

Rollema: What is the correlation between tumor grade and
elevation of PSA?

Cooper: I cannot tell you at this stage. All we know is that
all patients in this study are metastatic.

Fosså: Dr. Bauer and yourself have shown that PSA and PAP
are good markers to follow patients with primary endocrine
treatment. Is there any evidence that these markers are also
suitable for secondary treatment, namely chemotherapy?

Cooper: Dr. Bauer quoted to you the experience from the
United States where chemotherapy as a second line treatment
was used. This group thinks that PSA has an advantage over
other markers in following such patients.

Chodak: I am curious about the patients that have not been
treated. Did you follow them periodically to see whether PSA

would indicate progressive disease?

Cooper: We have done that. In patients who remain stable as far as clinical findings is concerned, we often saw that PSA would rise from initial values around 2 to values around 8 within 3 or 4 years. In patients who were eventually shown to have local or distant spread, the rate of change was much faster. Based on this I think that 3 to 4 months is an adequate time interval to make these measurements when there is no evidence of clinical progression.

Dubernard: Thank you for this nice discussion. We have to get on with the next presentation.

EORTC Genitourinary Group Monograph 5: Progress
and Controversies in Oncological Urology II, pages 57–65

TRANSRECTAL ULTRASONOGRAPHY AND CT SCANNING OF THE PRIMARY
TUMOUR IN THE FOLLOW-UP OF PATIENTS WITH PROSTATIC CARCINOMA

Peter G. Ryan[o], David R. Jones,[o+] W. Brian Peeling[o]
Ernest E. Roberts[+]
[o]Department of Urology, Gwent Urological Centre,
St. Woolos Hospital, Newport, U.K.   NP9 4SZ
[+]Academic Department of Radiology, University
Hospital of Wales, Cardiff, U.K.

INTRODUCTION

It is generally accepted that estimation of prostatic
volume by per-rectal digital palpation is unreliable, as
was shown by Meyhoff & Hald (1978), and of the several options for ultrasound transrectal axial scanning of the
prostate has emerged as the most accurate and applicable
process to measure prostatic volume (Declerq & Denis, 1980;
Hastak et al, 1982). Computerised tomography (CT) is also
capable of demonstrating and measuring the prostate and has
proved to be useful for planning radiotherapy treatment
(Pilepich et al, 1980). At the present time these are the
imaging techniques that might be used to follow up patients
with prostatic cancer and it is therefore appropriate to
review their relative merits firstly as methods for the
measurement of prostatic volume and then to consider their
application to monitoring of treatment.

1. Measurement of volume of prostatic tumour

In an ideal world, imaging techniques such as ultrasound or CT should be able to differentiate clearly between
a prostatic cancer and the benign tissue that surrounds it
and so be capable of measuring actual tumour size. Unfortunately that is not so, particularly for CT which cannot
even demonstrate the capsule and internal architecture of
the prostate so that with this imaging process it is not
possible to distinguish benign from malignant tissue within
the gland (Gore & Moss, 1983; Denkaus et al, 1983; Dobbs &
Husband 1985).

In contrast, the internal structure of the prostate and its capsule can be demonstrated by transrectal ultrasound but even when the cancers appear as apparently well defined hypoechoic lesions within the gland, measurement of its volume by ultrasound will be imprecise because the infiltrating nature of the periphery of the tumour (Lee et al, 1985). Therefore, measurement of TOTAL VOLUME of the prostate is usual, which can be done by both CT and transrectal ultrasound.

But how accurate are these procedures in real terms at measuring total prostatic volume? There are no objective data concerning CT in this regard, whereas for transrectal ultrasonography the situation has recently been clarified by a study on cadaver prostates. Jones and his colleagues (1987) examined 100 cadaver prostates to compare the actual size of each gland in direct comparison with the size measured by transrectal ultrasonic scanning of the cadaver specimen. The technique for this procedure has previously been described by Brooman et al (1981) whereby the rectum, prostate and bladder of the excised specimen from the cadaver were mounted in a specially designed water tank that could be placed upon an Aloka chair probe, so that the prostate could then be scanned as in a living patient. Of 100 specimens examined, 3 had extensive cancer whose volumes could not be measured because the margins were not definable by ultrasound. Of the remaining 97 prostates there was a close correlation between the physical volume of the gland with the volume measured ultrasonically, particularly for 71 prostates with benign hyperplasia (r=0.98); for 26 prostatic cancers studied the correlation was slightly less (r=0.85). This was affected adversely by 3 large unconfined cancers that were difficult to measure ultrasonically. (Fig 1).

It is evident from this work that total prostatic volume can be measured reliably by transrectal ultrasonic scanning except for larger unconfined (T3/T4) cancers. However, such tumours are suitable for imaging by CT which can show particularly well the irregular and malignant extension of such tumours into surrounding tissue (Denkaus et al, 1983; Dobbs & Husband 1985). Therefore the imaging technique of choice for routine follow-up of prostatic cancer would seem to be transrectal ultrasonic scanning, rather than CT.

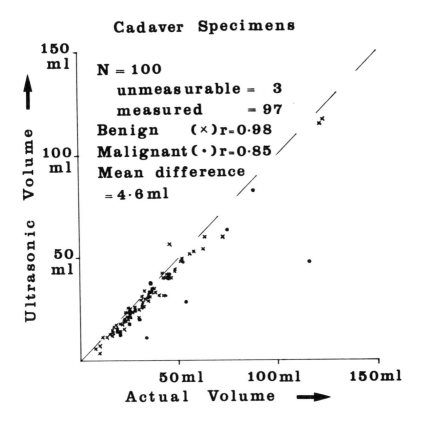

Fig. 1 Correlation between Ultrasound and Physical Volume in Cadaver Prostates

2. Application of prostatic volume measurements

In principle, measurement of prostatic volume through-out the management of a patient with prostatic cancer might provide an indicator of the responsiveness of the primary tumour to treatment, from which prognostic deductions might be made depending upon the rate of response of the tumour

to treatment. Continued monitoring of treated primary
prostatic cancers might also provide an early warning system
of relapse and re-activation of disease in a previously
controlled tumour, if it enlarges or if its character, such
as staging, increases secondarily. Can transrectal ultrasonography help urologists with those important aspects of
management of prostatic cancer?

a) Measurement of response to treatment. Urologists
who have experience with transrectal ultrasound have found
it to be of value for relating total volume changes of the
prostate, with other parameters such as plasma levels of
prostatic acid phosphatase (PAP), testosterone, and prostatic
specific antigen (PSA). This can be illustrated by a series
of observations made over 27 months in a recent study of 38
patients treated either by subcapsular orchidectomy or with
the depot formulation of LHRH analogue "Zoladex". There was
a progressive mean reduction of prostatic volume after treatment that stabilised at about 40% of the pre-treatment volume
and this occurred in association with suppression of plasma
testosterone levels to castrate ranges and a fall of plasma
prostatic acid phosphatase. (Fig 2).

Other workers have reported similar findings but
Carpentier et al, (1984) suggested that rates of change of
prostatic volume within the first six months of starting
endocrine treatment for disseminated prostatic cancer could
predict prognosis, with the greater slope of the volume reduction curve being associated with longer survival.

We have looked for a similar trend in 48 men treated by
subcapsular orchidectomy or with "Zoladex" depot. (Fig 3).
They were subdivided into 20 patients who showed objective
signs of progression within 12 months of first treatment,
and the second group of 28 patients who showed complete or
partial response, but no progression, during the first 12
months of their treatment. At the 6 months stage, there was
no statistical difference between the rates of volume reduction of these groups and we must conclude tentatively,
at least in our study, there was no evidence of a prognostic
factor related to the volumetric response of the primary
tumour to endocrine treatment.

b) Prediction of relapse. Just as reduction of prostatic volume in response to treatment seems to be a good sign,
is a secondary enlargement of a previously controlled prostatic cancer a reliable indicator of impending relapse and
re-activation of disease? We considered this in 65 patients

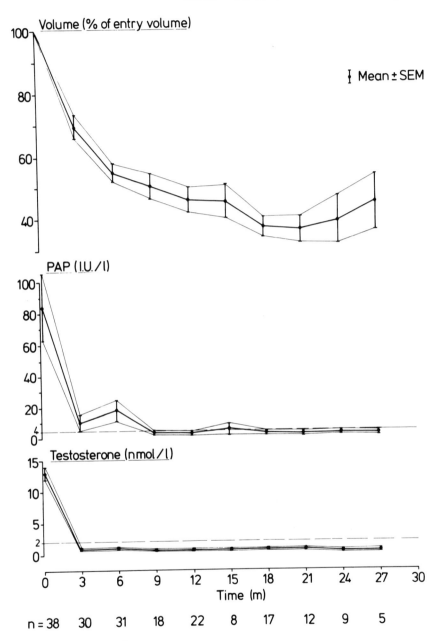

Fig. 2 Change in Prostatic Volume, Prostatic Acid Phosphatase, and testosterone with Time in Treated Prostatic Carcinoma.

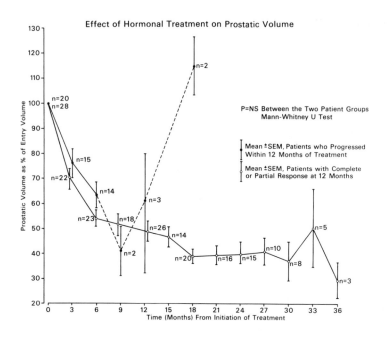

Fig. 3 Effect of Hormonal Treatment on Prostatic Volume for Patients who showed progression within 12 months of treatment and Patients with Complete or Partial Response at 12 months.

who had been treated either by orchidectomy or with depot "Zoladex". Most of the volume reduction of the prostate in these patients occurred within the first 6 months of treatment, although rarely this continued for as long as 36 months. Whilst being monitored, 37 patients showed signs of objective progression of cancer which sometimes occurred even though the primary tumour was apparently decreasing in size at the same time. So it is evident that volume responses of primary prostatic cancer is no indicator of the future behaviour of the disease as a whole.

It might be expected that ultrasonic monitoring of the STAGE, rather than the volume, of primary prostatic cancer would provide early information about re-activation of a previously controlled tumour. This idea was examined in

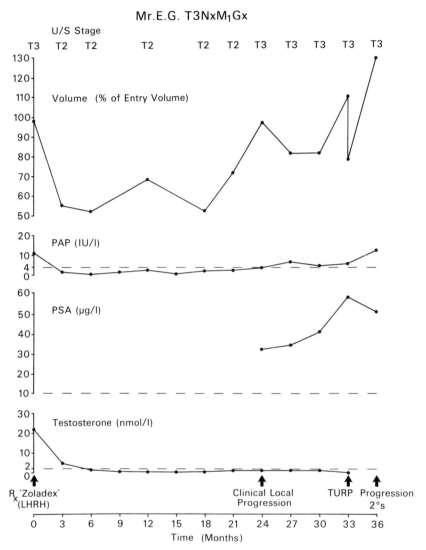

Fig. 4 An example of ultrasound monitoring of prostatic cancer in an individual case. Initial response of volume and stage to primary treatment. After 18 months increase in prostatic ultrasound volume. By 24 months clinical local progression and ultrasonic upstaging of primary tumour. Local progression continued. (TURP at 33 months). Progression of secondaries at 36 months.

34 patients with progressive disease. Seventeen showed no
change of ultrasonic stage at the time of progression and
in fact 6 had confined cancers that remained so throughout
the course of their illness. In 6 patients, down-staging
to confined disease occurred, in 6 the tumour became unconfined, and in 5 there was an initial down-staging to
confined disease that later reverted to an unconfined state.
Therefore, only 11 of 34 (32%) of these patients showed an
increase of ultrasonic staging at, or preceding, the time
of progression of their disease as determined by other criteria such as bone scan. Clearly, monitoring the STAGE of
primary prostatic cancer is of limited value in predicting
relapse, but may be evident in individual patients.
(Figs. 3, 4).

CONCLUSIONS

The best option for routine follow-up of primary pros-
static cancer is in our opinion transrectal ultrasound
rather than CT. Although total prostatic volume rather than
actual tumour volume is measured in monitoring, transrectal
ultrasound has proved itself of value to monitor volume
changes associated with treatment of prostatic cancer, including policies of deferred treatment, and is therefore
ideally suited for use in clinical trials. With regard to
continued monitoring of primary prostatic cancer in our
experience transrectal ultrasound cannot predict prognosis
or relapse and would seem therefore to be of no value as a
monitoring procedure in clinical trials once the initial
response of the primary tumour has been established. Nevertheless, in some individual patients, transrectal ultrasound may give advanced warning of re-activation of a previously controlled primary tumour.

REFERENCES

Brooman P J C, Griffiths G J, Roberts E, Peeling W B, Evans
K T (1981). Per-rectal ultrasound in the investigation
of prostatic disease. Clin. Rad. 32 : 669-676
Carpentier P J, Schroeder F H (1984). Transrectal ultrasonography in the follow up of prostatic carcinoma
patients : new prognostic parameter? J. Urol 131 903-905
Declercq G, Denis L (1978). Ultrasonic assessment of prostatic mass. Acta Urol. Belg. 46 : 74-79

Denkaus H, Dierkopf W, Grabbe E, Donn F (1983). Comparative study of suprapubic sonography and computed tomography for staging of prostatic carcinoma. Urology : Radiology 5 : 1-9

Dobbs H J, Husband J E (1985). The role of CT in staging and radiotherapy planning of prostatic tumours. Brit. J. Radiol. 58 : 429-436

Gore R M, Moss A A (1983). Value of computed tomography in interstitial 125I brachytherapy of prostatic carcinoma. Radiology 146 : 453-458

Hastak S M, Gammelgaard J, Holm H H (1982). Transrectal ultrasonic volume determination of the prostate - a pre-operative and post-operative study. J. Urol 127 : 1115-1118.

Jones D R, Griffiths G J, Parkinson C, Roberts E E, Evans K T (1987). Unpublished data

Lee F, Gray J M, McLeary R D, Meadows T R, Kumasaka G H, Borlaza G S, Straub W H, Lee F Jr., Solomon M H, McHugh T A, Wolf R M (1985). Transrectal ultrasound in the diagnosis of prostatic cancer : location, echogenicity, histopathology and staging. Prostate 7 : 117-129

Meyhoff H H, Hald T (1978). Are doctors able to assess prostatic size? Scand. J. Urol. Nephrol. 12 : 219-221

Pilepich M V, Percz C A, Prasad S C (1980). Computed tomography in definition radiotherapy of prostatic carcinoma. Int. J. Radiat. Oncol. Bio. Phys. 6 : 923-926

Rickards D, Gowland M, Brooman P, Mamtora H, Blacklock N J, Isherwood I (1983). Computed tomography and transrectal ultrasound in the diagnosis of prostatic disease - a comparative study. Brit. J. Urol 55 : 726-732

EORTC Genitourinary Group Monograph 5: Progress
and Controversies in Oncological Urology II, page 67
© 1988 Alan R. Liss, Inc.

Discussion: Transrectal Ultrasonography and CT Scanning of
the Primary Tumour in the Follow-up of Patients With
Prostatic Carcinoma

Fritz H. Schroder, Rotterdam, The Netherlands.

Dubernard: Are there any remarks? Does everybody agree with
the comment on ultrasound and CT-scanning?

Fosså: You said that ultrasound does not predict the prognosis. How about CT. Do you have any data showing whether
changes on CT will correlate with prognosis?

Peeling: This is an area that certainly needs to be looked
at, unfortunately, I do not have the answer.

Watanabe: Based on our data on measurements of the prostate
under treatment, I think these data to some part do indicate
the prognosis of the patient. We measure the prostatic size
after castration very frequently, some times 4 times a day.
If you plot prostatic volume against time you see that the
reduction of the volume is very sharp, especially in the
beginning, right after treatment. We have performed such
measurements on some 40 patients with stage D cancer. We
calculate a factor "tau" which is representative for the
volume decrease and which correlates with the prognosis of
the patient. Unfortunately, the time is limited, so I cannot
explain the whole procedure. At least in my opinion it is
possible to use prostatic volume to predict the prognosis of
stage D patients under endocrine management.

Dubernard: Thank you for this discussion. It is time to
close the session.

EORTC Genitourinary Group Monograph 5: Progress
and Controversies in Oncological Urology II, pages 69-70
© 1988 Alan R. Liss, Inc.

COMPARISON OF TRANSRECTAL ULTRASONOGRAPHY AND MAGNETIC
RESONANCE IMAGING FOR DIAGNOSIS OF PROSTATIC CANCER

Herman J. de Voogt, Erik P. v.d. Weijer, Thea E.G.
van Zanten, Richard P. Golding and Jaap Valk

Departments of Urology and Radiology, AZVU,
Amsterdam, The Netherlands

So far a number of studies on the value of transrectal
ultrasonography or of M.R. imaging of the prostate for diagnosing prostatic diseases have appeared (Egender et al,
1986; Peeling and Griffiths, 1984; Hamm and Wolf, 1986;
Chechile et al, 1986). The number of comparative studies of
these imaging modalities is however very small (Bartsch et
al, 1985).

This study was undertaken to see whether M.R. imaging
is of additional value in diagnosing prostatic cancer when
compared with Transrectal Ultrasound (TUS), of which we had
already determined sensitivity and specificity for that purpose in a previous study (De Voogt, 1986).

36 patients with prostatic enlargement entered the
study in which they underwent TUS and MRI in addition to
routine urologic examination including digital rectal palpation. From 25 patients histological diagnosis became available, 12 having benign prostate hypertrophy (BPH) and 13
having prostatic cancer (PCA). From 11 patients no histological confirmation of our diagnosis could be obtained for
various reasons.

For MRI sharp delineation of the gland and homogeneous
signal intensity were agreed upon as criteria for BPH whereas ill-defined glandular borders and inhomogeneous signal
intensity were considered as coinciding with prostate cancer.
For TUS we agreed on sharp delineation of the prostatic
capsule, homogeneous density distribution and symmetric seminal vesicles as criteria for BPH and irregular or broken-up
capsule, hypodense areas and asymmetry of seminal vesicles
as criteria for prostate cancer.

However, in MR images the criteria for BPH were only present in 5 of 12 patients, while 7 had either inhomogeneous signal intensity or an ill-defined capsule. In patients with prostatic cancer correlation with 2 criteria existed in 2 patients and with one criterion in another 6 patients. In 5 patients there was no correlation at all. In contrast, with respect to TUS, 9 of 13 patients with BPH had all 3 criteria and in 4 patients a suspicion of cancer on 1 criterion arose but could not be proven by biopsy (false negative). From the 12 patients with PCA the criteria of TUS were present all 3 in 5 patients, 2 criteria in 5 patients and 1 criterion in the remaining 2 patients.

From these data, although the relatively small numbers preclude statistical analysis, we concluded that MRI does not yet yield any additional specificity in identifying neoplasia from benign hyperplasia of the prostate. Future technical developments might improve this but are still in the experimental phase at present. Transrectal ultrasonography does provide additional diagnostic value to digital rectal palpation and should be used more routinely for diagnosis and monitoring conservative therapy.

REFERENCES

Bartsch G, Janetschek G, Zurnedden D (1985). Comparison of rectal sonography, CT-scan and NMR in prostatic cancer. J Urol 135:147A-176 (abstract).

Chechile G, Zungri E, Mallo N, Sanz M, Setocin J, Diaz I, Voldez L (1986). Nuclear magnetic resonance in advanced prostatic cancer. Urol Int 41:279-283.

Egender G, Furtschegger A, Schachner W, Pirker E, Bartsch G (1986). Transrectal ultrasonography in diagnosis and staging of prostatic cancer. World J Urol 4:159-162.

Hamm VB, Wolf KJ (1986). Bildgebende Diagnostik des Prostatacarzinoms. Röntgenpraxis 39:187-195.

Peeling WB, Griffiths GJ (1984). Imaging of the prostate by ultrasound. J Urol 132:217-224.

De Voogt HJ (1986). Ultrasonography of the prostate. In Jardin A (ed): "Proceedings XX Congres SIU 1985", Paris: pp 105-107.

EORTC Genitourinary Group Monograph 5: Progress
and Controversies in Oncological Urology II, pages 71-86
© 1988 Alan R. Liss, Inc.

ROUND TABLE DISCUSSION: THE VALUE OF BIOPSY TECHNIQUES, ACID
PHOSPHATASE AND THE IMAGING OF THE PRIMARY TUMOR FOR DIAGNO-
SIS AND RESPONSE TO TREATMENT (Chairmen: G. Rutishauser and
E.H. Cooper).

F.H. Schröder

Department of Urology, Erasmus University Hospital, Rotterdam, The Netherlands

RUTISHAUSER

In this round table we will be mainly concerned with
the primary tumor. We will further illuminate some of the
facts that have already been mentioned in the presentations.
This means that we will speak about the relative value of
biopsy techniques, marker substances and imaging methods for
diagnosis and follow-up of prostatic cancer patients. The
aim of our discussion will be to point out where we can
agree and to show where we do not agree and why we do not
agree on certain points.

Let us first speak about aspiration cytology and core
biopsies. Let us discuss this problem on the basis of the
assumption that the sampling error is excluded and that
equal quality of assessments resulting from both techniques
is provided. Some relevant questions could be formulated as
follows: Is either one of those biopsy techniques better
than the other? Is there still a place for transrectal core
biopsy?

FROHMÜLLER

The first question actually has been answered already in
the sense that if optimal quality of the specimen can be
assumed, the techniques are probably equal. Concerning your
second question, the answer should be no, there is no place
for transrectal core biopsy anymore. It is true that some

people are still practising this technique as is evident from a recent publication by Huland in a German journal. However, the complication rate is so much higher that the technique does not seem to be justified anymore. The results with the transperineal core biopsy are the same. Also, with the perineal approach you develop the same feeling where you have to stick your needle to obtain a proper specimen. So I think that the transrectal biopsy is out.

RUTISHAUSER

The next question would be: is fine needle aspiration biopsy sufficient for planning radical surgical treatment?

CHODAK

Especially for people who are still getting used to the fine needle aspiration biopsy it may be useful to obtain a core biopsy whenever well-differentiated tumor is diagnosed by cytology. This will add some confidence. Since most of the patients we discover are not potentially operable, I think there will be a small percentage of patients requiring this extra procedure. So I believe that the aspiration biopsy is ideal as a first step and of course there will be patients that still warrant a core biopsy.

RUTISHAUSER

The next question would be: is there a need for repeated fine needle or core biopsy in the follow-up of prostatic cancer patients? If that would be the case, why should such biopsies be done, which modality should be prefered and in what kind of treatment would it be useful?

CHODAK

I think it has already become evident that follow-up biopsies are very useful after radiotherapy where a positive biopsy may be associated with a poor prognosis as pointed out by Dr. Scardino. A positive biopsy may warrant some further therapy. I think that the aspiration biopsy is ideal for this purpose. If you would follow such patients with core biopsies and there is nothing palpable, I think it would be very hard for you to know whether you are biopsying the suspicious areas. The aspiration biopsy allows better sampling and this problem is prevented. In reviewing our material we have come accross cases that had a positive aspiration biopsy after radiotherapy in spite of the fact that you could not feel anything on rectal palpation. If at the end it turns out that we have to recommend additional radiotherapy to these people, then this technique will be very helpful.

FROHMÜLLER

Yes, I agree. In the follow-up the aspiration biopsy has it's place. Once you have to do the biopsy more often the simplicity and the practically painless procedure of the aspiration biopsy becomes more advantageous. One of the best papers on this subject has been written by Dr. Scardino, maybe he can say a few words about it.

RUTISHAUSER

I should like to ask first if there are any questions from the floor and then Dr. Scardino could sum up and give his opinion.

FAIR

I have a question to Dr. Chodak and maybe also to Dr. Collste. Dr. Chodak, I was more impressed by your data until you told me that you looked at all the slides yourself. I always thought this was exclusively done by the cytopathologist. If you, prior to looking at slides, feel a prostate and you feel a hard nodule, this must have some influence on your interpretation of the cytology. So my question is: have you looked at the results of the cytopathologist and compared those to the results obtained from the review of the cytopathologist with you together? Are there any differences?

CHODAK

The cytopathologist will give me a grading that will say: highly atypical cells, rule out malignancy. The specimen is looked at by the cytopathologist according to highly restrictive criteria. He may see 20 per cent of malignant cells, they may not call this cancer because they want to see a predominance of malignant cells. They do this because they want to be conservative and they do not want to see us get into trouble. So by reviewing those slides together and realizing that 20 per cent of the cells are malignant, you can encourage the cytopathologist by bringing in the whole clinical information to say that this is really cancer, it is just that I am uncomfortable for you doing a radical prostatectomy on this finding. What I would like to emphasize with this is that there really has to be dialogue between the two and that this is a good way to avoid missing the cancers. I believe that in the past people have ignored those specimens that showed very atypical cells because they may not have fitted entirely the criterium of malignant cells.

FAIR

I would like to ask an additional question. One way to quantitate this a little more accurately would be by means of flowcytophotometry. Can you or anybody else share with us any experience on the use of flowcytometry techniques on aspiration biopsies?

CHODAK

We do not have a flowcytometer. The pathologists at our institution have developed a system that they call the Titas system. With this system you can do DNA analysis on fixed specimens. We have looked at this system and found it very helpful. It allows to pick out patients that have more than 5 n DNA content as being the ones that are indicating malignancy. Yet, as time goes on, the system will be more automated and that will help further.

PEELING

One of the problems I find with patients who have had radiotherapy to their prostate is outlining the prostate itself because there is a lot of induration and thickening around it. For this reason I sometimes wonder how easy it is to biopsy the organ with the standard digital techniques. For this reason we have been recently using ultrasound guidance for both, the core and the aspiration biopsy. This has been very useful to us. I am wondering whether with the more widespread use of ultrasound more people are considering using that technique?

RUTISHAUSER

It is quite a procedure to do this ultrasound guided biopsy, is it not?

PEELING

No, it is an outpatient procedure.

RUTISHAUSER

Is it not rather time-consuming?

PEELING

Well, I do not know, it may take 15 minutes.

RUTISHAUSER

Mr. Scardino, would you sum up?

SCARDINO

The discussion suggests that in the presence of an adequate technique and a capable cytopathologist aspiration biopsy is comparable to core biopsy as far as sensitivity and specificity is concerned and that both techniques are available and will probably continue to be used. For following patients under treatment reports have been published on aspiration and on punch biopsy. For instance following the patients after radiotherapy has proven to be effective by both techniques. It is a secondary question whether one needs to do any additional therapy on the basis of the results. It is, however, fair to say that the treatment has failed locally if positive biopsies either by means of the punch or the aspiration cytology are obtained a reasonable period of time after radiotherapy. As far as the type of core biopsy is concerned, transperineal or transrectal, there seems to be agreement among the panelists that the transperineal approach is preferable, however, if we should ask a show of hands about this question, I am not so sure that we would obtain the same consensus from the audience. Certainly in the United States the transrectal approach seems to be prefered by most urologists in spite of the septic complications.

DEBRUYNE

I have a question for Dr. Scardino. You have published on quite a number of radical prostatectomies for relapse after radiotherapy. Would you rely on a fine needle aspiration biopsy prior to such a procedure?

SCARDINO

Not up to now. We are presently reviewing our biopsy material, which is obtained simultaneously by means of fine needle aspiration and core biopsies. My impression is that one could rely on the cytology alone. A radical prostatectomy after radiotherapy is, however, such a high risk operation that I have not been willing to put any patient through it without double confirmation of the diagnosis.

RUTISHAUSER

Our next problem are the biochemical marker substances, acid phosphatase, alkaline phosphatase and prostate specific antigen. The first question would be whether we can still rely on enzymatic determinations or whether an immunochemical form of determination of prostatic acid phosphatase is compulsory.

FROHMÜLLER

The enzymatic assay of acid phosphatase depends on temperature and time. For that reason I would consider the determination in itself by means of immunochemical techniques as more reliable. Your choice should, however, depend on what you really want. The immunochemical assay is more specific and only the prostatic acid phosphatase is measured. With the biochemical assay you also measure other phosphatase activities. So if you want to know the total amount of prostatic acid phosphatase in the serum, the immunochemical assay is more reliable.

COOPER

I agree that there is a difference concerning the immunochemical measurement in the sense that particularly close to the normal value you have a more reliable measurement. But I think that another point to be born in mind is the introduction of this test into hospitals in general while the test is frequently ordered by people who are not involved in the care of prostatic cancer patients. This exercise is somewhat doubtful from an economic point of view. The prostatic acid phosphatase and the determination of PSA, the new test we are going to hear about, now is particularly useful in the hands of those colleagues who are educated to use it. In the hands of colleagues who are not specialists in using these results, both tests are very likely to be misused.

BAUER

I can only agree with this, only the economics speak against this new test. In the hands of people who know how to use these results the increase of specificity and sensitivity and overall accuracy speak for the immunochemical tests.

SPLINTER

If one of the markers is rising during progression of this disease, does it rise exponentially?

BAUER

No, why should a marker rise exponentially?

SPLINTER

Because the tumor is growing in an exponential fashion.

BAUER

No, I cannot agree with this. Often enough you have a very slow rise of any of these markers. Sometimes even the rise is so borderline that it can only be detected by the immunochemical test.

SPLINTER

Actually, did you look at the changes on semiloga-rithmic papers with a linear time scale?

BAUER

Yes, I have done that and there was no exponential change.

SPLINTER

Then the next question. What is the relationship between these tumor markers and the tumor mass?

CHODAK

I suppose it would be fair to say that not the whole tumor is growing at the same rate. We know that there are multiple grades of malignancy present in the same tumor. The idea that if you have two cells now you have four cells the next time you look is probably false.

BAUER

Also, a lot of cells are known not to possess this antigen, especially the poorly differentiated ones.

KURTH

Suppose you are using both markers and you are looking for the prediction of progression. How does your predictive value increase if you combine both markers? Can the predictive value in identifying progressing patients be increased in this way?

BAUER

This is an important question. As you know, the predictive value depends on the prevalence of the disease in the collective you are studying. Depending on the prevalence of the disease the predictive value will be either positive or negative. These studies have not been done for PSA and also not for the combination of PAP and PSA. They have only been done for PAP, where the predictive value is about 60 per cent, which unfortunately is very low. If you, however, compare this to other clinical markers, their predictive value would be very similar.

COOPER

I think this question has not completely been answered. Where you know that a patient has the disease and where you know that by some form of treatment he is in remission, then using both markers would give you a small advantage in the sense that probably you could pick up one progressing patient in 50, who you would not pick up by either one of the markers alone. PSA is an expensive laboratory determination but of course if you need to know about that one individual being in progression or not, then the expense may be irrelevant and you should use both markers.

KURTH

This is a little bit the answer I expected. As we know PAP and PSA may be produced in different compartments of the tumor and this may result in a situation where in some cases you will only have an increase of the PAP and in others an increase of the PSA. Could you give an indication of what may be the frequency of this particular situation and how much the sensitivity may increase through this phenomenon?

COOPER

From what I have seen in terms of patients in whom only the PAP or only the PSA was elevated as a sign of progression after remission I would expect the diagnostic gain from using both procedures to be only a few per cent.

PAULSON

The question I have may be very simple-minded but Brenckman demonstrated that prostatic acid phosphatase as measured by the enzymatic assay has a marked biological variability in its release or at least in its detection, which could be roughly 50 per cent above or below a mean level over an extended period of observation. I believe it was Maatman who demonstrated the identical phenomenon with the immunochemical assay. The two questions I have for the panel are: Does PSA have the same variation when a series of observations are made in the same patient over a period of time and two, is the panel suggesting that a presistant elevation of PSA under treatment indicates progression of the disease or does this just mean that the disease has extended beyond the prostate and that it really cannot be used to measure the true extent of the disease?

COOPER

I can answer about the longitudinal measurements. We have followed patients that did not go into progression. In this way an individual may have been measured 10 or 12 times. His individual level may be 2.0 ng $\pm$ 0.5. That is the sort of variation we find. You also have to take into account that laboratories who are repeating measurements have an intrinsic error of themselves. If, in using PSA, you see little variation up and down you should not worry. If, however, you see PSA going up successively at the time of repeated determinations, you should begin to strongly think that the patient has developed more progressive disease.

SCARDINO

Dr. Paulson, I would like to refer to your second question about the significance of the elevated markers. Does an elevation mean disease just outside the prostate or more extensive disease? In our own work, using the enzymatic acid phosphatase assay, we looked at patients who had localized disease and were lymph node negative and split them into groups with an elevated and a normal acid phosphatase. The patients with an elevated acid phosphatase and negative nodes have the same rate of development of the metastases as those with positive nodes. For these reasons I believe that an elevated enzymatically determined acid phosphatase indicates metastatic disease. I am not so sure whether this is true with the immunoassay and it certainly is not true with the PSA.

FOSSÅ

I have a question about PAP and PSA in relation to the grade of differentiation. I learned previously that with increasing dedifferentiation of the tumor the PAP production may decrease and that may be the reason why we do not see elevation of PAP in some patients with progression. I think Dr. Bauer also indicated that. On the other hand, Dr. Cooper showed us that with decreasing grade in the N-plus patients he would still see an increase of the number of those with an elevated PSA. This may be at variance with the PAP observations. In my experience 20 per cent of all patients with metastatic disease do not have an elevated PAP. I always thought this is because the cancer has become so dedifferentiated. Is PSA more frequently elevated in hormone refractiory prostatic cancer patients?

COOPER

The answer is yes. I can find more patients who have an elevated PSA when they become hormone-resistent, then have a corresponding increase of PAP. Even if the PAP is negative, you can find the PSA rising.

RUTISHAUSER

Thank you for this nice discussion. Let us move on. Let us speak briefly about the role of alkaline phosphatase in prostatic cancer.

DE VOOGT

In a recent study of prognostic factors of two major EORTC studies of prostatic cancer patients the alkaline phosphatase seems to be a more important prognostic factor than the acid phosphatase. The acid phosphatase was prognostic only if the elevation was more than two times the normal value, whereas any elevation of the alkaline phosphatase correlated with survival. The least that can be said is that the alkaline phosphatase can be looked at as an important factor together with the acid phosphatase.

DEBRUYNE

We have done a similar review on our own material and I must confirm that the alkaline phosphatase is very important with relation to prognosis and even to treatment decisions. I have another question to Professor De Voogt. Have you looked at the iso-enzymes? Iso-enzyme 5 could be more predictive with regard to prognosis.

DE VOOGT

No, we have not looked at the iso-enzymes of alkaline phosphatase.

BERKOVIC

You are using alkaline phosphatase to monitor bone metastases. Since alkaline phosphatase may also originate from other organs and other metastases, would it not be more useful to use the hydroxyprolineurea as a marker? Can you compare the value of hydroxyprolineurea and alkaline phosphatase in patients with bony metastases?

BAUER

Alkaline phosphatase is only of importance for monitoring skeletal metastases. What we actually need is a good marker for metastatic carcinoma of the prostate wherever it occurs, in lymph nodes, lungs or other soft tissues. It may be in certain patients that bony metastases remain the only metastases and then you have a good marker by the use of alkaline phosphatase. If one, however, considers the whole biological spectrum of metastatic prostatic cancer, alkaline phosphatase is not a good marker of this disease.

BERKOVIC

I should still like to insist on the second part of my question about the hydroxyprolineurea. Does anyone of the panel have any experience with this marker?

RUTISHAUSER

No, apparently no member of the panel has experience with this marker. I shall ask Dr. Cooper to sum up what has been said about the marker substances.

COOPER

The first statement, Mr. Chairman, is that the markers you have today are far from being ideal. Some of you have pointed out small differences between the different products on the market. These are typical problems one runs into during the period of development of a new marker. The second question would be that you as surgeons define clearly what you want from a marker. This must be seen on the background that in prostatic cancer you do not have a whole series of effective alternative ways of management. And this is in contrast with testicular tumors where alphafoetoprotein and beta-HCG serve as markers. In some ways you like to apply what you know about testicular disease to this non-ideal situation around carcinoma of the prostate. And already you have seen this afternoon that numerous magic numbers have been mentioned, fives and tens and things, and this becomes part of the folklore of the marker. This is a dangerous thing. After all, the markers do not have an absolute value but help you in estimating probabilities. All you are doing all the time is taking all the probabilities into consideration. The marker is only one among a vast number of other factors that you integrate every time you see the patient and before you make a decision. So I think in that context we have got a little way further forward.

The other important thing is always to bear in mind the time scale of the disease you are dealing with. As you all know, prostatic cancer is a relatively slowly developing disease. Therefore, to read too much into one point of time is probably stupid. I urge you to make not one but two measurements three months apart and if you get a slope then this is much more meaningful than having one value.

RUTISHAUSER

Thank you very much, there is one more comment.

MOSTOFI

I should like to make two comments. If one looks at tissue with immunoperoxidase staining of PSA and PAP, one finds out that you actually have to do both stains. We have found that PSA in a way is more emotional than PAP. You must be sure that the PSA antibody you are using is really active.

RUTISHAUSER

Thank you very much. We now come to the third subject of this round table, which is the imaging of the prostate by means of ultrasound, the value of ultrasound guided biopsies and the value of NMR in imaging the prostate. We should answer the questions: What is the place of ultrasound in the evaluation of the primary tumor and what route should be prefered. Is the transrectal access really preferable?

CHODAK

I think the rectal ultrasound surpasses the suprapubic application. In 1987 in the United States if a patient walks into your office being worried about prostatic cancer, you really have to do a rectal examination and a transrectal ultrasound study because with the rectal examination you can miss tumors that can be picked up by the ultrasound and vice versa. The use of both techniques together will augment your ability to detect this tumor. Either one can be used for screening, but I think that we can really offer the patient an increased opportunity for making a diagnosis.

N.N.

I have a question to Dr. Scardino. In doing transrectal ultrasonography one can find either hypo-echoic or hyper-echoic areas. Which nodule will you biopsy? Tissue characterization by means of ultrasound at this moment seems to be rather impossible, does that mean that you will biopsy every suspicious finding on ultrasound?

SCARDINO

Thank you for this question. It gives me an opportunity to respond. I am not entirely sure whether I agree with Dr. Chodak on the role of ultrasonography in diagnosis. Our data on the use of ultrasound in follow-up in determining the extent of the disease makes me doubtful about the use of ultrasound for the diagnosis. We had much trouble in identifying tumors that actually were not palpable and this makes me wonder what the role of this modality will be in diagnosing non-palpable cancer. I am worried about the present radiological literature in the United States, where the implication under the line seems to be that with transrectal ultrasound you can diagnose many tumors that cannot be diagnosed otherwise. On the other hand, I am missing good data in these reports that indicate how many of these tumors have really been palpable and how many have not been. My view at this moment is that the value of ultrasonography in the diagnosis of prostatic cancer still remains to be proven. I would not recommend it for routine clinical use and not even for a routine requirement in a study. I would say it has to be looked into. It has the possibility but I think it is unproven.

PEELING

One of the problems is that the technology is certainly moving on. The type of pictures we are getting now are not the same ones we got ten years ago. The use of the chair probe has very great qualities, but one thing you cannot do is to manipulate the probe in such a way that you can get the optimum resolution. By using modern equipment and moving the probe into the most adequate position it has certainly been possible to diagnose very small cancers as Lee has described. My radiological colleague, Dr. Griffith, has recently analysed 221 cases of proven cancer that we have seen in recent years. He found that of the confined cases 92 per cent were echo-poor, 4 per cent were iso-echoic and therefore could not show up on ultrasound, so you would not diagnose them anyway, 4 per cent were hyper-echoic as Dr. Watanabe mentioned earlier today. These were looked at in the cadaver study I mentioned in my talk and it was shown that the hyper-echoic pattern is due to microcalcifications similar to those seen in breast cancer. This is an observation which was reported in 1981 by Peter Brooman as a result of a pilot study that we did in those days. The detection of early cancer is difficult because a few of them will not be picked up by this technique. But I still would not entirely agree with Dr. Scardino that transrectal ultrasonography should not be a routine procedure in the diagnostic work-up of prostatic cancer in a department. We do not screen patients but we scan patients that come up with some indication for a work-up.

CHODAK

I should like to get back to the role of ultrasound. I think it is fair to see that we all differ in our ability to diagnose prostate cancer. I for example have a short finger. The size of your finger, your sensitivity to what you are looking for, all these factors play a role. In our own department we have seen the different capabilities of different persons in detecting prostate cancer. The ultrasound seems to help us move away from some of that subjectivity. Another subjectivity comes in concerning the interpretation of the scan. The ultrasound, however, enables me to walk with the scan to another colleague and ask him what he thinks about it. This obviously cannot be done with a rectal examination. Perhaps this will allow us to detect more tumors. We know that we are missing a lot of tumors currently. For these reasons I believe that ultrasound is going to play a role in improving our abilities to make the diagnosis.

EORTC Genitourinary Group Monograph 5: Progress
and Controversies in Oncological Urology II, pages 87–95
© 1988 Alan R. Liss, Inc.

ROUTINE SCREENING FOR PROSTATE CANCER USING THE DIGITAL
RECTAL EXAMINATION

Gerald W Chodak, Paul Keller and Harry Schoenberg

Section of Urology, Department of Surgery, The
University of Chicago and the Pritzker School of
Medicine, Chicago, Illinois   60637

INTRODUCTION

Carcinoma of the prostate is currently the second
most common cancer in men in the United States and the
third most common cause of death from cancer. Despite
some advances in the past thirty years, the mortality rate
from this disease has continued to rise. One explanation
is that a majority of patients already have extracapsular
extension of tumor at the time the tumor is diagnosed
(Murphy et al., 1982). Once this has occurred, a cure is
difficult to attain.

Prompted by the high mortality rate from this
disease, we initiated a prostate cancer screening program
using the digital rectal exmination based on the
hypothesis that early detection would reduce mortality
from this disease.

MATERIALS AND METHODS

A description of the screening methods has been
previously described (Chodak and Schoenberg, 1984).
Briefly, beginning in 1981, a free digital exam was
offered to men over the age of 40 regardless of their
symptoms. Prior to the exam, a symptom questionnaire was
obtained that inquired about voiding patterns, nocturia,
hematuria and dysuria. The screening exam was performed
by either of two staff urologists at The University of
Chicago Hospitals and a prostate biopsy was recommended to
any patient if the prostate was slightly indurated or if

palpable nodules or stony hardness were present.

Initially biopsies were performed using the transperineal core method. In order to provide anesthesia, patients were usually hospitalized for one or two nights and administered general or spinal anesthesia. A prerequisite for anesthesia included a chest X-ray, electrocardiogram, complete blood count, kidney profile, and urinalysis. More recently, an aspiration biopsy was performed as an out-patient procedure as previously described (Chodak et al., 1984).

If the biopsy was positive for adenocarcinoma, a staging work-up was performed which included a complete blood cell count, an acid and alkaline phosphatase, a bone scan, a chest X-ray, and in some cases, a CT scan or transrectal prostate ultrasonogram.

The cost of screening was derived as follows. The staff costs were determined based on a cost of $50/hr for the physician and $25/hr for the clinic coordinator. On the average, 12 exams were performed per hour. For each hour of exams, the coordinator worked an additional two hours to register patients, make appointments, send correspondence and manage the data. The charges for the in-patient biopsies were taken from the hospital charts of patients requiring the procedure and the cost for the aspiration biopsy was a standard amount.

RESULTS

Since our program was initiated, we have examined 2,101 men over the age of 40. A biopsy was performed on 121 (5.8%) of these men because the digital exam was abnormal, and cancer was detected in 32. Thus, the positive predictive value of the digital exam was 26.4% (32/121). Two additional cases of prostate cancer were detected following a transurethral prostatectomy. In both patients, the digital exam was normal. Based on the clinical staging, 68% (N=23) of the tumors were Stage B compared to only 12% (N=4) for patients with Stage D disease (Table I).

TABLE 1: CLINICAL STAGE OF PROSTATE CANCER
IN MEN DETECTED BY ROUTINE SCREENING

CLINICAL STAGE	INCIDENCE OF PROSTATE CANCER No. (%)	
A	2	(6%)
B	23	(68%)
C	5	(14%)
D	4	(12%)

Pathologic staging was obtained on 13 patients with clinical Stage B disease; 7 (54%) were upstaged to C, and one (8%) to Stage D1 disease. Thus, only 5 (38%) of the surgically staged patients had pathologically proven Stage B disease. Eight patients in this group had a Gleason sum greater than 6, yet only 1 patient had positive lymph nodes. Presently, it is too early to report on overall survival, however, two patients have already died. One man was 66 at the time of diagnosis and he died of a heart attack while receiving radiotherapy, and a second patient who was 79 died of a stroke within two years of diagnosis.

The detection rate for each age group is shown in Table 2. An increase in the frequency of prostate cancer was observed with increasing age. The overall incidence of prostate cancer for men between the ages of 50 and 80 was 1.8% (34/1866).

TABLE 2: DETECTION RATE OF PROSTATE CANCER
IN SCREENED POPULATION

AGE	NO. CANCER/NO. SCREENED (%)	
41 - 50	0/235	(0)
51 - 60	7/923	(0.8%)
61 - 70	19/726	(2.6%)
71 - 80	8/217	(3.2%)
TOTAL	34/2101	(1.6%)

The detection rate for each year of the exam is shown in Table 3. Thirty-four tumors were diagnosed during the initial exam, and although 1,234 men had a second exam and 353 men had a third exam, we did not detect any additional cases of prostate cancer in these latter 2 groups. None of the patients diagnosed with prostate cancer presented because of urinary symptoms.

TABLE 3:   PROSTATE CANCER DETECTION RATE
                        BY YEAR OF EXAM

EXAM NO.	NO. CANCERS DETECTED/NO. SCREENED	
1	34/2101	
2	0/1234	
3	0/353	
4	0/81	
5	0/10	
TOTAL	34/3779	(0.9%)

    The approximate cost for the program was $140,656 which was primarily due to the costs from performing core biopsies (Table 4).

TABLE 4:   APPROXIMATE COST
                OF PROSTATE CANCER SCREENING PROGRAM

ITEM	TOTAL COST
Project staff	53,300
In-patient core biopsy	51,750
Aspiration biopsy	16,950
Pathology	13,100
Supplies	3,804
Miscellaneous	1,702
TOTAL EXPENSE	$140,606

During the early part of the program, transperineal core biopsies were performed when an abnormal exam was detected. At that time, general anesthesia was used and the patient was hospitalized for one or two nights. Because many of the prostatic lesions were small, we could not be sure that an adequate sample had been taken from the proper location. Thus, we began to use transrectal aspiration which cost $150 for the procedure and $100 for the cytology interpretation. Presently, the costs associated with a core biopsy would be much lower than those incurred earlier in our program because we now use out-patient surgery without hospitalization, and fewer routine pre-anesthesia tests are ordered. Based on the expenses that were incurred when the program was initiated, the cost per exam was approximately $37, and the cost per prostate cancer detected was approximately $4,135.

DISCUSSION

The annual death rate from prostate cancer has continued to rise during the past thirty years. One reason may be the inability to diagnose the disease at an early stage. In one U.S. survey, only 57% of the patients had clinically localized disease at the time of diagnosis (Murphy et al., 1982). Because many patients are understaged, the actual number of patients with potentially curable tumors is actually very low.

These disturbing statistics prompted us to determine if routine screening by the digital exam is beneficial. Although more data are needed before we can make firm conclusions, several observations can be made. It appears from our results that routine screening may increase the percentage of patients who are diagnosed with clinically localized disease, and it may decrease the percentage of patients diagnosed with pelvic lymph node metastases. In previously published reports, pelvic lymph node metastases were found in 50% of patients with a Gleason sum of 7, and in 75% of patients with a Gleason sum of 8 (Stamey, 1983). Yet, in our small group of surgically staged patients, only 13% of the patients with high Gleason sums had tumor in the lymph nodes.

A surprising finding from our study is that all of the tumors were suspected on the first digital exam. In contrast other investigators reported that 0.2% - 1% of the screened patients had tumors detected in subsequent exams after a normal exam in the previous year. There are two possible explanations for this result. First, some of our patients may have developed cancer in subsequent years, but the diagnosis was made by other physicians at other hospitals. Because only 59% of the total population returned for a second exam, these other men must be contacted before any firm conclusions can be made. A second explanation is that a more aggressive attitude toward prostate biopsy combined with the use of the transrectal aspiration biopsy method may have resulted in our detecting some small tumors in the first year of our program that were not usually detected until subsequent exams in other programs. Overall, only one program had a higher cancer detection rate than ours (Thompson et al., 1984), which would strongly suggest that we are not missing more tumors than other programs. If these data can be confirmed, then perhaps an annual digital exam may not be necessary.

If less frequent exams are sufficient, the cost of a screening program could be greatly decreased. Yet, even in its present form, routine screening by the digital exam is a reasonable cost. Furthermore, substantial cost reductions can be made by performing biopsies using the transrectal aspiration rather than the transperineal core method. We and others have found that aspiration biopsy is a more sensitive method for detecting prostate cancer than the core method (Chodak et al., 1984, Kaufman et al., 1982). This may be especially true when a biopsy must be performed on a very small lesion.

Although our data suggest that routine screening may enable us to diagnose patients when the disease is less extensive, there is presently no good evidence that screening is beneficial to patients. Other screening programs conclude, however, that screening is valuable because they find a higher overall survival rate in screened men than in patients with prostate cancer who are diagnosed by routine methods (Mariani et al., 1982, Gilbertson, 1971, Jenson et al., 1981). Gilbertson claimed that the 5 and 10 year survival rates in their screened men who had prostate cancer approximated the actual survival rate for the rest of the population (Gilbertson, 1971). These conclusions are invalid, however, because they ignore lead and length time biases. The only appropriate method for analyzing the results of a routine screening program must use mortality as the end point for evaluation. The lead time bias may appear to increase the length of survival because tumors are diagnosed before symptoms develop (Love and Camilli, 1981). Yet, if the screened men eventually die of the disease without a prolongation of life, then screening offered no benefit.

Similarly, screening benefits from length time bias by resulting in the detection of slower growing or less aggressive tumors, whereas, the more rapidly metastasizing tumors result in symptoms that cause a patient to seek medical attention before he can be screened (Love and

Camilli, 1981). Thus, if the two groups are compared, the screened men will appear to have a better outcome. Proving that routine screening is justified may be possible only by performing a randomized trial that includes a control group of either unscreened or untreated men. In the absence of such a study, there is no evidence to support the establishment of routine screening programs for prostate cancer.

Another requirement that must be satisfied to recommend routine screening is that the screening test must have a high sensitivity and specificity. Although the digital exam may be the best test available for detecting prostate cancer (Guinan et al., 1980), it appears to be too insensitive to be used as a basis for routine screening. Based on autopsy series, the incidence of prostate cancer has been reported to be 29% for men over 50 and it increases thereafter (Franks, 1954). In previous screening studies, the cancer detection rate by the digital exam for men in this age group ranged from 0.6% - 2.8% (Mariani et al., 1982, Gilbertson, 1971, Chodak and Schoenberg, 1984, Thompson et al., 1984). Thus, the calculated sensitivity of the digital exam may only be approximately 2% - 9%. These results indicate that before a screening program for prostate cancer can be recommended, a more sensitive test must be developed.

Another potential screening method is transrectal ultrasonography which detects some tumors missed by the digital examination (Watanabe et al., 1980). Presently, however, there is no evidence that the sensitivity of TRS for detecting prostatic carcinoma is significantly higher than the digital exam to warrant its use as a routine screening procedure. Furthermore, screening by transrectal sonography would be far more costly.

Although a prostate cancer screening test must have a higher sensitivity to justify its routine use, a more sensitive test could create a greater problem. Based on autopsy studies, only one man will die of prostate cancer for every 380 men who have histologic evidence of the disease (Stamey, 1983). Thus, diagnosing and treating most of the other patients would not be beneficial and it would be very costly.

Furthermore, most prostate tumors are less than 1 cc

in volume (McNeil, 1986) and they may not require treatment. At the same time, however, once a tumor is larger than 1 cc it may have already extended beyond the capsule (Scott et al., 1969) which would make it difficult to cure. Ironically, many of the tumors that may be curable at the time of diagnosis are also the ones that probably do not require treatment. Until a marker is found that identifies tumors with a high metastatic potential, screening could result in treating many men who would never develop symptoms. Although the complication rates associated with treatment for localized prostate cancer may be very low, unnecessarily treating a large number of patients will still result in morbidity to a substantial number of men. This problem would seem to support not recommending routine screening until more proof is available that patients actually derive a clear benefit from this procedure.

A final issue that receives little attention is the adverse effects of screening. These include the psychological trauma of a false positive digital exam, the added cost of additional tests, and most importantly, the psychological and physical effect of detecting a tumor if there is no clear benefit from treatment. These potential problems have never been evaluated for prostate cancer screening, but they could present a problem if mass screening programs were to be established.

In summary, early detection of prostatic cancer by routine screening may result in diagnosing less extensive tumors, however, there are no data to show that screening will have any impact on mortality. Before mass screening programs are established, additional data are needed to determine if patients will derive any real benefit.

REFERENCES

Chodak GW, Bibbo M, Straus FH II, Wied GL (1984). Transrectal aspiration biopsy versus transperineal core biopsy for the diagnosis of carcinoma of the prostate. J Urol 132:480.
Chodak GW, Schoenberg HW (1984). Early detection of prostate cancer by routine screening. JAMA 252:3261.
Franks LM (1954). Latent carcinoma of the prostate. J Path Bact 68:603.

Gilbertsen, V.A. (1971). Cancer of the prostate gland. JAMA 215:81.

Gilbertson VA (1971). Cancer of the prostate gland. JAMA 215:81.

Guinan P, Bush I, Ray V, et al. (1980). The accuracy of the rectal examination in the diagnosis of prostate carcinoma. NEJM 303:499.

Jenson CB, Shahon DB, Wangensteen OH (1960). Evaluation of annual examinations in the detection of cancer. JAMA 174:91.

Kaufman JJ, Ljung BM, Walther P, Waisman J (1982). Aspiration biopsy of the prostate. Urology 19:587.

Love RR, Camilli AE (1981). The value of screening. Cancer 48:489.

Mariani AJ, Tom C, Hariharan A, Stams UK (1982). Prostate Cancer: The paradox of early diagnosis, Hawaii Med J 34.

McNeil JE, Bostwick DG, Kindrachuk RA, Reswine E, Freika FS, Stamey TA (1986). Patterns of progression in prostate cancer. Lancet I:60.

Murphy GP, Natarajan N, Pontes JE (1982). The national survey of the prostate cancer in the United States by the American College of Surgeons. J Urol 128:928.

Scott Jr. R, Mutchnik DL, Laskowski TZ, Schmalhorst WR (1969). Carcinoma of the prostate in elderly men: Incidence, growth characteristics and clinical significance. J Urol 101:602.

Stamey TA (1983). Cancer of the prostate. Monographs in Urol 4:68.

Thompson IM, Ernst JJ, Gangai MP, Spence CR (1984). Adenocarcinoma of the prostate: Results of routine urological screening. J Urol 132:690.

Watanabe H, Date S, Ohe H, Saitoh M, Tanaki S (1980). A survey of 3,000 examinations by transurethral ultrasonography. The Prostate 1:271.

EORTC Genitourinary Group Monograph 5: Progress
and Controversies in Oncological Urology II, pages 97–98
© 1988 Alan R. Liss, Inc.

Discussion: Routine Screening for Prostate Cancer Using
the Digital Rectal Examination

Herman J. de Voogt, Amsterdam, The Netherlands

Collste: Thank you Dr. Chodak for stating your case so very
firmly. We have time for a couple of questions.

Whitmore: About the figures from Leasdale. Were the patients
who were detected by transrectal ultrasound patients who had
a palpable nodule? In other words, is it possible that he
detected another 3%, a different 3% than you were detecting?

Chodak: That is a possibility although they claim that it
seems to be a mixture. So the primary problem of doing only
the ultrasound examination is that it is hard to determine
how many of those people also had a palpable lesion. I
believe that here some cancers are detected that we would be
missing by digital palpation. But a disturbing thing is that
the detection rate is not much higher and that even if it is
another 3%, it still means you are only detecting 6% of the
cases. In fact, there is a study done in the fifties, a
prospective study in which an open core-biopsy was done on
men who randomly came to the clinic and they found an alar-
ming incidence of 13 or 14% of prostate cancer. What we
really want to do is screening. We ought to consider using
an open biopsy as a more effective way of doing it. So
ultrasound could be hopeful but by itself will not be enough
of advantage.

Scardino: I just like to express ones concerns about what
you said, because I am not so sure that, just because you
detect only 3% or 6%, that is a problem. You may be
detecting the 3 or 6%, that are most likely to have progressive cancer. The difficulty are the extremely small tumors
found at autopsies, which we are not detecting by rectal
examination, by ultrasound or other techniques and which may
just be the ones we do not want to detect because they do
the patients no harm. So I think I would not condemn
screening because we are not picking up all of the tumors we
would see on serial sections in a prostate autopsy. What we

want to do is detect the ones that are going to be a threat to the well-being of the patient and maybe these are just the ones that we are detecting, because they are large enough to be visible or palpable.

Chodak: We are obviously not doing a very good job of picking up a lot of the cancers that we would ultimately go on to treat. It is true some of the cancers we missed are very small. If we go ahead in screening without any proof that it makes a difference whether we treat or not treat these patients, I think that we are not offering any benefit. If we are going to prove that screening offers a benefit we have to show that the patients with early cancers we detected, actually do better. It may be alright to miss some, at least we are believing that these people with very small tumors are at very low risk of progression. So I think that the problem is really a complex one and screening really does not have any real validity at the present time.

Collste: We have plenty of time to discuss these very important things in the round table. Thank you very much Dr. Chodak. We go on to hear about the Japanese experience. Dr. Watanabe.

EORTC Genitourinary Group Monograph 5: Progress
and Controversies in Oncological Urology II, pages 99–107
© 1988 Alan R. Liss, Inc.

SCREENING FOR PROSTATIC CANCER IN JAPAN

Hiroki Watanabe

Department of Urology, Kyoto Prefectural
University of Medicine
Kawaramachi-Hirokoji, Kyoto, Japan 602

PREVENTIVE ONCOLOGY PROJECT

In general, preventive oncology consists of
two areas, namely, primary and secondary prevention. The former is the prevention of the generation of disease, which is achieved by avoiding
risk factors revealed through epidemiologic investigations. The latter is the prevention of the
progression of disease, which is achieved by detecting patients in the pre-clinical stage and
treating them before onset.

For primary prevention, we made an epidemiological study to clarify the high risk group for
prostatic cancer (Mishina et al, 1985). An original
questionnaire, consisting of 111 questions, was designed in 1976. A case-control study by matched-
pair analysis was conducted on 100 prostatic cancer
cases and 100 controls matched for age and residence.

In summary, the high risk group for prostatic
cancer belongs to blue collar people in the lower
income brackets, living on a Western diet rather
than a traditional Japanese one, and having an
active sexual life in younger years and an inactive sexual life in advanced years.

We have published information regarding the
risk factors of prostatic cancer for people's
awareness in newspapers, magazines, on television

and in films as widely as possible. According to
our estimate, awareness has been achieved for a
total of over 10 million people in Japan up to 1984.

TABLE 1. High risk group of prostatic cancer

Occupation and income

	Odds ratio
No involvement with administrative job*	3.24
Contact with dyes at work	11.00
Lack of military service*	2.23
Present annual income less than ¥1,200,000	1.70

Diet

Not taking sea food everyday*	1.97
Not taking green and yellow vegetables everyday	1.97
Preference for spices*	1.78
Preference for salty things*	1.94

Sexual habit

Marriage younger than age 24*	2.50
Marriage lasting for more than 40 years	1.57
First sexual intercourse at less than age 19	3.37
Frequency of sex.int.over 1/month from age 15 to 20*	2.19
Frequency of sex.int.less than 1/month from age 61 to 70*	2.17
Earlier cessation of sexuality*	3.57

$*p < 0.05$ others : $p < 0.1$

HISTORY AND SYSTEM OF MASS SCREENING PROGRAM

For the secondary prevention of the preventive oncology project for prostatic cancer, an original mass screening program for prostatic diseases has been established by our laboratory.

We originally developed transrectal sonography (TRS) in 1967 and found that this new diagnostic means is suitable for the screening of prostatic cancer and benign prostatic hypertrophy. For that reason, we organized a new mass screening program for prostatic diseases, using transrectal sonography as the primary study of the program in 1975 (Watanabe et al, 1977a).

TRS is a simple and non-invasive examination with an excellent diagnostic ability, indicating a sensitivity of 96.6% and a specificity of 81.8% for prostatic cancer (Watanabe et al, 1980a). It takes less than 3 minutes to carry out for each person including preparation time.

The system of the mass screening program is as follows: As a rule examinees are limited to males over 55 years of age. Each examinee is first asked to supply details of his medical history by a questionnaire and then examined using TRS for the primary study. In some necessary occasions digital palpation is combined. Sonograms are evaluated carefully, taking the data from the questionnaire into consideration. When the findings warrant it, some screened subjects are requested to submit to a secondary study which consists of an ordinary urological examination including digital palpation, measurement of residual urine, X-ray procedures, and/or prostatic needle biopsy, if necessary.

Model trials of the screening system were initially performed on 180 males between January, 1975 (Watanabe et al, 1977a), and April, 1977 (Watanabe et al, 1977b). In the next stage, we advanced to field trials on 145 males from November, 1977, to September, 1979, in two small towns near Kyoto (Watanabe et al, 1978). In all of these trials the equipment necessary for the studies was transported by motor vehicle and set up at each location.

Based on the data obtained in these trials, a proto-type mobile unit for the primary study was developed in January, 1980 (Watanabe et al, 1980b). This was followed by the development of a practical mobile unit, the "Dolphin", in December, 1980 (Watanabe et al, 1984). The name "Dolphin" was chosen because of the connection with that animal's use of ultrasound for communication.

The floor area of the bus is about 8 m^2, with an operation console in the center where two chair-type transrectal scanners are fixed one on either side. During the examination of one person on one side, the next person is in preparation on the other side. No undressing area is required inside the unit because examinees only have to lower their trousers to the knee for examination. The capacity of the unit is approximately 20 examinees per hour, which amounts to some 150 examinees every day.

RESULTS OF MASS SCREENING PROGRAM

Up to March, 1986, 5,070 males from various areas in Japan were submitted to the mass screening program. The final diagnoses are given in Table 2. After the primary study, the prostates of 1,484 males were diagnosed ultrasonically as abnormal. By the secondary study, 1,179 males (23.3%) were diagnosed as having benign prostatic hypertrophy and 24 males (0.5%) as having prostatic cancer. The detection rate of 0.5% is significantly high as compared with other screening systems e.g. for gastric cancer (0.1%), uterine cancer (0.15%) or breast cancer (0.06%)(Watanabe, 1985).

In 46% of the patients in whom prostatic cancer was detected, the malignancy belonged to Stage B. This rate for detection in the early stages is much larger than that in general urological clinics, indicating a proportion between 10 and 20%.

TABLE 2. Result of mass screening
(January, 1975-March, 1986)

Examinees	5070
Average age	65.2 y.o.
Cases for secondary study	1484 (29.3%)
Final diagnosis	
BPH Stage I	930 (18.3%)
BPH Stage II	249 (4.9%)
Prostatic cancer	24 (0.5%)
Prostatitis	63 (1.2%)
Miscellaneous	77 (1.5%)

Some typical cases will be demonstrated. The sonogram shown on Fig. 1 is of a case having a tiny nodule of cancer in the left lobe of the prostate. The section is slightly asymmetric and a hypoechoic area is seen in the left lobe.

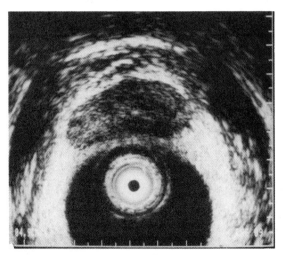

Figure 1. Prostatic cancer in Stage B_1.
Hypoechoic area in the left lobe.

Fig. 2 is also a case of prostatic cancer in Stage B. A deformity of the section is observed.

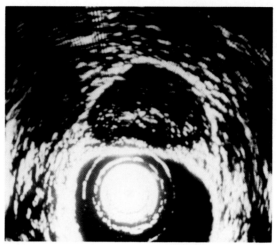

Figure 2. Prostatic cancer in Stage B_2.
Deformity of the prostatic section.

COST-BENEFIT ANALYSIS OF MASS SCREENING PROGRAM

Now for a balance sheet showing income and expenditure relating to the mass screening system. The mobile unit "Dolphin" belongs to a mass screening company in Kyoto. They request $20 per case as an examination fee for the primary study. Since the detection rate of prostatic cancer in the primary study was 0.5%, it costs $4000 to find one case of prostatic cancer at this step.

In the secondary study, ordinary urological examinations are performed for which the fee is $50 per case on average. Since the detection rate of cancer in this study is approximately 5%, an additional $1000 are required to detect one case. In total, accordingly, it costs $5000 to detect one cancer case. However, since cases in an early stage represent 40% of all detected cases, the total cost per case in an early stage becomes $12500.

On the other hand, patients with prostatic cancer in an early stage are usually treated with radical prostatectomy resulting in a complete cure.

An average treatment fee for such cases is approximately $10000 in our clinic. When the patients are in an advanced stage, however, the average fee goes up to $30000 or $40000 though the patients of course finally succumb.

Therefore, if we assume a difference in treatment fee between an early and an advanced stage case as $20000 or $30000, then the cost-benefit balance of our mass screening program may be approximately $10000 positive for every early cancer case detected. This account includes neither benefits relating to the quality of life nor benefits connected with the detection of benign prostatic hypertrophy. If such benefits were included in the account, the positive balance would be considerably greater.

PROSTATIC MASS SCREENING IN OTHER INSTITUTIONS IN JAPAN

Following our project, a mass screening for prostatic cancer has been starged in 12 other institutions in Japan up to July, 1986, according to a survey by the Foundation for Prostate Research (Director: Emeritus Professor K. Shida). The screening system was basically similar, consisting of a primary and secondary study, employing digital palpation and/or transrectal sonography for the screening modality (Table 3).

Final diagnosis was made by needle biopsy in the majority of the institutions (Table 4).

Summing up the results, a total of 118 cases (0.7%) of prostatic cancer was screened out of 16,645 examinees in these 13 institutions including ours. Approximately half of the patients belonged to the early stages of prostatic cancer (Table 5).

TABLE 3. Number of institutions concerned with prostatic mass screening in Japan (1986)

Primary study		Secondary study	Number
Q+P	→	PAP+B	2
	↘	TRS+PAP+B	1
Q+P+TRS	→	B	2
	↘	PAP+B	1
Q+P+PAP	→	B	2
	↘	TRS+B	2
Q+P+TRS+PAP	→	B	3
Total			13

Q: History taking,   P: Palpation,   B: Biopsy,
TRS: Transrectal sonography,
PAP: Prostatic acid phosphatase

TABLE 4. Procedure for final diagnosis

Needle biopsy	10
Aspiration biopsy	2
Others	1
Total	13

TABLE 5. Results of prostatic mass screening in 13 institutions in Japan (July, 1986)

Number of examinee   16,645

Final diagnosis:

PC	Stage	A - B	54		
	Stage	C - D	53	118	(0.7%)
	Stage	unknown	11		
BPH				1,034	(6.2%)

Prostatic mass screening is thus being appreciated very much even in Japan, where the incidence of the disease is only one tenth of that in Western countries. There is no doubt that this type of intervention in preventive oncology would be very effective especially in Western countries. We strongly recommend such countries to consider the possibility of adopting the system.

REFERENCES

Mishina T, Watanabe H, Araki H, Nakao M (1985). Epidemiological study of prostatic cancer by matched-pair analysis. Prostate 6:423-436.

Watanabe H, Saitoh M, Mishina T, Igari D, Tanahashi Y, Harada K, Hisamichi S (1977a). Mass screening program for prostatic diseases with transrectal ultrasonotomography. J Urol 117:746-748.

Watanabe H, Saitoh M, Ohe H, Tanaka S, Itakura Y (1977b). A mass screening program for prostatic diseases by means of transrectal ultrasonotomography in two homes for the aged. Proc Jap Soc Ultrasonics Med 32:123-124.

Watanabe H, Saitoh M, Ohe H, Tanaka S, Itakura Y, Yamanaka Y, Ohta Y (1978). A first experiment of field mass screening program for prostatic diseases by means of transrectal ultrasonotomography. Proc Jap Soc Ultrasonics Med 33:151-152.

Watanabe H, Date S, Ohe H, Saitoh M, Tanaka S (1980a). A survey of 3,000 examinations by transrectal ultrasonotomography. Prostate 1: 271-278.

Watanabe H, Ohe H, Mishina T, Tanaka S, Kaneko Y, Ohta Y (1980b). A mass screening program for prostatic diseases (1st report) -- Development of a prototype mobile unit for mass screening of prostatic diseases --. Proc Jap Soc Ultrasonics Med 36:381-382.

Watanabe H, Ohe H, Inaba T, Itakura Y, Saitoh M, Nakao M (1984). A mobile mass screening unit for prostatic disease. Prostate 5:559-565.

Watanabe H (1985). Secondary prevention in preventive oncology. Oncologia 12:54-68.

EORTC Genitourinary Group Monograph 5: Progress
and Controversies in Oncological Urology II, pages 109–110
© 1988 Alan R. Liss, Inc.

Discussion: Screening for Prostatic Cancer in Japan

Herman J. de Voogt, Amsterdam, The Netherlands

Rollema: I wonder how you got to this high sensitivity of
your method of 96%? Yesterday we heard that there was 20%
false positive diagnosis in ultrasound and only 50% of the
tumors are hypoechoic, so how do you explain your high
sensitivity rate?

Watanabe: I would think that the hypoechoic area is the only
sign for the prostatic cancer. From the beginning stages of
my developing of transrectal sonography we have always emphasized that not only the inside echos but also the
deformity and the asymmetry of the whole section of the
prostate is very important in the diagnosis of prostate
cancer and I assure you that the sensitivity of 96% is true.
This is based upon data from out-patient clinics which the
patients are visiting from their own living area. This is
not so adaptable for general condition. We made a brilliant
reading camera, and we gave 100 pictures including normal
prostatic hypertrophy and prostatic cancer pictures to 20
urologists. In this way we did a test which resulted in a
sensitivity of this group of excellent urologists of over
80% and of the most excellent urologists of 86% and a specificity of just below 80%. So I think that transrectal sonography is a very suitable method for screening.

N.N.: In my country we have a lot of ultrasound people that
detect nodules, the are called nodule-hunters. We are called
to biopsy all these nodules. Would you comment on this
discrepancy between nodules and capsule deformity and can
you comment on tissue characterization by ultrasound?

Watanabe: Whether it is important to distinguish between a
nodule or deformity, depends on the case. In a very early
case we may find small hypoechoic areas in such a prostate
as shown on my last slide. In that case I showed that palpation was ineffective. They cannot palpate a nodule in that
case, but only transrectal sonography detected that case.

Some other   cases the deformities were more important   than the nodule.

Chodak: I wonder if you can comment on how many biopsies you would have to do in order to find one cancer.

Watanabe: About 10.

EORTC Genitourinary Group Monograph 5: Progress
and Controversies in Oncological Urology II, pages 111–120
© 1988 Alan R. Liss, Inc.

BACKGROUND FOR SCREENING - EPIDEMIOLOGY AND COST
EFFECTIVENESS

Martin I. Resnick

Division of Urology, Case Western Reserve
University School of Medicine, Cleveland,
Ohio 44106

BACKGROUND

Surveys indicate that in 1987, cancer of the prostate
will be the second most common malignancy to be diagnosed
in men (96,000)and that it will account for more than
27,000 deaths (American Cancer Society, 1987). In the
past the physician has relied mainly on digital examination
of the prostate for diagnosis and staging purposes but this
has often led to misdiagnosis and understaging of the
disease. It is well established that more than 75% of
patients have metastatic or locally infiltrative disease at
time of diagnosis. Additionally, studies have shown that
12 to 66% of patients with seemingly localized disease will
demonstrate extension into the seminal vesicles and peri-
prostate tissue at the time of radical prostatectomy and a
comparable number will have metastatic disease that is
undetectable without the aid of additional clinical studies
(Jewett et al., 1974; Walsh and Jewett, 1980; Elder et al.,
1982; Spirnak and Resnick, 1984).

Studies have also indicated that when detected early
the cure rate for carcinoma of the prostate is potentially
improved. Though only limited studies have been carried
out screening programs appear to be effective in this
regard (Vihko et al., 1985; Chodak and Schoenberg, 1984;
Guinan et al., 1980). A recent autopsy study indicated
that 1 cc of tumor volume was associated with the capacity
to metastasize and tumors of lesser volume did not appear
to have acquired this ability (McNeal et al., 1986). Other
investigators have not quantified the volume as accurately

but have made similar observations in that larger tumors were associated with a higher incidence of local invasion and metastases (Cantrell et al., 1981).

Improvement in the specificity, sensitivity and predictive values of non-invasive imaging modalities and biochemical markers would provide the clinician with considerable assistance in the early diagnosis of patients with carcinoma of the prostate. Additionally, extension and combination of currently available non-invasive procedures and techniques and the development of new methodology would improve the whole range of effort from diagnosis to treatment monitoring in patients with carcinoma of the prostate. Finally it is important to emphasize that no test currently in use allows for the reliable separation of specifically progressive tumors from those with a less aggressive potential.

THE IDEAL TEST

The ideal test for screening a patient population in an attempt to detect potentially curable disease should be non-invasive, preferably on an easily obtainable body fluid (urine, blood, prostate fluid) and be inexpensive. It would be desirable if the test was not only highly specific and sensitive but also reliable in predicting either the presence or absence of the disease in a specifically designated population. Finally, the test should not only identify patients with the disease but also differentiate those individuals whose disease is potentially progressive and lethal in contrast to those having indolent or dormant tumors that will not progress and therefore not be life threatening. Obviously those patients in the former category require further evaluation and therapy and those in the latter would neither benefit from nor require other therapeutic approaches. Three studies will be reviewed: physical findings; an imaging study; and laboratory determinations.

RECTAL EXAMINATION

Rectal palpation is the single most important step in the physical examination for detecting carcinoma of the prostate and it is well recognized that there is an

increased incidence of early disease detection when it is
done routinely (vanBuskirk and Kimbrough, 1954; Kimbrough
and Rowe, 1951). Although small nodular or indurated areas
in the prostate may be readily palpable the differentiation
between benign and malignant lesions cannot be made by
physical examination alone (Jewett, 1956; Grabstald, 1955).
Interestingly the value of the routine rectal examination
in an attempt to screen an asymptomatic population is
somewhat controversial and its value and frequency has yet
to be clearly established (Vihko et al., 1985; Chodak and
Schoenberg, 1984). It has also not been established as to
the optimum age to begin screening and a recent retrospective study of asymptomatic patients with confirmed prostatic
carcinoma revealed that prostatic nodules were detected in
27% of younger (those less than 55 years of age) patients
compared to an incidence of only 5% in an older group
(greater than 65 years of age) (Resnick, 1986).

Many clinicians follow the dictum "every hard prostate
is cancer until proven otherwise" and that the only certain
method of establishing the proper diagnosis is with adequate
biopsy. It must be remembered that small early infiltrating
prostatic tumors can be confused with a variety of different
diseases of the prostate. Several studies have shown that
approximately 50% of nodules or indurated areas of the
prostate are malignant and most reports emphasize that there
is little or no correlation between the clinical impression
as determined by rectal palpation and the results of
surgical biopsy (Barnes and Okamato, 1961; Emmett et al.,
1962; Goldstein and Weinberg, 1954). Benign prostatic
nodules may be secondary to benign prostatic hyperplasia,
acute prostatitis, chronic prostatitis, (non-specific,
tuberculous, granulomatous, abscess), calculi, vascular
injury (prostatic infarct, periprostatic venous thrombosis)
or hormonal influences (squamous metaplasia) (Grabstald,
1965). Prostatic malignancies causing nodules include
adenocarcinoma, squamous cell carcinoma, transitional cell
carcinoma, sarcoma, lymphoma and metastatic tumors. Recent
evidence suggests that the positive predictive value of an
abnormal rectal examination (the per cent of patients with
a positive examination having the disease) ranges from
11-26 percent.

As noted previously, digital palpation of the prostate
is not accurate in determining the local extent of disease
and from 12-16 percent of patients with seemingly localized

tumors have involvement of the seminal vesicles and periprostatic tissues at the time of radical prostatectomy.
Studies indicate that more than half of patients with B2
nodules have microscopic evidence of capsular invasion or
penetration (Elder et al., 1982). Errors in staging also
occur because a significant number of patients have lymphatic metastases in the absence of either local extention of
the primary tumor or metastatic bony involvement
(McCullough et al., 1974; Arduino and Glucksman, 1966;
Pistenma et al., 1976). Finally, rectal examination to
detect tumor regression after initiation of endocrine
therapy or use of cytotoxic chemotherapy is not completely
objective and often it is difficult to monitor tumor
response accurately (Resnick and Grayhack, 1975). Similarly tumor reactivation or growth following an initially
satisfactory response to endocrine therapy is usually
apparent at metastatic sites and changes in the primary
tumor are often not evident.

ULTRASONOGRAPHY

Though transabdominal ultrasonography has been shown
to be an adequate method of measuring prostate size most
investigators believe that a more accurate examination
of the prostate can be obtained with rectal studies.
Though initially believed to be useful as a screening
modality, some studies indicate that because of the lack
of sensitivity the false-positive and false-negative rates
are unacceptably high (Watanabe et al., 1984; Resnick,
1985). The positive predictive value of a transrectal
ultrasound examination is in the range of 30-35 percent.
Further carefully controlled clinical studies are needed
to assess the true role of transrectal ultrasonography
as a screening modality in the early detection of prostatic
carcinoma. Consequently digital rectal examination
continues to be the modality of choice in the screening
of an asymptomatic population over a specific age range.
The original concept that prostatic carcinoma was characterized by enhanced echogenicity on ultrasound
evaluation is inaccurate. Not only are high intensity
areas non-specific because of their association with
other pathologic changes such as prostatitis, prostatic
calculi and infarcts but tumors and other pathologic
processes will appear as hypoechoic areas as well
(Lee et al., 1986; Rifkin et al., 1986). Ultrasound

appears useful as a staging modality though as expected microscopic invasion of the prostatic capsule is difficult if not impossible to identify, as is diffuse disease, and specificity of abnormal findings is limited (Pontes et al., 1985). Tumor response can also be monitored with this examination in that following an adequate response to endocrine manipulation (estrogen, orchiectomy) a reduction in prostatic size and diminution in echogenicity is observed. Problems occur because tumor reactivation cannot be detected with this technique in the majority of patients (Fujino and Scardino, 1985).

BIOCHEMICAL MARKERS

Reliable biochemical markers could, and in some instances do, contribute significantly to the diagnosis, staging, assessment of treatment and follow-up evaluation of patients with carcinoma of the prostate. In the absence of these markers, recognition of significant risk of carcinoma of the prostate is usually dependent on discovery of a palpable abnormality of the gland on rectal examination. The limitations of this latter technique are well recognized. If a biochemical marker could substitute for or add significantly to the rectal examination as a screening tool to identify patients at increased risk of the disease earlier in its course, the options for management of a greater number of patients could be expanded. These markers would likely have a role in assessing tumor burden or extent of disease because the existing imaging modalities have significant false-positive and false-negative rates making them unreliable in many instances. The difficulty in assessing treatment response, viability of post-treatment residual tumor and similarly recognizing treatment failure is evident in trials of chemotherapy and hormonal therapy. The availability of biochemical markers with a high degree of sensitivity and specificity would likely assist in all of these endeavors. Recognized biochemical markers exist in serum, urine and prostatic fluid (Ban et al., 1984; Schacht et al, 1984). Serum markers include acid phosphatase, alkaline phosphatase, lactic dehydrogenase, phosphohexose isomerase, carcinoembryonic antigen, alpha-fetoprotein polyamines, ribonuclease, seromucoid creatinine kinase BB (CK-BB) and specific prostate tissue and tumor antigens; others have been recently reported (Kaneti et al., 1984; Kuriyama et al.). Biochemical and immunologic methods have been applied to the detection of these markers but improved isolation and detection techniques in addition to the identification of new markers are required. Biochemical markers in urine have been identified and these represent substances presumably produced by the tumor (cholesterol, specific amino acids, polyamines-spermidine, carcinoembryonic antigen, fibronectin, prostatic cancer antigen) and non-specific substances, which are a response of tumor grown either within the prostate or in metastatic sites (hydro-doxyproline). As with serum markers other substances need to be isolated and identified because these studies offer potential for not only detecting the disease early but assessing its extent and response to treatment. Finally, markers have been identified in prostatic fluid and acid phosphatase, (leucine aminopeptidase), proteins (transferrin, complement C_3, complement C_4, ferritin) and a variety of other substances (immunoglobulins IgA, IgG, IgM, polyamines-spermine spermidine putrescine, cholesterol, zinc). As with markers in other body fluids the role of biochemical and immunologic markers must be defined in the management of patients with carcinoma of the prostate. Currently, because of the high false positive rates with many of the markers their role as a screening study is limited. Serum determinations of prostatic specific antigen appears promising but further studies are required to assess its role as a screening study.

CRITERIA FOR SCREENING

When considering screening in asymptomatic population with the intent of diagnosing a disease in an early form it is important to consider the age of the patients that should be evaluated in this manner. Few would disagree that thirty year old men should not be included in a screening survey for early detection of carcinoma of the prostate. Additionally, men greater than 80 years of age probably also should not be evaluated in a routine manner. The important question however is which age range should be included. Obviously it is important to choose an age range that will detect the disease prior to the development of symptoms so that it would have a high likelihood of being localized. Additionally, the upper limits of the age range should be in a group of patients that would be amenable to treatment should the disease be detected. Probably an age range from 40 to 75 years of age would

not be unreasonable but certainly others might want to
expand or contract this group for various reasons.

Another concept that is important relates to the determination of the optimum interval that should be used in the
screening survey. For carcinoma of the prostate a yearly
examination does not seem unreasonable. An important factor
relates to the cost effectiveness of the study and the cost
benefit of the study. Models can be developed which show
the relationship between cost of the screening program and
lives saved per patients screened (Figure 1) (Love, 1985).

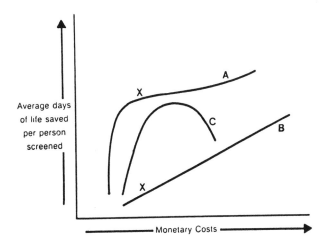

For a financial investment in a person screened the
average days of life saved for screening for cancer A is
obviously greater than for screening cancer B. In cancer A,
with increasing costs a point (X) is reached where increased
frequency and subsequent increase in costs result in minimal
benefit of life saved. For cancer A it would be most beneficial
to identify point X and base costs on this point. For cancer
B increasing cost continues to show increased life saved.
Another model relates to cancer C in which increasing costs
can have a negative effect and actually result in decreased
life savings. This may occur for example with use of
cytological examinations for bladder cancer or cervical
cancer where the laboratories could not handle the case load
and increasing error would result in wrong interpretation.

Though it is difficult to judge screening in terms of

costs, unfortunately these considerations are real and are required. Additionally, one must also consider the cost of the study. For example, screening for carcinoma of the prostate by rectal examination is certainly more inexpensive than screening with transrectal ultrasonography. This is further emphasized when one considers that it is yet to be determined that screening with transrectal ultrasonography is any more effective than with routine digital rectal examination.

In summary, screening for early detection of carcinoma of the prostate is likely best done with routine digital rectal examination. When an abnormal examination is found further studies including biopsy, serum acid phosphatase and ultrasonography would be of benefit. Though no definite guidelines have been established it does not seem unreasonable to screen a population of men ranging from 40 to 75 years of age by digital rectal examination on a yearly basis. This should yield a significant number of individuals with early tumors that would be candidates for curative radiotherapy or radical prostatectomy.

The development of new studies to accurately identify and quantify carcinoma of the prostate would be invaluable in patient evaluation and assessment of subsequent treatment. Improved, non-invasive techniques to assist in diagnosis and clinical staging are goals that should be pursued with the highest priority. Additionally, accurate methods to monitor treatment response and tumor viability are required. Addition of this methodology to the clinician's armamentarium would significantly add to the entire range of our current management efforts in patients with carcinoma of the prostate and could provide information that would guide the search for new therapeutic opportunities.

REFERENCES

American Cancer Society (1987). Cancer Statistics. Ca - A Cancer Journal for Clinicians 37:2.
Arduino LF, Glucksman MA (1966). Lymph node metastases in early carcinoma of the prostate. J Urol 88:91.
Ban Y, Wang MC, Chu TM (1984). Immunologic markers and the diagnosis of prostate cancer. Urol Clin NA 11:269.
Barnes RW, Okamato S (1961). Diagnosis of prostatic carcinoma: A statistical study. West J Surg 9:362.

Cantrell BB, deKlerk DP, Eggleston JC, et al (1981). Pathological factors that influence prognosis in stage A prostatic cancer. J Urol 125:516.

Chodak GW, Schoenberg HW (1984). Early detection of prostatic cancer by routine screening. JAMA 252:3261.

Elder JC, Jewett JH, Walsh PC (1982). Radical perineal prostatectomy for clinical stage B2 carcinoma of the prostate. J Urol 127:704.

Emmett JL, Barber KW Jr, Jackman RJ (1962). Transrectal biopsy to detect prostatic carcinoma: A review and report of 203 cases. J Urol 87:460.

Fujino A, Scardino PT (1985). Transrectal ultrasonography for prostatic cancer: its value in staging and monitoring the response to radiotherapy and chemotherapy. J Urol 133:806.

Goldstein AE, Weinberg T (1954). The importance of correct diagnosis of carcinoma of prostate: Clinical application. Amer Surg 20:971.

Grabstald H (1955). Further experience with transrectal biopsy of the prostate. J Urol 74:211.

Grabstald H (1965). The clinical and laboratory diagnosis of cancer of the prostate. Cancer 15:76.

Guinan P, Bush I, Ray V, Vieth R, Rao R, Bhatti R (1980). The accuracy of the rectal examination in the diagnosis of prostate carcinoma. N Eng J Med 303:499.

Jewett HJ (1956). Significance of the palpable nodule. JAMA 160:838.

Jewett HJ, Eggleston JC, Yawn DH (1974). Radical prostatectomy in the management of cancer of the prostate: Probable causes of some therapeutic failures. J Urol 107:1034.

Kaneti J, Winikoff Y, Zimlichman S, Shainkin-Kestenbaum R (1984). Importance of serum amyloid A (SAA) level in monitoring disease activity and response to therapy in patients with prostate cancer. Urol Res 12:239.

Kimbrough JC, Rowe RB (1951). Carcinoma of the prostate. J Urol 66:373.

Kuriyama M, Takeuchi T, Shinoda I, Okano M, Nishiura T (in press). Clinical evaluation of alpha-seminoprotein in prostate cancer.

Lee F, Gray JM, McLeary RD, Lee F, Jr, McHugh TA, Solomon MH, Kumasaka GH, Straub WH, Borlaza GS, Murphy GP (1986). Prostatic evaluation by transrectal sonography: Criteria for diagnosis of early carcinoma. Radiology 158:91.

Love RR (1985). Principles of cancer screening. In Stoll BA (ed): "Screening and Monitoring of Cancer.

New Horizons in Oncology. Vol LV," New York: John Wiley
& Sons.

McCullough DL, Prout GR Jr, Daly JJ (1974). Carcinoma of
the prostate and lymphatic metastases. J Urol 111:65.

McNeal JE, Kindrachuck RA, Freiha FS, Bostwich DG,
Redwine EA, Stamey TA (1986). Patterns of progression
in prostate cancer. Lancet 1:60.

Pistenma DA, Ray, GR, Bagshaw MA (1976). The role of
megavoltage radiation therapy in the treatment of prostatic carcinoma. Semin Oncol 3:115.

Pontes JE, Eisenkraft S, Watanabe H, Ohe H, Saitol M,
Murphy GP (1985). Preoperative evaluation of localized
prostatic carcinoma by transrectal ultrasonography.
J Urol 134:289.

Resnick MI (1985). Use of transrectal ultrasound in
evaluating prostatic cancer. J Urol 134:314.

Resnick MI (1986). Personal observations.

Resnick MI, Grayhack JT (1975). Treatment of stage IV
carcinoma of the prostate. Urol Clin NA 2:141.

Rifkin MD, Freidland GW, Shorliffe L (1986). Prostatic
evaluation by transrectal endosonography detection
of carcinoma. Radiology 158:85.

Schacht MJ, Garnett JE, Grayhack JT (1984). Biochemical
markers in prostatic cancer. Urol Clin NA 11:253.

Spirnak JP, Resnick MI (1984). Clinical staging of
prostatic cancer: New modalities. Urol Clin NA 11:221.

vanBuskirk KE, Kimbrough JC (1954). Carcinoma of the
prostate. J Urol 71:742.

Vihko P, Kontturi M, Lukkarinen, Ervasta J, Vihko R (1985).
Screening for carcinoma of the prostate. Rectal examination and enzymatic and radioimmunologic measurements
serum acid phosphatase compared. Cancer 56:173.

Walsh PC, Jewett HJ (1980). Radical surgery for prostate
cancer. Cancer 45:1906.

Watanabe H, Ohe H, Inabe T, Itakura Y, Saitoh M, Nakao M
(1984). A mobile mass screening unit for prostatic
disease. Prostate 5:559.

EORTC Genitourinary Group Monograph 5: Progress
and Controversies in Oncological Urology II, pages 121–122
© 1988 Alan R. Liss, Inc.

Discussion: Background for Screening - Epidemiology and
Cost Effectiveness

Herman J. de Voogt, Amsterdam, The Netherlands

Collste: Again we have to cut down the number of questions
but we do have time for a couple of questions.

Schröder: Both you and Professor Watanabe are very experienced ultrasound people. Could you offer an explanation why
the sensitivity might be so much higher in Japan?

Resnick: No, I cannot.

Schröder: Could it be because rectal examination is not
carried out very carefully in Japan?

Resnick: Maybe.

Watanabe: Also it was shown that with reading cameras two
months ago that some experience is necessary to obtain a
good sensitivity and specificity. On the results of sensitivity and specificity we had a very clear demonstration of
people having experience with about three thousand cases.
Their results were all similar to the data just shown here.
I think it is only natural because of their very large
experience. So to improve the sensitivity and specificity in
diagnosing prostate cancer by transrectal sonography, we
must do our best to improve our ability to read the sonograms.

Chodak: We did a study with Dr. Watanabe in which we took
the ultrasounds from our screened patients to Dr. Watanabe's
group to have them read these and they detected accurately
and identified 86% of the patients we had with palpable
abnormalities. So I think this again indicates that the
ultrasound is able to detect 86%. But the ones we had most
difficulties with were the smallest tumors and although that
was not a perfect study it did give some indication that the
ultrasound by itself is not going to be good enough either.

Resnick: But you also have to consider the false-negatives which are lacking in many of the reports that are in the literature.

Watanabe: I have to say that the meaning of screening is different in Japan and the western countries. In Japan the usual screening program is: field trials. We are going to the field to address people in little towns and to collect data from the examinees addressed. In the western countries the meaning of screening is just waiting in some laboratory or hospital. That is the difference! So the basis of the population of the examinees is different. For doing a field study which includes a complete urological examination we need too many experienced urologists. It is impossible. By using our system we can give everything to the engineers or drivers of a mobile unit and just after recording we only read the results. That describes the different ideas of screening between the two countries!

Collste: Thank you Dr. Resnick. The last of the formal presentations this morning is by Dr. Whitmore on the natural history and the effect of treatment.

EORTC Genitourinary Group Monograph 5: Progress
and Controversies in Oncological Urology II, pages 123–130
© 1988 Alan R. Liss, Inc.

BACKGROUND FOR SCREENING: NATURAL HISTORY AND TREATMENT

Willet F. Whitmore, Jr.

Memorial Sloan-Kettering Cancer Center, New York
New York   10021

A motivation for screening derives from two elementary observations: 1) the advanced stage of prostatic cancer in a significant proportion of patients at the time of its clinical recognition. Illustrated by data from the patterns of care study of the American College of Surgeons: approximately 50% of patients present with clinically advanced (stage C or D) disease; 2) the better survival rates of patients with prostatic cancer in stage A or B than of patients with stage C or D lesions, illustrated by data from the same study (Murphy et al, 1982). To what extent the respective survival rates are consequences of treatment rather than of tumor natural history is impossible to quantify in the absence of satisfactory controls.

Assuming that screening will improve identification of patients with stage A or B_1 prostatic cancer and that such recognition will lead to treatment, interpretation of end results will be difficult due to the confounding effects of tumor and host natural histories and of treatment. These considerations will be briefly examined.

Both clinical and pathologic evidence supports the potential possibilities of stage progression of prostatic cancer shown in Figure 1 (Whitmore, 1973), variations in the rate and pattern of such evolution being functions of the growth rate and metastatic potential of individual tumors.

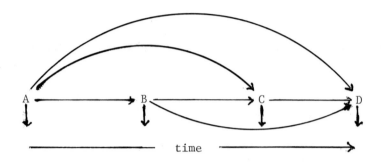

Figure 1

The local manifestations of progression are not well
documented. Metastatic progression, especially relative to
regional lymph node metastases, has been characterized
on the basis of experience with pelvic lymph node staging
(Donohue et al, 1982). Interpretations of such data on
metastatic progression are qualified by the selection
criteria for staging laparotomy (e.g., exclusion of
patients with distant metastasis), the usually restricted
nature of the pelvic lymphadenectomy vis a vis the more
extended lymphadenectomy utilized by Golimbu et al (1979),
the accuracy of the pathologic assessment of removed lymph
nodes, and the patients with apparently uninvolved pelvic
lymph nodes who later develop evidence of distant metastases
(presumably by-passing regional lymph nodes). The proportion
of individuals with prostatic cancer presenting in each
stage and the pattern and rate of stage progression for
individual stages (and grades) of prostatic cancer are being
progressively better defined, but the pattern and rate of
progression for an individual patient's tumor remains
uncertain. This is especially true for patients with the
A or B_1 cancers detected by "effective" screening. The
earlier the stage at diagnosis, the greater the number of
progression possibilities, the broader the range of management options, and the less certain the relevance of treatment
to survival.

Justification for treatment rests upon both of two considerations, namely, a demonstrated risk from the untreated disease and an established efficacy of the projected treatment in reducing such risk. Rich (1935) and Moore (1935) were principally responsible for calling the attention of clinicians and pathologists to the prevalence of clinically unrecognized prostatic cancer (stage A). To what extent the latter lesions are representative of the prostatic cancers incidentally found by pathologists during examination of tissue removed for the relief of bladder outlet obstruction remains uncertain but will become of immediate importance when a screening technique capable of recognizing all stage A lesions is developed. Bauer et al (1960) were among the first to point out the association of the grade and volume of stage A lesions to subsequent progression. Jewett (1975) subsequently suggested dividing A lesions into two categories, A_1 and A_2, on the basis of grade and volume criteria. No universally accepted definitions of A_1 and A_2 lesions exist but most agree that high grade lesions of any size and all lesions of more than "limited" volume have relatively increased progression probabilities. Cantrell et al (1981), in prostates operated for clinically benign obstruction, found that 2% of untreated patients with less than 5% cancer and none with Gleason scores of 4 or less (A_1) progressed within 4 years, whereas 32% of untreated patients with more than 5% cancer and 17% with Gleason scores greater then 4 (A_2) progressed within 4 years. Epstein et al (1986), among a group of 94 men with A_1 lesions defined according to the Cantrell et al criteria, reported that 26 died of other causes without progression less then 4 years after diagnosis and 18 were living without progression 4 to 8 years after diagnosis. However, 8 of 50 at risk 8 years or longer from the time of diagnosis had disease progression. Intervals from diagnosis to progression ranged from 3.5 to 8 years and 6 of the 8 patients died of cancer. Among the latter 8 tumors, 4 had originally involved less then 1% of the removed tissue and 6 had been of low grade. The remaining 42 patients were without evidence of progression 8 to 18 years from diagnosis.

Blute et al (1986) reviewed 23 men less then 60 years of age at diagnosis and at risk for 10 to 25 years with untreated stage A cancer. The overall survival for the first 10 years was comparable to that of an age and sex matched group of Mayo Clinic patients and no progression was noted before 9 years. Among 8 with $A2_3$ lesions (A_1 is $< 1cm^3$ and well differentiated; A_2 is $\geq 1cm^3$ or poorly differentiated), 2 progressed, one of whom died of prostatic cancer. Among 15 with A1 lesions, 4 progressed an average of 10 years after diagnosis but none had died of prostatic cancer. In addition to one death from prostatic cancer there were 3 from cardiovascular causes, 4 from colorectal cancer, 1 from brain tumor, and 1 from a gun shot. Three patients were lost to follow up after 3,10 and 11 years, respectively.

In addition to the unequivocal risks of disease progression indicated by these two illustrative but not necessary typical experiences, there was a significant mortality from unrelated causes, and a notable unreliability of the respective definitions of A_1 and A_2 lesions in anticipating progression.

Comparison of the autopsy prevalence of clinically unrecognized prostatic cancer to the corresponding age specific prostatic cancer mortality rates suggests prevalence to mortality ratios approximating 1000 between the ages of 50 and 60 years and falling to less than 100 after the age of 80 (Whitmore, 1963). Morbidity amd mortality from prostatic cancer appear to increase more rapidly with age than does the prevalence of clinically unrecognized carcinoma. Ashley (1965) calculated the incidence of clinically unrecognized prostatic cancer to be a function of the 2nd power of the age and the death rate for carcinoma of the prostate to be a function of the 7th power of the age. Halpert et al (1963) pointed out that the observed death rate from prostatic cancer at the age of 80 years corresponds to the observed prevalence of prostatic cancer in the decade 30-39; literally interpreted, this would suggest a 40-50 year course of the disease. Inferences from such analyses must be guarded, but the discrepancy between the pathologic prevalence of clinically unrecognized cancer and the incidence of clinically recognized cancer supports the concept that "although big oaks from little acorns grow, not all little acorns develop into big oaks".

The majority of B1 cancers progress although the time course may be protracted. Among 14 histologically proved and untreated B_1 lesions, 9 progressed over follow up intervals ranging to more than 12 years: five progressions were local and 4 involved bone metastases, 1 in association with and 3 after local progression (Whitmore et al, in press).

McNeal et al (1986) in examination of 100 prostate glands containing adenocarcinoma at autopsy and 38 containing cancer at radical prostatectomy found capsular invasion in 1 of 56 tumors under 0.46ml and in 17 of 33 larger than 0.46ml in volume. The correlations with grade, volume and metastasis noted in McNeal's study are consistent with multiple clinical experiences relating invasion and metastasis to tumor volume and grade, and with modern concepts of tumor biology. Nevertheless, the apparent "cure" of some stage B_2 or C prostatic cancers by irradiation or surgery and the absence of evidence of metastasis at autopsy in a small proportion of patients dying with stage C prostatic cancer (Arnheim, 1948; Schoones et al, 1972) suggest that the relationship between tumor volume and metastasis is not categorical.

Natural history of the host. Although average overall life expectancy is increasing, it remains finite and is diminishing relatively rapidly at the time when the incidence of prostatic cancer is steeply increasing. Relevance of natural life expectancy to treatment is nicely illustrated in the Epstein et al (1986) and Blute et al (1986) series wherein mortality from causes other than prostatic cancer considerably exceeds that from prostatic cancer.

The effectiveness of current treatments in the control of stage A lesions remains to be demonstrated, although it seems reasonable that such management will be as relevant to stage A cancers as to more advanced stages. Some 25-30% of patients with A2 lesions subjected to staging laparotomy have regional node metastases (Donohue et al, 1982) and this may account for the "progressors" among untreated patients with A_2 lesions; an analogous possibility exists for A_1 lesions. Such considerations add to the uncertainties relative to treatment rationale and to interpretation of end results in patients with A lesions.

Two important biases may confound interpretations of the effects of screening (and treatment) on survival in patients with stage A or B_1 prostatic cancer. One is lead time bias or zero time shift: this results from earlier diagnosis and yields a greater duration of life (after diagnosis and treatment) without extension of survival. The other is length bias: this results from the detection (and treatment) of cancers which are not progressing or which are progressing or which are progressing extremely slowly; inclusion of such

lesions automatically improves survival rates by diluting
the potential adverse survival impact of more aggressive
lesions. Given the enormous discrepancy between the pathologic prevalence of stage A cancers and the age specific
morbidity and mortality of prostatic cancer, the potential
for length bias in an "effective" screening for stage A
lesions looms especially large. There seems no doubt that
earlier diagnosis and treatment will improve survival rates
but to what extent this will be a consequence of such
potential screening biases will be difficult to define.
Proof of a reduction in prostatic cancer mortality as a
consequence of "effective" screening may well depend upon
a controlled study of a screened versus an unscreened risk
population. Such would require a large "at risk" population
and a protracted period of follow up.

Conclusions: Effective screening would by definition
diagnose more stage A and B1 lesions. Treatment of such
patients would improve overall survival rates in patients
with prostatic cancer but to what extent this would be a
function of lead time and length biases would be uncertain.
The potential protracted course of early stage prostatic
cancer and unrelated mortality imposed by the natural history
of the host introduce significant risks of therapeutic
overkill. The absence of prognostically reliable definitions
of A1 and A2 makes criteria for identification of biologic
potential an arguably more urgent need than "effective"
screening. Even in currently recognized patients with
stage A or B_1 cancers, clinical judgement remains a key
element in selection of patients for treatment and in choice
of treatment. More quantitative and reliable assessments
of host life expectancy relative to age and recognized
medical problems (e.g. diabetes, arteriosclerosis, etc.),
of tumor growth rate and metastatic potential, of extent
of the neoplasm (clinical staging), and of the responsiveness
of a particular tumor in a particular patient to a particular
treatment may enable computer applications of decision
theory to replace clinical judgement (Pauker and Kassirer,
1987).

REFERENCES

Arnheim FK (1948). Carcinoma of the prostate: A study of
    the postmortem findings in one hundred and seventy-six
    cases. J Urol 60:599-603.

Ashley DJB (1965). On the incidence of carcinoma of the prostate. J Pathol Bacteriol 90:217-224.

Bauer WC, McGavran MH, Carlin MR (1960). Unsuspected carcinoma of the prostate in suprapubic prostatectomy specimens. A clinicopathological study of 55 consecutive cases. Cancer 13:370-378.

Blute ML, Zincke H, Farrow GM (1986). Long-term followup of young patients with stage A adenocarcinoma of the prostate. J Urol 136:840-843.

Cantrell BB, DeKlerk DP, Eggleston JC, Boitnott JK, Walsh PC (1980). Pathological factors that influence prognosis in staging A prostatic cancer: the influence of extent versus grade. J Urol 125:516-520.

Donohue RE, Mani JH, Whitesel JA, Mohr S, Scanavino D, Augspurger RR, Biber RJ, Fauver HE, Wettlaufer JN, Pfister RR (1982). Pelvic lymph node dissection. Guide to patient management in clinically locally confined adenocarcinoma of prostate. Urology XX:559-565.

Epstein JI, Paull G, Eggleston JC, Walsh PC (1986). Prognosis of untreated stage A1 prostatic carcinoma: A study of 94 cases with extended followup. J Urol 136:837-839.

Golimbu M, Morales P, Al-Askari S, Brown J (1979). Extended lymphadenectomy for prostatic cancer. J Urol 121:617-620.

Halpert B, Sheehan EE, Schmalhorst WR, Scott R Jr (1963). Carcinoma of the prostate. A survey of 5,000 autopsies. Cancer 16:737-742.

Jewett HJ (1975). The present status of radical prostatectomy for stages A and B prostatic cancer. Urol Clin North Am 2: 105-124.

McNeal JE, Kindrachuk RA, Freiha FS, Bostwick DG, Redwine EA, Stamey TA (1986). Patterns of progression in prostatic cancer. Lancet 60-63.

Moore RA (1935). The morphology of small prostatic carcinomas. ibid 33:224-234.

Murphy GP, Natarajan N, Pontes JE, Schmitz RL, Schmidt JD, Mettlin C (1982). The national survey of prostate cancer in the United States by the American College of Surgeons. J Urol 127:928-934.

Pauker SG and Kassirer JP (1987). Medical progress. Decision analysis. The New England Journal of Medicine 250-258.

Rich AR (1985). On the frequency of occurrence of occult carcinoma of the prostate. J Urol 33:215-223.

Schoones R, Palma LD, Gaeta JR, et al (1972). Prostatic carcinoma treated at categorical center. NY State J Med 1: 1021-1027.

Whitmore WF Jr (1963). The rationale and results of ablative
  surgery for prostatic cancer. Cancer 16:1119-1132.
Whitmore WF Jr (1973). The natural history of prostatic
  cancer. Cancer 32:1104-1112.
Whitmore WF Jr, Rosenberg S, Chopp R (in press). Wait and see:
  Experience with B1 lesions. Progress and Controversies in
  Oncological Urology. Alan R. Liss, New York.

EORTC Genitourinary Group Monograph 5: Progress
and Controversies in Oncological Urology II, pages 131–137
© 1988 Alan R. Liss, Inc.

SCREENING FOR PROSTATIC CARCINOMA - USEFUL OR NOT?

G.P. Murphy

Department of Urology, State University of New
York at Buffalo, School of Medicine and Urologic
Cooperative Oncology Group, Room 139 Parker Hall,
Buffalo, New York 14214

ABSTRACT

Screening of asymptomatic males for prostatic cancer by
any means has not shown to date any benefit. There is a need
to evaluate prostatic ultrasound with new equipment combining
transaxial and sagittal rectal ultrasound with some markers
and rectal exam in asymptomatic men between the ages of 55-
70, with appropriate biopsy based on suspicious findings.
Such a multicenter study has been organized in the United
States. Based on such limited studies, results can be
evaluated in 5 years - and then the true place of screening
for prostatic cancer tested if such pilot detection projects
suggest sufficient merit.

INTRODUCTION

The question the participants of this section of the
program are addressing concerns the status of the present
possibility of screening for prostatic cancer. At present
with available tested technology, be it rectal exam or serum
markers, there is no objective evidence that such exists
(Guinan et al., 1985; Chodak and Schoenberg, 1984; Spiegelman
et al., 1986). No satisfactory study of a true high risk
group of asymptomatic males has been identified and followed
for a long period of time, and on these strict requirements,
rectal ultrasound has not yet shown objective improvement
(Chodak et al., 1986).

Sponsored in part by Cancer Research Fund, University at
Buffalo Foundation.

PROSPECTS FOR THE FUTURE

On the other hand, it has been accepted, based on an international consensus meeting that I chaired in July 1985, that in the posterior prostatic zone decreased or hypoechoic areas suggest in over two-thirds of the cases an early localized adenocarcinoma (Lee et al., 1986). It is in the earlier detection of such lesions, confirmed by ultrasonic guided biopsy and aspiration, that the future depends. We know that even without such techniques a national survey in the United States has recently suggested a relative increase in localized, occult, or unsuspected non-clinical adenocarcinoma of the prostate (Young et al., 1981; Schmidt et al., 1986) (Figure 1).

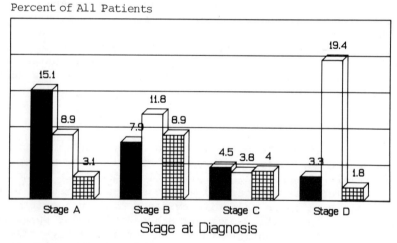

Figure 1. A recent study from the American College of Surgeons confirming the high rate of so-called A_1 lesions found in the most recent national study.

NATIONAL PROSTATIC CANCER DETECTION PROJECT

To attempt to provide such objective data at 7 centers geographically spread over the United States, such a project has been organized. Firstly, we recognize, based on available data in the USA, the significant relative rise in incidence of prostatic cancer in asymptomatic U.S. males ranging in age from 55-70 (Figure 2).

Prostate Cancer Incidence And Age

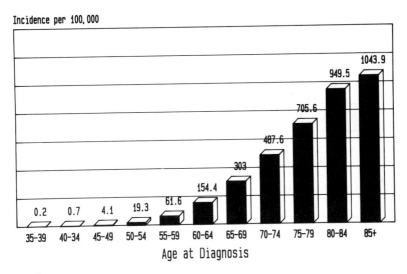

Incidence per 100,000

Source: SEER

Figure 2. The relative range of increasing incidence in asymptomatic U.S. males seen from ages 55 to 70.

In order to study such an asymptomatic population as described, we wish to evaluate men who have no prior history of diagnosis or treatment for BPH (benign prostatic hypertrophy), inflammation, or cancer. Each person who volunteers will receive a selective history, urological examination, a prior blood specimen for prostatic antigen, and a rectal ultrasound examination (trans-axial and sagittal) each year

for 5 years. If a suspicious area is seen or palpated, a
biopsy will be performed and the patient followed as shown
in Figure 3 for the course of treatment and follow-up.

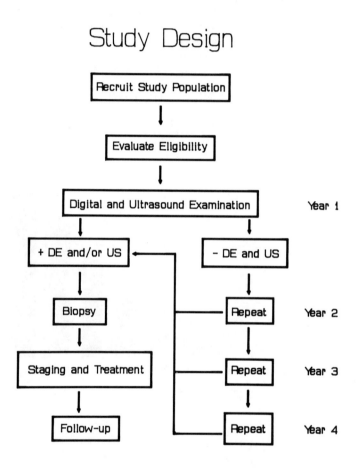

Figure 3.   The manner in which the National Group will
follow with rectal exam, PSA, and rectal ultrasound,
asymptomatic men aged 55-70 for five years or for subsequent follow up and treatment.

For completeness' sake, a quality control center will be
maintained for recording and secondary reviewing of all
ultrasound examinations as recorded on video tape, the clinical data, and pathological slide review (Figure 4).   Such a

NPCDP Organization

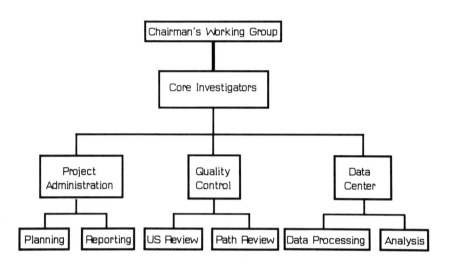

Figure 4. The group organizational structure for a U.S. national ultrasound detection project.

study may establish in a sufficient number, e.g. 5,000 suitable men, an idea of the detection capacity of prostatic rectal ultrasound in combination with blood testing, history, and prostatic examination. In general, a variety of possibilities exist (Figure 5). A positive US (ultrasound) exam versus, for example, a negative or positive concurrent rectal exam, as shown, could raise a variety of results (Figure 5). Realistically, no knowledge of what will be seen in this multicenter study is yet known. Obviously, more studies are also needed everywhere.

Based on such data, then, larger studies which would incorporate significant numbers of at-risk males (e.g. Black U.S. males) can be accomplished and the results truly evaluated as prostatic screening. Also, at present, the equipment has greatly improved. Further technical advances may occur, but these would not lessen in any way this widespread need for progressive evaluation.

Hypothetical Outcomes

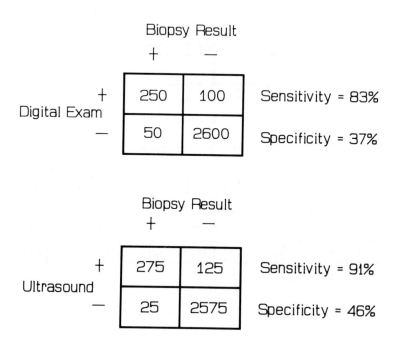

Figure 5. Some possible hypothetical outcomes of the National Prostatic Cancer Ultrasound Detection Project.

REFERENCES:

Chodak GW, Schoenberg HW (1984). Early detection of prostate cancer by routine screening. JAMA 252:3261–3264.
Chodak GW, Wald V, Parmer E, et al (1986). Comparison of digital examination and transrectal ultrasonography for the diagnosis of prostatic cancer. J Urology 135:951–954.
Guinan P, Gilham N, Nagubadi SR, et al (1985). What is the best test to detect prostate cancer? CA-A Cancer Journal for Clinicians 31:141–145.
Lee F, Gray JM, McLeary RD, Murphy GP, et al (1986). Prostatic evaluation by transrectal sonography: criteria for diagnosis of early carcinoma. Radiology 158:91–95.

Schmidt JD, Mettlin C, Natarajan N (1986). Trends in patterns of care for prostate cancer, 1973–1983: results of surveys by the American College of Surgeons. J Urology 136:416–421.

Spiegelman SS, McNeal JE, Freima FS, Stamey TA (1986). Rectal examination of carcinoma of the prostate: clinical and anatomical correlations. J Urol 136:1228–1230.

Young JL, Percy CL, Asire AJ (1981). Surveillance, epidemiology, and end results: Incidence and mortality data, 1973–1977. Natl Cancer Inst Monograph 57.

EORTC Genitourinary Group Monograph 5: Progress
and Controversies in Oncological Urology II, pages 139-145
© 1988 Alan R. Liss, Inc.

ROUND TABLE DISCUSSION: SCREENING FOR PROSTATIC CARCINOMA –
USEFUL OR NOT?   (Chairmen: L. Collste and F.H. Schröder)

H.J. de Voogt

Department of Urology, Free University Hospital,
Amsterdam, The Netherlands

COLLSTE

May I ask the panelists to come up here? Dr. Denis will
start. Can I ask you to be as short as possible please since
we are running over time.

DENIS

The Chairman gave me the permission to show you 6
slides on a pilot study that we do in Flanders on the early
detection of prostatic cancer. We are dealing with 6 million
people and have to do the study with 30,000 dollars per
year. In the complex world of screening or early detection
of prostatic cancer like others we have elected to focus on
the ultrasound machine and our finger. But the problem is
far more difficult than that and I think several speakers
have pointed this out. To give you an example: In breast
cancer the reward for screening was that the breast could be
kept intact. But early detection of prostate cancer means:
take the prostate out and down is the patient's sex-life. We
think that the General Physician should learn rectal examination and should do it! Look for the men of 60-75 years
with pulmonary obstructive disease and other diseases and we
will find more BPH and bladder cancer in addition to prostate cancer!

MURPHY

Under people of 55-75 years screening could only be cost-effective if we are looking at people at high risk, like the older age groups and the blacks in the U.S.A.

COLLSTE

We have been listening to a lot of nice papers. Could we ask each of the panelists to give a short statement on screening?

RESNICK

Screening for PCA should start with rectal palpation.

CHODAK

Unless we do a randomized study of screened, unscreened or untreated populations, we will not know whether or not screening is justified in the next 30 years.

SCHRÖDER

I do agree that such studies are necessary and I do agree with Dr. Whitmore's view of feasibility.

JACOBI

Advertising is very important to get people to go to a screening program, which should employ rectal palpation.

WHITMORE

I have not yet seen any screening program that fulfills all criteria.

MURPHY

Hypo-echoic areas are only seen in peripheral parts of the prostate with ultrasound and not always in all nodules.

WATANABE

Perhaps the best method is combining ultrasound and rectal digital examination. Very often rectal palpation was proven to be incorrect by ultrasound and after ultrasound you probably can palpate more or better. It is also very necessary to document ultrasound findings in screening.

PAVONE-MACALUSO

I have a question. It has been pointed out that screening should be useful to detect a disease that might be a threat to the well-being of a given individual. We learned what the possible benefit can be. We did not hear anything about it being detrimental for some of these people, in particular regarding the data Dr. Watanabe gave to us. If my recollection of his results is reliable, of 1000 individuals tested 5 had cancer. Certainly a larger number, maybe 100, got biopsies, only 5 had cancer which means that 95 got biopsies without having cancer. I am not speaking about the complications but the well-being of a person can also be influenced by the psychological impact of all this. I wonder what were these people told? Were they told they might have cancer? I think there is a possibility of suicide or of severe depression or other psychological problems in those 300 people who went to secondary studies. Five had cancer but 295 had further studies but had no cancer. What were these people told in the rural areas in particular? Were they told they might have cancer? How did they react?

WATANABE

Usually we are doing the prostatic biopsy by ultrasound guidance and it takes only 3 or 5 minutes for one person and we never use an anaesthesia. Only local anaesthesia is injected and the injection is performed also under the ultrasound guidance. It is very easy to take prostatic tissue. According to our method the biopsy is not so troublesome and we have encountered no complications by that method. So I think the 5 positive patients in 100 biopsy persons is not so bad.

COLLSTE

Thank you, we have one further remark on this particular question.

CHODAK

We have been aware of this psychological problem. Many patients are very upset when we tell them that we need a biopsy. We have to tell them that there is a lesion of which we do not know if it is cancer. I would say on our 100 or so men we biopsied it is probably 10% who refused biopsy because they were concerned. I think it is a real problem in doing a mass screening program, to deal with these adverse psychological effects.

COLLSTE

Thank you. Any more questions?

KHOURY

Given the present economic condition I am afraid that to work on the concept of mass-screening is becoming a utopia as well in cancer as in any other disease. I think if you want to think of screening today we are compelled to define the population. We cannot screen mass populations today. We only can screen high risk populations. The same is true in prostatic cancer. For patients who might benefit from discovering prostatic cancer and as Professor Denis said we have to couple several things that we can investigate at the same time so that the yield would be better. But I think the very concept of mass detection of prostatic cancer is a utopia and is not a practical thing. Thank you.

PAULSON

The concept of screening a population is discussed very adequately by the speakers in the panel today. It raises the issue of the current concept between stage A and stage B or T1 and T2 disease and almost all of the speakers have made allusions to the volume of the disease as being the important predictor in the ultimate outcome whether they are observed or actively treated. Perhaps the panel would like to comment on whether or not we should perhaps begin to think about T1 and T2 disease as a common entity and begin to segregate in low volume disease and high volume disease being defined as you decide. But there seems to be no significant difference in the outcome of treatment for patients who have their disease identified by say transurethral resection or needle biopsy who subsequently undergo definitive therapy. Similarly there seems to be a great parallel between the observed response to observation alone in the very low volume nodules and the observation alone in the low volume "stage A" disease which is probably only having about 8% progression over a period of time.

CHODAK

The dilemma is the following: The tumors that we can truly cure are the ones that are less than 1 cm in cubic volume. And those are the ones who are most difficult to diagnose by screening. At the same time if we were to find them we would be uncertain whether to treat most of them anyway, because we know that most of them will not progress. So I would submit that we really have a dilemma: we can cure some people but I am not sure that we want to treat them.

WHITMORE

There are two questions that need to be answered. One is, is cure necessary and who knows in whom it is possible? and is cure possible and who knows in whom it is necessary? We really do not have any answer to either one of those questions.

RESNICK

Well, Mr. Chairman, I think that for those 8% patients from Baltimore we also do not know whether they are multi-focal or otherwise, that their cancer that arrived over a period of time was the same A1 cancer that they were initially seen with. Of course, had they been to Dr. Watanabe and had they had ultrasound, maybe we would not be arguing about that. But hopefully we will no argue too much longer about proper prospective trials, randomized or not, which need to be conducted to answer the pending questions.

WHITMORE

One of the disconcerning observations, at least to me, is a fact that although Steamy and McNeal have suggested from their data in radical prostatectomy studies that volumes greater than 1 cc are those with associated metastatic disease, we know that some patients with stage C disease are apparently cured by appropriate therapy without evidence of metastatic disease. Furthermore, in the definition of stage A if you control the TUR material by the method which is pretty widely adopted, I believe, if you take 5% of the resected tissue as the upper limit for stage Al lesion, if you have 5% of a 100 gram gland it is a 5 gram tumor. I you have 5% of a 10 gram gland it is a 0.5 gram tumor and yet a direct question was that they could not see any difference, based on this volume of tissue resected. So this volume concept is not perfectly clear and of course what the cancer biologist tells us is simply that as the cancer gets larger the possibility of genetic instability leading to metastatic clones gets greater. It is not so much the volume, it is the change in tumor biology as tumors expand in size that determines the outcome.

COLLSTE

We have one final question.

FOSSÅ

It is more a comment than a question. I am left with the impression that screening - I mean: the politics of screening - might be quite different in Japan, Germany and for example in the Scandinavian countries. When we set up screening - mass screening especially - we will have to know more about psychological aspects of what we are really doing. For example Dr. Jacobi told us that in Germany they now will avoid the word "cancer" in the invitation to the patient. I really want to know how do we know that this will increase the compliance? Is there any evidence that this is relevant for the German population? I think in the Scandinavian countries it would be the opposite. We tell our patients that we do this to avoid or to detect cancer and we get more patients. In Japan, well I do not think we can have this type of mass screening. In Japan it looks to me a little bit unhuman, at least in my western European way of thinking and so I think it is very difficult to compare the results from such different populations and at least the politics of setting up such mass screening in such different countries.

COLLSTE

Thank you Dr. Fosså. I think we have to conclude that we have had a great morning, at least I did. We have an excellent and expert panel, on a very difficult subject and I am sorry that we have to finish it here.

EORTC Genitourinary Group Monograph 5: Progress
and Controversies in Oncological Urology II, pages 147-155
© 1988 Alan R. Liss, Inc.

IS THERE A BEST ENDOCRINE MANAGEMENT OF PROSTATIC CARCINOMA?

M.R.G. Robinson

Department of Urology, The General Infirmary,
Friarwood Lane, Pontefract, West Yorkshire,
WF8 1PL, England

INTRODUCTION

Endocrine therapy of carcinoma of the prostate has been
practised for the whole of this century. In 1895, White advocated castration to relieve prostatic obstruction and in 1942,
Randall reported the results of the first large series of patients with carcinoma of the prostate treated by orchidectomy.
Shortly before this, in 1941, Huggins and Hodges established
the rationale for both orchidectomy and oestrogen therapy.
Since then the endocrine therapy of prostatic cancer has become established and has been intensively investigated in
clinical trials. Until the Veterans Co-operative Urological
Research Group reported the results of their studies in 1967,
emphasizing the often lethal cardiovascular side effects of
oestrogens, most patients were treated with differing, often
very large, doses of diethylstilboestrol.

The majority of prostatic cancers remain, like normal
prostatic tissue, for a variable period of time dependant
upon androgens for cell secretory activity, growth and multi-
plication. All endocrine therapy is based upon the removal or
suppression of the sites of androgen production. The principle
androgen influencing prostatic function and growth is testosterone, which is converted in the gland to the more active
dihydrotestosterone. The principle source of testosterone is
the testes and thus castration or suppression of testicular
production of testosterone by oestrogen therapy were the
first two forms of endocrine management to be practised. In
much smaller quantities, other androgens such as androstene-
dione and dehydroepiandrosterone are produced by the adrenal

cortex. These weak androgens are converted to testosterone and dihydrotestosterone peripherally in the prostate and other target organs. Secondary endocrine therapy by the removal or suppression of the adrenal glands by adrenalectomy (Huggins and Scott, 1945), pituitary ablation (Fergusson and Hendry, 1971) or medical adrenalectomy (Robinson, Shearer and Fergusson, 1974) has been practised with relief of symptoms but with little in the way of objective tumour response or prolongation of survival. More recently, Labrie, Dupont and Belanger (1985) have advocated complete androgen blockade using a luteinising hormone releasing hormone (LHRH) analogue and Flutemide and have claimed improved results. LHRH analogues given in supraphysiological doses are effective as a form of medical orchidectomy because they paradoxically suppress the secretion of luteinising hormone and thus the production of testosterone by the interstitial cells of the testes.

Other hormonal drugs with progestational and anti-androgen activity have been used in the management of prostatic cancer. Cyproterone acetate acts by blocking the uptake of dihydrotestosterone by receptor proteins in the prostatic cell cytoplasm. In addition it suppresses the pituitary production of luteinising hormone and the adrenal synthesis of androgens. Medroxyprogesterone acetate and megestrol acetate are progestational agents which compete for cytosol receptor and block the conversion of testosterone to dihydrotestosterone by suppressing 5-alpha-reductase activity. Flutamide is a non-steroidal pure anti-androgen which also acts through the cytosol androgen receptors.

The simplest and least expensive endocrine management of carcinoma of the prostate is by surgical orchidectomy or by the administration of the synthetic oestrogen diethylstilboestrol. Unfortunately, orchidectomy produces psychological trauma in many men and stilboestrol has a high incidence of cardiovascular toxicity. Both, as do most other forms of endocrine therapy, produce impotence and neither suppress the production of androgens by the adrenal gland.

This brief review of the rationale for and the methods of endocrine therapy of carcinoma of the prostate raises the question of which is the most effective form of endocrine management in this disease. For this reason, the Urological Group of the European Organisation for Research and Treatment of Cancer (EORTC) are investigating hormonal therapy in an on-going series of Phase III Clinical Trials. The first of these randomised Phase III studies, Protocol 30761, compared diethylstilboestrol (DES) 1 mg three times a day with Cyproterone acetate (CPA) 250 mg a day and Medroxy-progesterone acetate (MPA) given in a loading dose of 500 mg intramuscularly three times a week for eight weeks followed by 100 mg orally three times daily. Two hundred and ten eligible patients were entered: 75 received CPA, 71 MPA and 64 DES. The second study, Protocol 30762, compared DES 1 mg three times a day with Estramustine phosphate (Estracyt) 280 mg twice daily for eight weeks followed by 140 mg twice daily. Two hundred and twenty-seven patients were eligible for analysis: 112 received DES and 115 Estracyt. Final clinical analyses of these two studies have been reported by Pavone Macaluso et al (1986) and Smith et al (1986). A third study, Protocol 30805, fully recruited but not finally analysed, compared bilateral orchidectomy with bilateral orchidectomy plus CPA 50 mg three times a day and DES 1 mg daily. Three hundred and fifty patients have been entered into this study, but not all are yet fully evaluable.

Patients entered into Protocol 30761 and 30762 had either locally advanced (T3, T4, M0: TNM classification) disease or metastatic disease (M1). Those entered into Protocol 30805 all had metastatic disease (M1). Response criteria for Protocol 30761 and 30762 included local and distant objective response, time to progression and survival. Because of the difficulties in prostatic carcinoma of measuring true local and distant responses, Protocol 30805 is only being evaluated for time to progression and survival. Two other EORTC Phase III Protocols are evaluating the LHRH analogues Buserelin and Zoladex. At the present time it is too soon to comment on these studies.

There are many ways of assessing the best form of endocrine treatment. Among the important factors to consider are objective tumour regression, the time interval until there is tumour progression, length of survival, subjective relief of symptoms and performance status, treatment toxicity and the quality of life as expressed by the patient himself. The completed EORTC studies have considered all these aspects of endocrine therapy with the exception of The Quality of Life, the study of which is included in the current trials.

OBJECTIVE TUMOUR REGRESSION

Tumour regression has proved difficult to assess in these studies. Rectal ultrasound was not widely available to measure the volume of primary disease when these protocols were activated and it is extremely difficult to quantitate the appearances seen on scintigrams and x-rays of the common bone metastases. Therefore, no attempt was made to measure tumour regression in Protocol 30805. Objective tumour regression for Protocol 30761 and 30762 is summarized in Table 1.

Table 1: Complete plus Partial Regression (%)

		LOCAL	DISTANT
	(CPA	40	13.3
30761	(MPA	25.8	2.9
	(DES	54.4	17.9
30762	(DES	57.5	31.4
	(ESTRACYT	35	24.4

It can be seen that in Protocol 30761 there is no significant difference in tumour regression for CPA and DES. MPA is less effective but the dosage that was given in this study is now considered very low. In Protocol 30762 there are no significant differences between DES and Estracyt but again it has been suggested that the dosage of Estracyt employed was too low. It would appear from these studies that the objective response rate to DES of the local tumour is of the order of 50-55% and of distant metastases of 20-30%. This is much less than the formerly widely held view that 80% of prostatic tumours "respond" to oestrogen therapy.

TIME TO TUMOUR PROGRESSION

In Protocol 30761 the time to tumour progression was shorter for patients receiving MPA than those receiving either CPA or DES. This was more marked for patients who had metastatic disease at the time of entry to the study. Protocol 30762 demonstrated no difference in the time to progression for patients receiving DES or Estracyt. The time to progression, however, for patients with non-metastatic disease at the time of entry into the study was much longer than for patients with metastatic disease. The preliminary analysis of Protocol 30805 (Robinson and Hetherington, 1986) shows no difference in time to progression in patients with metastatic disease who were treated either by orchidectomy alone, orchidectomy plus CPA or DES 1 mg only per day.

LENGTH OF SURVIVAL

Patients treated on MPA in Protocol 30761 had a significantly shorter length of survival if they entered the study with metastatic disease. There was no significant difference if they entered without metastases. In Protocol 30762 and so far in Protocol 30805, there are no significant differences in overal survival rates and death from prostatic cancer for any of the treatment regimes used (Pavone Macaluso et al, 1986; Smith et al, 1986; Robinson and Hetherington, 1986).

SUBJECTIVE RELIEF OF SYMPTOMS AND PERFORMANCE STATUS

The patient with prostatic carcinoma judges his treatment on relief of symptoms and his personal level of general activity or performance status. These important aspects of the response to therapy have not yet been fully analysed for the EORTC Trials of Hormonal Therapy. It is, however, well established that effective hormonal therapy relieves, often dramatically, pain from metastases and improves performance status. Conversely, failure to relieve symptoms is associated with disease progression and a poor prognosis. There is no evidence that any of the effective hormonal therapies that have been studied is more effective than the others in relieving symptoms.

TREATMENT TOXICITY

The most serious toxicity which has caused concern in the EORTC studies has been cardiovascular. For Protocols 30761 and 30762 this has been reported in detail by De Voogt (1986). The observed cardiovascular complications have been fluid retention, hypertension, electrocardiographic changes, myocardial infarction and thromboembolic disease. They occur more frequently during the first six months of treatment and are much more common in patients with cardiovascular disease prior to therapy. Increasing age and obesity are adverse factors. Cardiovascular toxicity is highest with DES therapy and least with CPA therapy. It is hoped that the analysis of Protocol 30805 will demonstrate a lower toxicity with DES 1 mg daily in comparison to DES 1 mg three times a day. So far cardiovascular toxicity has not been a problem in this study.

With respect to less serious toxicity all the endocrine therapies investigated by the EORTC have produced impotency. Apart from the psychological trauma of castration, the only other toxicity observed with orchidectomy is hot flushes. On rare occasions these are severe and require treatment with oestrogens. Gynaecomastia occurs with DES, CPA, MPA and Estracyt. It is much more prevelant and severe with DES. Gastrointestinal symptoms have been reported with Estracyt and to a lesser extent with DES.

DISCUSSION

The current results of the EORTC Urological Studies in Endocrine Treatment of Prostatic Cancer demonstrate that the effective therapies they have used, i.e. DES, CPA and Estracyt, are all equally proficient in relieving symptoms and producing tumour regression. There is also no difference between them in prolonging the time to progression or the length of survival. Contrary to the experience of Benson (1983) the combination of a cytotoxic agent and an oestrogen (Estracyt) has not proved more effective than DES. The dose of Estracyt used in the EORTC studies was, however, less than that used by Benson and his associates.

Bracci (1972) advocates the combination of orchidectomy and CPA to improve the results of the hormonal therapy of prostatic cancer. This is based upon the concept of total androgen blockade. So far the results of Protocol 30805 have not supported Bracci's results. Labrie (1985) has claimed that the combination of an LHRH analogue and a pure anti-androgen, such as Flutemide or one of its analogues, is more effective than conventional endocrine therapy. He prefers this to the combination of orchidectomy and CPA because CPA

has a progestational-like action which, because there are pro-
gestin receptors in the prostate, may have a stimulatory effect.
Labrie's hypothesis is being tested in the current EORTC Protocol 30805 which compares Zoladex (a depot LHRH preparation) plus
Flutamide with orchidectomy. At the present time, however, it
seems unlikely that total androgen blockade or any other form
of combined endocrine therapy is likely to be significantly
more effective in prolonging survival and producing subjective
and objective responses.

It is, therefore, apparent that selection of the best endocrine treatment for carcinoma of the prostate depends on other
factors which have to be taken into consideration. These include
patient selection, the timing of treatment with respect to disease stage (i.e. defered versus immediate treatment), patient
compliance with treatment, treatment toxicity, cost and availability of the drugs and most important the quality of life
during treatment.

The results of Protocol 30762 for patients with non-
metastatic disease have demonstrated that the time to progression is very similar to that reported for patients with
VACURG Stage III (advanced non-metastatic) disease treated by
placebo in the initial VACURG study (Smith et al, 1986). This
would suggest that endocrine therapy is best reserved only for
patients with metastatic disease. Recently Klotz et al (1986)
have advocated intermittent endocrine therapy for patients
with bone pain and positive radionuclear scans. They administered
DES to 19 patients and Flutemide to 1 patient until a clinical
response was clearly demonstrated and then the treatment was
withheld until symptoms recurred. All the patients who subsequently relapsed had a rapid clinical response following
the resumption of endocrine therapy. Patients with impotency
following intermittent endocrine therapy resumed sexual activity within three months of stopping treatment. Therefore, the
concept of only treating patients with symptomatic metastatic
disease by hormonal therapy needs further investigation.

Serious toxicity, especially cardiovascular toxicity,
remains a problem especially with oestrogen therapy and there
is no doubt that if patients will accept castration,
orchidectomy is the cheapest and least toxic endocrine therapy.
DES remains the cheapest alternative. There is no doubt that
endocrine therapy has profound psychological effect on patients
which cannot be measured simply in terms of performance status,

relief of symptoms and treatment toxicity. This is why the Quality of Life studies which are being employed in the current EORTC Protocols will produce further information about the best choice of endocrine therapy. At the present time, however, no treatment seems to be superior to simple total or subcapsular orchidectomy.

REFERENCES

Benson RC, Gill GM, Cummings KB (1983). Randomised double blind cross over trial of diethylstilboestrol (DES) and Estramustine phosphate (ENCYT). The stage D Prostatic Cancer Seminar in Oncology, Volume 10, Suppl. 3, p 43-45.
Bracci U (1977). Our present procedures in the treatment of prostatic cancer. In Bracci U, Sylvesteria FD (eds): "Hormonal Therapy of Prostatic Cancer," Cohese, Palermo.
Fergusson JD and Hendry WG (1971). Pituitary irradiation in advanced carcinoma of the prostate: Analysis of 100 cases. Br J Urol 43:514-519.
Huggins C and Hodges CV (1941). Studies of prostate cancer: effective castration, estrogen and androgen injection serum phosphatase in metastatic carcinoma of the prostate. Cancer Res 1:293-294.
Huggins C and Scott WW (1945). Bilateral adrenalectomy in prostatic cancer, clinical features and urinary excretion of 17-ketosteroide and estrogen. Annals of Surgery 122: 1031-1044.
Klotz LH, Herr HW, Morse MJ, Whitmore WF (1986). Intermittent endocrine therapy for prostatic cancer. Cancer 58:2546-2550.
Labrie F, Dupont A, Belanger A (1985). Complete androgen blockade for the treatment of prostatic cancer. In DeVita VT, Helman S, Rosenberg SA (eds): "Important Advances in Oncology", Lippincott Company, Philadelphia.
Pavone Macaluso M, de Voogt HJ, Viggiano G, Barasolo E, Lardennois B, de Pauw M, Sylvester R (1986). Comparison of diethylstilboestrol, Cyproterone acetate, Medroxyprogesterone acetate in the treatment of advanced prostatic cancer: final analysis of the randomised Phase III Trial of the European Organisation for Research on Treatment of Cancer Urological Group. J Urol 136:624-631.
Randall A (1942). Eight year results of castration for cancer of the prostate. J Urol 48:706-709.
Robinson MRG and Hetherington J (1986). The EORTC studies: Is there an optimal endocrine management of M1 prostatic cancer? World J Urol 4:171-175.

Robinson MRG, Shearer RJ, Fergusson JD (1974). Adrenal suppression in the treatment of carcinoma of the prostate. Br J Urol 46:555-559.

Smith PH, Suciu S, Robinson MRG, Richards B, Bastable JRG, Glashan RW, Bouffioux C, Lardennois B, Williams RE, de Pauw M, Sylvester R (1986). A comparison of the effect of diethylstilboestrol with low dose Estramustine phosphate in the treatment of advanced prostatic cancer: final analysis of a Phase III Trial of the European Organisation for Research on Treatment of Cancer. J Urol 136:619-623.

Veterans Administration Co-Operative Urological Research Group (1967). Treatment and survival of patients with cancer of the prostate. Surg Gyn Obst 124:1011-1017.

Voogt HJ de, Smith PH, Pavone Macaluso M, de Pauw M, Suciu S and members of the European Organisation for Research on Treatment of Cancer Urological Group (1986). Cardiovascular side-effects of diethylstilboestrol, Cyproterone acetate, Medroxyprogesterone acetate and Estramustine phosphate used for the treatment of advanced prostatic cancer: results from European Organisation for Research on Treatment of Cancer Trials 30761 and 30762. J Urol 135:303-307.

White JW (1895). The surgery of the hypertrophied prostate. Annals of Surgery 17:70-75.

EORTC Genitourinary Group Monograph 5: Progress
and Controversies in Oncological Urology II, pages 157–158
© 1988 Alan R. Liss, Inc.

Discussion: Is There a Best Endocrine Management of
Prostatic Carcinoma?

Karl H. Kurth, Rotterdam, The Netherlands

Pavone Macaluso: I only have a small addition to what Robinson said regarding protocol 30761, which I coordinated. The
patients were allocated randomly to receive either 250 mg
oral Cyproterone acetate per day, 500 mg Medroxy-progesterone acetate intramuscularly daily for 8 weeks followed by
an overall dose of 200 per day thereafter, or 3 mg Diethylstilboestrol daily orally. We recently had the possibility
to analyse the plasma testosterone level of patients treated
with the 3 different regimes. All patients were down to
castration levels, independent whether they were treated
with DES, CPA or MPA. So with regard to endocrine efficacy
MPA was not used in too low a dose as reflected by the
plasma testosterone levels. It is very hard to understand
why the survival rate and the time to progression were worse
in the MPA arm compared to the other treatment arms. It is
difficult to tell, whether the differences in survival might
be due to some endogenous stimulation produced by the compound as such, but this remains questionable in my point of
view.

Robinson: I agree with you. Another possibility may be,
because there is a progesterone receptor, the drug may
stimulate the prostate in some way.

Kjaer: I have repeatedly heard reports of the EORTC trials.
Every time there is much talk about response. In my opinion
phase III studies are meant for one thing: comparison of
survival. I cannot understand how you can set up a multicenter protocol aimed to study response in a phase III setting
where you really are looking for survival. Can you comment
on this.

Robinson: You are absolutely correct and I would agree with
what you said. We thought in 1976 that we could make an
attempt at measuring response. In 1980 when we did the 30805
protocol we said we could not measure response and it would

be much easier to measure time to progression in distant metastases, which in most cases means a new hotspot on the bone scan. But again it is not so easy to measure time to progression as it seems to be even in protocol 30805, where all patients had metastatic disease and progressed much more rapidly than the non-metastatic patients. Several patients were taken off study before there was a documented progression. The responsible physician felt, that if patients were having pain, loosing weight or becoming anaemic, they had to change the treatment. Thus even time to progression is not so easy to measure, but it is certainly easier to measure than response.

EORTC Genitourinary Group Monograph 5: Progress
and Controversies in Oncological Urology II, pages 159–173
© 1988 Alan R. Liss, Inc.

IS CHEMOTHERAPY READY FOR CLINICAL USE IN PROSTATIC
CANCER PATIENTS?

W G JONES
University Department of Radiotherapy
Cookridge Hospital
Leeds LS16 6QB
Great Britain

Cytotoxic chemotherapy has had a considerable impact on
the management of a small group of relatively rare
malignancies. Diseases such as Hodgkin's disease,
choriocarcinoma, the leukaemias, histiocytic lymphomas, germ
cell tumours and various solid tumours of childhood have not
only been shown to be chemo-responsive but chemo-curable.
Spurred on by these successes in the 1960's and 1970's,
clinicians have exhibited great enthusiasm in trying to
achieve similar results in the commoner adult solid tumours.
This has proved not to be possible and the bulk of cytotoxic
drug therapy given today is administered with palliative
intent. The decision to use this modality of therapy must
entail a consideration of the balance between likely
benefits and expected toxic effects of the therapy. The use
of cytotoxic chemotherapy in common adult malignancies has
been extensively discussed by Kearsley (1986), who stressed
the need for the therapist to be realistic in his aims of
palliation. Particular attention has to be paid to the
impact of toxicity on the patient, together with the impact
of investigations used in trying to assess response. Above
all it is necessary for the clinician to examine his own
motives, (and at times desperation "to do something"), which
might well do his patient more harm than good. These
concerns are also expressed by Mead and Whitehouse (1984).

Most aspects of the management of carcinoma of the
prostate are somewhat controversial. Kirk (1985)
highlighted the fact that this disease exhibits a wide
spectrum of natural history from a very virulent life-
threatening and unpleasant disease, to an almost "benign"

disease that may not inconvenience the patient at all.

Johnson and von Eschenbach (1980) suggest that the biological behaviour of carcinoma of the prostate can be characterised by a number of different biologicial patterns. Depending upon the tumour kinetics and pathology, the cancer either remains localised to the prostate or spreads either by the lymphatic route to the pelvic lymph nodes and thence to the skeleton, or directly by the haematogenous route mainly to the axial skeleton. Over 50% of patients with prostate cancer present with metastatic disease, predominantly in bone. Jones et al (1986a) have suggested that perhaps a fourth variety of disease exists, the patients developing soft tissue or visceral lesions as well. Such patients have a much poorer outlook than the others.

In 1975, Carter and Wasserman reviewed the status of chemotherapy in different urological tumours and concluded that the evaluation of non-hormonal chemotherapy in prostate cancer had been minimal up to that time. Torti and Carter (1980) attempted an assessment of the state of affairs while acknowledging that patterns of metastatic disease made classic response rates difficult to obtain and interpret. In 1979, in the first of the EORTC Chemotherapy Annuals, Stoter et al came to the conclusion that cytotoxic chemotherapy had not been adequately evaluated. One of the problems experienced in their attempt to decide which drugs were active was that the reported rates quoted for the same drug were often highly divergent. Different definitions of response had been employed in the various trials and often only small numbers of patients had been studied. Einhorn (1983) undertook an overview of chemotherapeutic trials in advanced cancer of the prostate and came to the following conclusions: a) that chemotherapeutic agents could be safely given to elderly patients in the presence of bone (and bone marrow) metastatic disease, and who showed a propensity for urinary tract infections; b) significant palliation and perhaps modest survival benefit could be achieved; c) likely active single agents included cyclophosphamide, methotrexate, adriamycin, 5-fluorouracil and perhaps DTIC; d) there was no reason to believe that combination chemotherapy was more effective than single agent therapy; e) a hope was expressed of the development of better methods of assessing response so that effective single agents could be identified and then combined in a rational way into regimes capable of producing a more substantial benefit.

The EORTC Genitourinary Cancer Group subscribe to this latter conclusion (Jones et al, 1986b). Yagoda (1983) presented a valuable review of the situation at that time, examining various problems with performing clinical trials in advanced prostate cancer and preparing clinicians to be able to critically analyse claims about the relative efficiency of chemotherapy. He shares the view of the EORTC Genitourinary Group (Jones et al, 1986a) that the only objective way to assess the efficacy of an investigational agent in advanced prostate cancer is to use bidimensionally measurable soft tissue and visceral lesions for this assessment. Others, however, (Citrin et al, 1984; Murphy, 1984) suggest that the results of studies employing such lesions may be misleading, since patients with non-boney metastases may have a poorer prognosis than those with bone-dominant disease. This criticism is accepted by the EORTC Genitourinary Group, but these studies may well give more meaningful results being a more stringent test of the agent.

There were a number of important publications in 1984 and 1985, but confusingly they expressed opposing views and controversies still exist. For example in November 1984, Murphy, in reviewing the studies of the National Prostatic Cancer Project (NPCP), stated that it had been shown that chemotherapy was effective when either single agent or combination therapy was administered. It was suggested that combining chemotherapy with hormonal agents as the initial treatment for metastatic disease may be more effective than delaying such therapy until later. In January 1985, Page et al concluded their paper on a randomised trial of combination chemotherapy, with the following sentence "the current role of chemotherapy in hormone resistant prostate cancer remains ill-defined, but this modality should be regarded as one of several therapeutic options offering palliation". Torti et al (1985), stated that although a number of drug combinations had been used in prostatic cancer, response rates and durations of response were not clearly superior to those of single agents alone, reiterating the view of Einhorn (1983). Paulson (1985) suggested that "although individual institutional multi-agent programmes may have shown enhanced response, it is uncertain whether or not this represents patient selection or the impact of treatment". Eisenberger et al, (1985) state quite categorically that "the palliative role of non-hormonal cytotoxic chemotherapy in the treatment of

endocrine resistant prostatic carcinoma has not been
established" and went on to suggest that for further Phase
III studies of chemotherapy in this disease a
no-chemotherapy control arm consisting of the best
symptomatic care, or a uniformly applied second line
endocrine manipulation, was essential. Tannock (1985) posed
the question whether there was evidence that chemotherapy
was of any benefit to patients with carcinoma of the
prostate, again undertaking a rather critical review of
published trials. He stressed the palliative nature of the
therapy, and examined the various criteria that had been
used in an attempt to assess response. He concluded that
chemotherapy had not apparently caused any meaningful
prolongation of survival, but that it could detract from the
quality of the patient's survival. He suggested that these
factors should be studied in future trials. The assessment
of quality of life is in itself rather difficult, although
simple techniques as suggested by Priestman and Baum (1976)
might be easily applicable in this disease. A more detailed
examination of quality of life assessment is found elsewhere
in this volume. Since the main aim of systemic therapy in
metastatic prostate cancer is palliation, it is difficult to
accept claims that a particular therapy is effective and
worthy of more extensive study, when that therapy involves
moderate to severe toxicity, life threatening morbidity and
mortality such as that reported in a Phase II study of
cyclophosphamide, adriamycin and cisplatinum by Drelichman
et al (1985), especially when only one of 21 patients
achieved a truly objective partial remission.

Active and Non Active Agents

In the light of the controversies regarding the
effectiveness of various agents either singularly or in
combination, the ways in which response to treatment is
assessed, and the adequacy of various studies in terms of
patient numbers (so that the probability that a correct
conclusion was reached was high), I have adopted a similar
critical standpoint as that of the various authors of the
chapters on "Genitourinary Tumours" in successive volumes of
the EORTC Chemotherapy Annual (Stoter et al, 1979; Stoter et
al, 1980; Stoter et al, 1981; Williams et al, 1982; Stoter
and Williams, 1983; Williams and Stoter, 1984 and Ozols and
Yagoda, 1985). It would be unhelpful for me to repeat the
details of their analyses of published works and I refer the

TABLE 1a
SUMMARY OF % RESPONSES SEEN IN
NPCP CHEMOTHERAPY STUDIES
IN ADVANCED PROSTATE CANCER PATIENTS

Patients without extensive prior irradiation

Protocol	Drug(s)	No of Patients	Reported Responses (%)				% Excluded from analysis after randomisation
			CR	PR	Stable	Prog.	
100	Cyclophosphamide	41	0	7	39	54	
	5-PU	33	0	12	24	64	)) 12)
	Standard treatment*	36	0	0	19	81	
300	Cyclophosphamide	35	0	0	26	74	
	DTIC	55	0	4	24	72	)) 22)
	Procarbazine	39	0	0	13	87	
700	Cyclophosphamide	43	2	5	28	65	
	Me-CCNU	27	0	4	26	70	)) 22)
	Hydroxyurea	28	4	4	7	86	
1100	Methotrexate	58	2	3	36	59	
	Cisplatin	50	0	4	32	64	)) 16)
	Estramustine	50	0	2	32	66	

* Supportive care, radiotherapy, hormones etc.
(after Tannock IF, 1985)

TABLE 1b

SUMMARY OF % RESPONSES SEEN IN
NPCP CHEMOTHERAPY STUDIES
IN ADVANCED PROSTATE CANCER PATIENTS

Patients with extensive prior irradiation

Protocol	Drug(s)	No of Patients	Reported Responses (%)				% Excluded from analysis after randomisation
			CR	PR	Stable	Prog.	
200	Estramustine	46	0	6	24	69	
	Streptozotocin	38	0	0	32	68	) 16
	Standard treatment*	21	0	0	19	81	)
400	Estramustine + Prednimustine	54	0	2	11	87	)
	Prednimustine	62	0	0	13	87	) 14
800	Estramustine	27	0	4	22	74	)
	Vincristine	34	0	3	12	85	) 26
	Both drugs	29	0	0	24	76	)
1200	Estramustine	40	0	0	18	82	)
	Cisplatin	42	0	0	21	79	) 17
	Both drugs	42	0	0	33	61	)

* Supportive care, radiotherapy, hormones etc.
(after Tannock IF, 1985)

interested reader to their various chapters where relevant references may be found.

Elder and Gibbons (1985) presented the results of the Chemotherapeutic Trials of the NPCP in sufficient detail to allow the analysis presented in Tables 1a and 1b. In a critical review of these studies, Tannock (1985) highlighted the high proportion of randomised patients excluded from the analysis for various reasons. The patients in these studies had failed hormone therapy, had metastatic disease and were assessed according to the NPCP criteria of response. The "stable disease category" used by the NPCP as an objective indicator of response is not accepted by many investigators. (See chapter on response criteria). If one examines the objective response rates of the patients shown in Tables 1a and 1b, in respect of complete and partial responders only, then none of the agents shown could be said to have any activity worthy of further study. In reviewing this work, confirming the opinions of the authors of the chapters in the EORTC Chemotherapy Annual up to 1985, and the data and results presented by Carter and Wasserman 1975; Braich et al, 1986; Moore et al, 1986; Dexeus et al, 1986 and Scher 1986, I have come to the conclusion that the 21 agents shown in Table 2 are apparently ineffective i.e. showing objective response rates (CR+PR only) <10%. It would appear there are very few active agents in this disease if it is expected that such agents should exhibit at least a 20% objective response rate, and those which do are presented in Table 3. There is considerable debate as to the effectiveness of cis-platinum. Doxorubicin is not thought to be as active as it was originally and concern must be expressed about the toxicity of these agents. Vindesine is neurotoxic in this rather elderly group of men, and the response rate quoted for vinblastine is for continuous infusion therapy (Dexeus et al, 1985). The most effective agent would appear to be mitomycin-C, which has been tested in combination with other agents, but with the same order of response as that observed by the EORTC Group in a single agent study with very strictly defined response criteria (Jones et al, 1986b). On the basis of this response rate, mitomycin-C has been incorporated into a randomised Phase III study by the EORTC GU Group, estracyt being in the other arm. The toxic effects of mitomycin-C include renal toxicity. This appears to be dose dependent as discussed by Jones et al, 1986b; Verwey et al, 1987; and Valavaara and Nordman, 1985. It is predicted that there will be an incidence of approximately

TABLE 2. APPARENTLY INEFFECTIVE CYTOTOXIC DRUGS IN
ADVANCED PROSTATE CANCER OBJECTIVE (CR+PR) RATES <10%

BCNU	Hydroxyurea	Neocarzinostatin
Busulphan	M-AMSA	Peplomycin
CCNU	Methyl-CCNU	Procarbazine
Cyclophosphamide	Melphalan	Spirogermanium
DTIC	Methotrexate	Streptozotocin
Esorubicin	Mithroymycin	Vincristine
5-Fluorouracil	Mitoxantrone	VP16-213

TABLE 3. CYTOTOXIC DRUGS SHOWING SOME
ACTIVITY IN ADVANCED PROSTATE CANCER

Drug	% Order of Objective Response (CR+PR)
Cis-platinum	Approx. 15-20%
Doxorubicin	Range 15-25%
Mitomycin-C	Approx. 30%
Vindesine	Approx. 20%
Vinblastine (infusion)	Approx. 20%

10% renal toxicity above cumulative dose levels of 30 to 50 mg/m^2 if the treatment is delivered in doses of 10 to 15 mg/m^2 at 6 to 8 weekly intervals. Mitomycin is commonly used at 6 weekly intervals because of a second nadir in blood count.

It is interesting to note that some investigators have used slightly unconventional approaches to overcome toxicity in their attempts to achieve palliation. Encouraging results were reported by Torti et al, (1983) when doxorubicin was administered at a dose level of 20 mg/m^2 on a weekly basis. An objective response rate of 33% was seen in patients with bidimensionally measurable tumours. (If the response criteria of the National Prostatic Cancer Project were applied, the response rate was 84%!). Robinson et al, (1983) using doxorubicin at a dose level of 10 mg/m^2 weekly in a study of palliation reported significant subjective improvement in their patients. Unfortunately an EORTC study using epirubicin, an analogue of adriamycin, at a dose intensity of 12 mg/m^2 weekly has not shown a useful objective response rate (12%), although the quality of the objective responses seen was excellent. Further studies with higher doses of this agent are suggested (Jones et al, 1987).

Könyves et al (1984) agreed that the interpretation of results with chemotherapy is greatly obscured by the incorporation into clinical trials of patients without evaluable disease and they suggest that for Phase II studies, entry should be restricted to patients with clearly measurable indicator lesions. They also suggested that there is a need for screening additional agents and that androgen priming techniques should be investigated. Concerning this latter suggestion, Stoter and Williams (1983) urged great caution about the possible deleterious effects to patients due to tumour stimulation. This obviously occurred in patients in a study reported by Manni et al, (1986), two patients developing reversible spinal cord compression during the androgen administration. The suggestion that patients should be subjected to a screening myelogram to rule out sub-clinical spinal metastasis before androgens, is directly opposite to the view of Kearsley (1986), in that such intensive investigation is often inappropriate to the patient's needs when the overall aim of therapy is palliation.

Although there are a number of laboratory models for the testing of chemotherapeutic drugs in urological malignancies, it would appear that in vitro chemotherapy sensitivity testing for prostatic cancer is unsuccessful (Chin et al, 1986).

An alternative approach to the management of patients with aggressive metastatic prostatic cancer would be to give chemotherapy before hormonal manipulation. In a recent study reported by Seifter et al, (1986) a disappointing response was seen to a combination of cyclophosphamide, doxorubicin and cis-platinum delivered in an aggressive manner prior to hormone therapy. The latter was much more effective when subsequently applied. This approach is not recommended.

Recommendations and Conclusions

Considerable controversy exists at the present time about the non-hormonal systemic therapy of metastatic prostate cancer. The results of studies performed in the last decade or so are disappointing despite considerable clinical research work. One of the biggest problems in this field is the ability to assess response objectively as discussed elsewhere in this volume.

Before we can go further, our aims and intentions must be defined more clearly. Until agents have been objectively proved effective in the advanced disease state, they cannot be incorporated into combination regimes with the ultimate and desirable intention of developing curative and adjuvant treatments. This will require well controlled Phase II studies in which a relatively small number of patients with bidimensionally measurable disease are studied. Only drugs with a response rate >20% should be considered for further study in comparative Phase III studies to see if they are of benefit to the patients. In these Phase III studies, attempts must be made to assess the quality as well as the length of survival and disease free interval. The nature of the study population must be defined very accurately. All patients entering clinical trials must be accounted for in the final analysis. For studies of chemotherapy, only patients who have received no previous chemotherapy should be included.

In answer to the question posed in the title of this chapter, I feel that despite frustration with the clinical situation, the enthusiasm to treat and an anxiety to do something when clinicians are faced with a patient who has become hormonally unresponsive, cytotoxic drug therapy cannot be recommended for the palliation of prostate cancer in routine practice outside the setting of a clinical trial. Patients will probably have a better quality of survival if alternative "standard" therapies are used such as: transurethral resection for obstructive symptoms; radiotherapy for painful deposits; the exhibition of second line hormone therapies or corticosteroids; symptomatic relief with sufficient analgesia to completely relieve pain, making use of anti-inflammatory agents as well as narcotic and non-narcotic analgesics. Chemotherapy should only be given as part of a well designed Phase II or Phase III study as outlined above.

Sadly, the conclusion that chemotherapy is at present unhelpful is not only confined to prostate cancer. Similar questions are being asked and conclusions drawn about the treatment of other adult solid tumours. To quote Kearsley (1986) "the use of toxic, and therefore potentially fatal, cytotoxic drugs should be seriously questioned unless they are likely either to yield a high incidence of durable complete remissions (some leading to ultimate cure) or to cause such a regression of advanced cancer that symptomatic relief affords a prolonged period of improved quality of life. Lamentably, however, not only is our ability to assess palliation and the quality of life rather rudimentary but the current proliferation of trial results that cannot be properly evaluated may lead both oncologists and non-oncologists to over-estimate the role of chemotherapy and at the same time to under-value the impact of toxicity related to treatment". This statement must be taken together with a consideration that patients with metastatic prostate cancer are mainly elderly, have other concurrent diseases and have disease related reduced function (e.g. reduced renal function due to pre-existing renal obstruction, and bone marrow depression due to bone marrow infiltration by tumour) which may contribute to the undesirable toxicity of the treatment. It may be that such patients are at less risk of dying from their prostatic tumour than from other conditions such as cardiovascular disease, even if their prostate cancer remains untreated   (Kirk, 1985).

REFERENCES

Braich T, Ahmann FR, Garewal HS, Robertone A, Salmon SE
(1986). Phase II trial of 4' - deoxydoxorubicin
(esorubicin) in hormone resistant prostate cancer.
Invest New Drugs, 4: 193-196.

Carter SK, Wasserman TH (1975). The Chemotherapy
of Urologic Cancer. Cancer, 36: 729-747.

Chin JL, Slocum HK, Bulbul MA, Rustum YM (1986). Current
status of chemotherapy sensitivity testing for urological
malignancies. J Urol, 136: 555-560.

Citrin DL, Elson P, DeWys WD (1984). Treatment of
metastatic prostate cancer - an analysis of response
criteria in patients with measurable soft tissue disease.
Cancer, 54: 13-17.

Dexeus FH, Logothetis C, Samuels ML, Hossan B (1986).
Phase II study of spirogermanium in metastatic prostate
cancer. Cancer Treat Rep, 70: 1129-1130.

Dexeus F, Logothetis CJ, Samuels ML, Hossan E,
von Eschenbach AC (1985). Continuous infusion of
vinblastine for advanced hormone-refractory prostate
cancer. Cancer Treat Rep, 69: 885-886.

Drelichman A, Oldford J, Al-Sarraf M (1985). Evaluation of
cyclophosphamide, adriamycin, and cis-platinum (CAP) in
patients with disseminated prostatic carcinoma. A Phase
II study. Am J Clin Oncol, 8: 255-259.

Einhorn LH (1983). An overview of chemotherapy trials in
advanced cancer of the prostate. In: Skinner DG (ed):
"Urological Cancer". New York: Grune and Stratton,
pp 89-100.

Eisenberger MA, Simon R, O'Dwyer PJ, Wittes RE, Friedman MA
(1985). A re-evaluation of nonhormonal cytotoxic
chemotherapy in the treatment of prostatic carcinoma.
J Clin Oncol, 3: 827-841.

Elder JS, Gibbons RP (1985). Results of Trials of the USA
National Prostatic Cancer Project. In: Schroeder FH,
Richards B (eds): "Therapeutic principles in metastatic
prostatic cancer". New York: Alan R Liss, pp 221-242.

Johnson DE, von Eschenbach AC, (1980). Prostatic carcinoma:
A Trilogy of clinical expressions. S Med J, 73:
1304-1307.

Jones WG, Bono AV, Verbaeys A, De Pauw M, Sylvester R
(1986a). Can the primary tumour be used as the sole
parameter for response in phase II chemotherapy studies in
metastatic prostate cancer? An EORTC Genitourinary Group
report. World J Urol, 4: 176-181.

Jones WG, Fosså SD, Bono AV, Croles JJ, Stoter G, DePauw M, Sylvester R (1986b). Mitomycin-C in the treatment of metastatic prostate cancer: Report on an EORTC phase II study. World J Urol, 4: 182-185.

Jones WG, Fosså SD, Bono AV, Klijn JGM, De Pauw M, Sylvester R. (1987). An EORTC Phase II study of low dose weekly epirubicin in metastatic prostate cancer - Submitted for publication.

Kearsley J (1986). Cytotoxic chemotherapy for common adult malignancies: "the emperor's new clothes" revisited? Br Med J, 293: 871-876.

Kirk D (1985). Prostatic carcinoma. Br Med J, 290: 875-876

Könyves I, Müntzing J, Rosencweig M (1984). Chemotherapy principles in the treatment of prostate cancer. The Prostate, 5: 55-62.

Manni A, Santen RJ, Boucher AE, Lipton A, Harvey H, Simmonds M, White-Hershey D, Gordon RA, Rohner T, Drago J, Wettlaufer J, Glode LM, (1986). Hormone stimulation and chemotherapy in advanced prostate cancer: Interim analysis of an ongoing randomised trial. Anticancer Res, 6: 309-314.

Mead GM, Whitehouse JMA (1984). Chemotherapy of solid tumours: Trials and tribulations. Br Med J, 288: 585-586.

Moore MR, Troner MB, DeSimone P, Birch R, Irwin L (1986). Phase II evaluation of weekly cisplatin in metastatic hormone-resistant prostate cancer: A South-Eastern Cancer Study Group trial. Cancer Treat Rep, 70: 541-542.

Murphy GP (1984). Chemotherapy: Is it effective in treatment of prostatic cancer. Urology, 24 (suppl): 41-47.

Murphy GP (1984). Workshop on response criteria and evaluation of the stable disease category in carcinoma of the prostate, breast and large bowel. Oncology, 41: 64-67.

Ozols RF, Yagoda A (1985). Genitourinary tumours. In: Pinedo HM, Chabner BA (eds): "Cancer chemotherapy/7". (The EORTC Cancer Chemotherapy Annual). Amsterdam, New York, Oxford: Elsevier, pp 347-365.

Page JP, Levi JA, Woods RL, Tattersall MN, Fox RM, Coats AS (1985). Randomised trial of combination chemotherapy in hormone-resistant metastatic prostate cancer. Cancer Treat Rep, 69: 105-107.

Paulson DF (1985). Management of metastatic prostatic cancer. Urology 25 (suppl): 49-52.

Priestman TJ, Baum M (1976). Evaluation of quality of life in patients receiving treatment for advanced breast cancer. Lancet,i: 889-900.

Robinson MRG, Chandrysekran S, Newling DWW, Richards B, Smith PH (1983). Low dose doxorubicin in the management of advanced carcinoma of the prostate. Br J Urol, 55: 747-748.

Scher HI, Sternberg C, Heston WDW, Watson RC, Niedzwiecki D, Smart T, Hollander P, Yagoda A (1986). Etoposide in prostatic cancer: experimental studies and phase II trial in patients with bidimensionally measurable disease. Cancer Chemother Pharmacol, 18: 24-26.

Seifter EJ, Bunn PA, Cohen MH, Makuch RW, Dunnick NR, Javadpour N, Bensimon H, Eddy JL, Minna JD, Ihde DC (1986). A trial of combination chemotherapy followed by hormonal therapy for previously untreated metastatic carcinoma of the prostate. J Clin Oncol, 4: 1365-1373.

Stoter G, Rozencweig M, Pinedo HM (1979). Genitourinary tumours. In: Pinedo HM (ed): "Cancer Chemotherapy 1979" (The EORTC Cancer Chemotherapy Annual 1). Amsterdam, Oxford: Excerpta Medica, pp 317-339.

Stoter G, Williams SD (1983). Genitourinary tumours. In: Pinedo HM, Chabner BA (eds): "Cancer Chemotherapy 1983" (The EORTC Cancer Chemotherapy Annual 5). Amsterdam, New York, Oxford, Elsevier, pp 357-368.

Stoter G, Williams SD, Einhorn LH (1980). Genitourinary tumours. In: Pinedo HM (ed): "Cancer Chemotherapy 1980". (The EORTC Cancer Chemotherapy Annual 2). Amsterdam, Oxford: Excerpta Medica, pp 306-320.

Stoter G, Williams SD, Einhorn LH (1981). Genitourinary tumours. In: Pinedo HM (ed): "Cancer Chemotherapy 1981". (The EORTC Cancer Chemotherapy Annual 3) Amsterdam, Oxford: Excerpta Medica, pp 317-332. Tannock IF (1985). Is there evidence that chemotherapy is of benefit to patients with carcinoma of the prostate? J Clin Oncol, 3: 1013-1021.

Torti FM, Aston D, Lum BL, Kohler M, Williams R, Spaulding JT, Shortliffe L, Freiha FS (1983). Weekly Doxorubicin in endocrine-refractory carcinoma of the prostate. J Clin Oncol, 1: 477-482

Torti FM, Carter SK, (1980). The chemotherapy of prostatic adenocarcinoma. Ann Inter Med, 92: 681-689.

Torti FM, Shortliffe LD, Carter SK, Hannigan JF, Aston D, Lum BL, Williams RD, Spaulding JT, Freiha FS (1985). A randomised study of doxorubicin versus doxorubicin plus cisplatin in endocrine unresponsive metastatic prostatic carcinoma. Cancer, 56: 2580-2586.

Valavaara R, Nordman E (1985). Renal complications of mitomycin-C therapy with special reference to total dose. Cancer, 55: 47-50.

Verwey J, de Vries J, Pinedo HM (1987). Mitomycin-C induced renal toxicity, a dose-dependent side effect? Eur J Cancer Clin Oncol, 23: 195-199.

Williams SD, Stoter G, Einhorn LH (1982). Genitourinary tumours. In: Pinedo HM (ed): "Cancer Chemotherapy 1982". (The EORTC Cancer Chemotherapy Annual 4). Amsterdam, Oxford: Excerpta Medica pp 298-308.

Williams SD, Stoter G (1984) Genitourinary tumours. In: Pinedo HM, Chabner BA (eds): "Cancer Chemotherapy/6". (The EORTC Cancer Chemotherapy Annual) Amsterdam, New York, Oxford: Elsevier pp 344-362.

Yagoda A (1983). Cytotoxic agents in prostate cancer: An enigma. Semin Urol, 1: 311-321.

EORTC Genitourinary Group Monograph 5: Progress
and Controversies in Oncological Urology II, pages 175–176
© 1988 Alan R. Liss, Inc.

Discussion: Is Chemotherapy Ready for Clinical Use in
Prostatic Cancer Patients?

Karl H. Kurth, Rotterdam, The Netherlands

Klijn: May I ask you a provocative question? Do you feel
that it is possible to combine in a phase II study testing
of a certain new drug and treating that particular patient?

Jones: I am afraid, the answer is no. A phase II study is a
test of a drug and is not treating the patient. This is in
contradiction to a phase III study where you are testing the
differences between 2 active therapies. The whole concept
behind a phase II study is to find active therapies.

Klijn: I disagree with you. Dr. Murphy has a comment on
this.

Murphy: I grant what you said, but let us look at the
future. In the urological cooperative oncology group Dr.
Scardino and others have just completed an assessment and we
do plan on randomized phase II studies where one can compare
statistically. So there is a disagreement, let us indicate
that.

Jones: This is an important point. Randomized phase II
studies are scientific studies of the drug, not a therapy.
Maybe we ought to talk over the oncologist's view of a phase
II study and the urologist's concept of treating a patient.
I think this is a very fundamental point.

N.N.: As medical oncologist we regularly see patients who
have been previously treated by urologists with all kinds of
endocrine therapy. When they became resistant to hormonal
therapy they were referred to medical oncologists. In those
symptomatic patients it seems reasonable to give two courses
of some combined chemotherapy and to reevaluate the patient
after these two courses. If the patient becomes free of
pain, or responds in another way, then one may go on with
further treatment. In many patients at least palliation is
achieved.

Jones: There are two comments. One is combination chemotherapy. There is no evidence that combination chemotherapy is
more effective than single agent treatment. The next comment
is, if you will give to your patient cytostatic drugs, why
do you not put this patient in a phase II clinical trial?
You cannot guarantee your patient any chance of response by
picking an agent out of the pharmacy code.

Rao: Dr. Jones I do agree with your definition of a phase
II study as a scientific study. I would like to come back to
your comment on that you are not able to test chemotherapeutic drugs in vitro. I would say drugs that are not active in
a patient would not be active in vitro. In other words, do
not knock off totally the in vitro results.

Jones: I would agree with that and I think that we have to
look at better methods of in vitro drug sensitivity testing.
In my own institution for example we are looking at multi-
cellular tumor spheroids: human tumors which I would suggest
may be more predictive than animal models under the types of
scientific laboratory assessments, but I agree with you, we
have got to carry on the research on all fronts.

Fosså: I have 2 questions: How do you qualify estramustine
phosphate? Treatment with this drug is sometimes called a
hormone treatment, sometimes its called a chemotherapeutic
agent and sometimes it is called a combination treatment. I
am always in doubt where I have to place this drug.

Richards: I do not think we have any evidence as to which of
these actions is the one that is effective. Experimentally
estramustine certainly has a cytotoxic activity separate
from its estrogenic activity, but when one compares it in
patients who are hormone sensitive, it doesn't appear to
contribute anything. When it is first used, probably the
hormone activity is predominant, but there is evidence, as
you know, that it seems to be active in hormone-resistant
cases and I think it must have some cytotoxic action.

Rao: I have just a comment, Dr. Richards. You stated very
clearly that prostatic carcinoma is a multiclonal tumor.
What has to be emphasized here is that we need information
on the conditions under which a given therapy failed and
what was the status of the tumor before initiating therapy.

Richards: I agree with that comment. The information is not
always available, of course.

EORTC Genitourinary Group Monograph 5: Progress
and Controversies in Oncological Urology II, pages 177–186

SIMULTANEOUS ENDOCRINE MANAGEMENT AND CHEMOTHERAPY AS
INITIAL TREATMENT IN M1 PROSTATIC CARCINOMA.

Brian Richards

Department of Urology, York District
Hospital, York, England.

INTRODUCTION

The logic of combining endocrine manipulation and
chemotherapy depends on one or other of two arguments
which conflict. Firstly, it is known that most
chemotherapeutic agents are more effective when the cells
are dividing, and it is possible that hormone stimulation
which encourages cell division might enhance the
effectiveness of chemotherapy. The second approach
depends on the fact that carcinoma of the prostate is
thought to be a multi-clonal tumour and that not all of
its components are necessarily hormone sensitive. Those
which are hormone insensitive might be sensitive to
chemotherapy, and the combination could have a greater
effect than either alone. The effects might be additive -
as though both modalities were acting independently; with
luck they might be synergistic; though of course it must
be accepted that they might be antagonistic to one another
and that their combined effectiveness could be less than
that of the two individual modalities alone.

TESTOSTERONE STIMULATION WITH CYTOTOXIC CHEMOTHERAPY

Chemotherapeutic agents have not been conspicuously
effective in the treatment of prostatic cancer (Torti and
Carter, 1980). This may in part be due to their slow rate
of growth, and it has been suggested that enhancement of
tumour growth prior to chemotherapy might increase its
effectiveness (Valeriote and Van Putten, 1975; Fowler and
Whitmore, 1982).

Experiments on androgen stimulated chemotherapy in the Dunning R - 3327 prostatic adenocarcinoma in the rat have shown that the combination of castration, testosterone and methotrexate inhibited the growth of transplanted tumours more than castration alone and more than castration combined with methotrexate (Grossman et al, 1981). The authors postulated that testosterone increased the effectiveness of the subsequent cell cycle specific chemotherapy.

Despite such theoretical considerations it is still not known if the action of chemotherapeutic agents will be enhanced clinically by concurrent androgen therapy. Fowler and Whitmore have warned that such investigations should be undertaken with extreme caution - the "flare phenomenon" which is now recognised in patients given LHRH agonists is not new (Donati et al, 1966; Fowler and Whitmore, 1982). They described unfavourable responses to testosterone stimulation among 52 cases treated at the Memorial Sloan Kettering Cancer Center and in a further 138 cases reported in the literature, emphasizing that they were particularly frequent in patients in symptomatic relapse following endocrine therapy and that serious morbidity occurred in almost 10% of these cases.

Most of the clinical studies of androgen stimulation have involved treatment with radioactive phosphorus. But there is some evidence involving cytotoxic agents. Kadia et al (1981) reported an 85% response rate (National Prostatic Cancer Project Criteria) in 30 men with advanced prostatic cancer who had been given testosterone for 3 days before treatment with cyclophosphamide, 5-fluorouracil and Cisplatin. However not everyone is so enthusiastic. Suarez and his colleagues reported a further study of 21 patients pre-treated with fluoxymesterone before being given cyclophosphamide and methotrexate. There was one complete response, three partial responses and disease stabilisation in five. They point out that these results are similar to those of other studies in which chemotherapy was used alone. As there was at least one case of spinal cord compression following androgen priming, the authors comment on the need for additional basic studies of the effect of testosterone on tumour cell kinetics before further clinical trials of this approach are initiated. Manni and her colleagues report a randomised trial in which 34 of the 67 patients received fluoxymesterone 3 days before the date of chemotherapy and the other 33 did not. 41% of the patients given the androgen were inevaluable, mostly as a result of toxicity from fluoxymesterone, and when the data including all randomised patients were analysed the response rate was found to be slightly higher in the control than in the stimulation arm (Manni et al, 1986).

At present, androgen stimulation prior to chemotherapy, though attractive in theory, should be undertaken only with extreme caution.

ANDROGEN SUPPRESSION AND CHEMOTHERAPY

As the majority of newly diagnosed tumours of the prostate regress on hormone therapy one would not expect cytotoxic drugs to be particularly effective in combination with endocrine management as initial treatment. The use of the combination as first treatment for advanced disease is based on two observations. The first is that prostatic cancer is a heterogeneous disease containing hormone sensitive and hormone insensitive cells. There is good evidence for this, at any rate in tumour models. Isaacs and Coffey (1981) point out that small trocar pieces containing identical numbers of cells of the Dunning R-3327 hormone sensitive rat adenocarcinoma grow at identical speeds in intact animals. If the tumour is heterogeneous, similar small pieces will contain differing proportions of androgen dependent and androgen independent cells. When transplanted into orchidectomised rats the rate of growth would depend on the number of androgen independent cells. The time taken to reach a specified size would vary - and in practice does vary - accordingly. The fluctuation in the time required for inoculations to grow to a volume of 1 ml in intact or castrate male rats is very convincing evidence for the heterogeneity of the original tumour.

The second observation is that chemotherapy may be more effective when given in the presence of a small tumour load. Hormone insensitive cells will not be eliminated by endocrine manipulation and might be destroyed by concomitant chemotherapy.

The Dunning R-3327-H tumour has been used to study the effect of combining chemotherapy and androgen deprivation experimentally. Rosenberg and her colleagues measured the survival of 6 groups of rats implanted with equal sized fragments of tumour and found that orchidectomy, cyclophosphamide + orchidectomy and cyclophosphamide + testosterone were each equally effective in prolonging survival and reducing tumour size. Cyclophosphamide alone reduced survival because of toxicity (Rosenberg et al, 1985). The deleterious effect of chemotherapy on the survival of experimental animals inoculated with Dunning adenocarcinoma was also noted by Grossman et al (1981).

The results of combination therapy in clinical studies are difficult to interpret and to compare because of the differences of criteria of response in different studies (Aabo 1987; Konyves et al, 1984).

Non-randomised studies

Merrin (1980) was the first to use the combination of orchidectomy and chemotherapy as initial treatment for advanced prostatic carcinoma. He treated 34 patients, with objectively measurable or evaluable lesions with bilateral orchidectomy, followed by Diethylstilboestrol 1 mgm daily and then by cisplatinum 1mgm/Kg once weekly for 6 weeks and 3 weekly thereafter. A partial objective remission was observed in 22 patients and included the decrease or disappearance of bone lesions on bone scan and Xray films in 15. He did not quote figures for survival. He concluded after comparing the response rate with that previously achieved by estrogens and cisplatinum alone that the combination was synergistic.

Rather similar, though probably less toxic, chemotherapy with 5-fluoro-uracil and cyclophosphamide following bilateral orchidectomy and estrogens was used on 24 patients by Servadio et al (1983), who reported a very good subjective response together with stabilisation or partial disappearance of osteoblastic lesions in bone in almost 80% of patients. There was complete disappearance of bone lesions in three patients. They quoted a median survival rate of 6 years. The difficulties in comparison are illustrated by a further study of 14 patients treated with orchidectomy and cyclophosphamide with 2 complete responses, 9 partial responses and a median survival of only 8.5 months (Lluch et al, 1982). Beckley and his colleagues treated 10 patients with newly diagnosed Stage D disease with Estramustine phosphate (EMP), cyclophosphamide, 5-fluoro-uracil and cisplatin, gaining 70% partial responses and 30% stabilisation (Beckley et al, 1981).

The Role of Conjugated Estrogens

The combinations of an estrogen with a cytotoxic agent in the same molecule has a number of theoretical advantages. The estrogen might act as a carrier which would bind to estrogen receptors and lead to a selective distribution of the combination. The synthesis of various alkylating agents with steroids as biological carriers has been carried out in a number of ways (Konyves et al, 1984). Estramustine phosphate (EMP)is one of these hormone-cytostatic combinations. The carbamate binding in this molecule is stable and the complex is able to reach the prostate with minimal hydrolysis. It has been demonstrated in experiments with rats and human subjects that there is a relatively high prostatic uptake of estramustine (Konyves et al, 1984). EMP is effective in previously untreated prostatic adenocarcinoma, though some of its action is due to androgen suppression as a result of its estrogen component and some studies have found it no more effective than the estrogen alone (Andersson et al, 1980; Nickel and Morales, 1983; Murphy et al, 1983; Smith et al, 1986), perhaps because G3 cases were excluded (Andersson et al, 1980), or because the dose of EMP was low (Smith et al, 1986). However, EMP has a cytostatic effect in experimental and clinical studies where estrogens are inactive (Edsmyr et al, 1982; Murphy, Slack and Mittelman, 1983), which indicates that it has some cytostatic activity as well as its hormonal effect, and the only double blind randomized comparison between EMP given in adequate dosage and estrogens has shown a significant delay in the time to progression in the EMP treated group (Benson and Gill,1986).

Randomised Trials

Unfortunately the early enthusiasm for combining endocrine and cytotoxic management as early treatment for newly diagnosed prostatic cancer has had to be modified in the light of a later generation of controlled studies. In a study reported from Stockholm in which EMP was compared with Estradurin combined with Ethinyloestradiol, no statistically significant difference between the two treatments with respect to rate or duration of response was evident, although it is noteworthy that in this study patients with poorly differentiated (G3) cancer were excluded (Andersson et al, 1980). The National Prostatic Cancer Project protocol 500 randomized untreated patients with metastatic prostatic cancer to 3 arms. The first was treated with orchidectomy or Stilboestrol 1 mgm. t.d.s.; the second with Stilboestrol + cyclophosphamide 1G/m2 q. 3 weeks and the third with EMP 600 mg/m2 and cyclophosphamide 1G/m2. q. 3 weeks. Response rates at 12 weeks were the same in the three treatment arms. Median survival times were similar in patients with no pain though there was some benefit noted in the subset of patients who presented with pain. The survival curves for the group given EMP and cyclophosphamide were the poorest of the three when there was no pain, but the best of the three when pain was present (Murphy et al, 1983). Rather similar results were obtained in NPCP Protocol 600 in which patients who had been stabilised on orchidectomy or hormone therapy for 3 months were randomized to receive additional DES alone or DES + cyclophosphamide or DES + EMP. Objective response rates, response duration and survival were not demonstrably different between treatment arms, either for all patients or within good or poor prognosis groups (Murphy, Slack and Mittelman, 1983). Another trial from the NPCP involving combination chemo- and hormonal therapy (protocol 1300) compares standard endocrine therapy with EMP used on its own, and with the combination of cyclophosphamide, 5-FU and stilboestrol or orchidectomy. Once again no major differences between the treatments have been reported (Murphy, Huben and Priore, 1986).

However, not all the results are as gloomy. In a double blind study comparing EMP with Diethylstilboestrol a significant advantage was evident in the group of patients treated with EMP. The primary determinant of efficacy was

the time between the start of therapy and progression, and
a significant advantage was seen not only in the group as
a whole, but in sub-categories with little pain, moderate
to severe pain, little reduction in activity, significant
reduction in activity, the presence or absence of
cardiovascular disease, age above or below 70 years, and
"good" or "bad" histology. Despite the convincing
evidence of a significantly longer duration of response in
these patients there was no difference in overall survival
between the two groups (Benson and Gill, 1986).

It seems that early treatment of advanced prostatic
carcinoma with a combination of hormone therapy and
cytotoxic chemotherapy, disappointingly, has not been
shown to give improved results when the agents are given
separately, as compared with androgen ablation alone.
Recent encouraging results with Estramustine phosphate
await confirmation. The approach remains theoretically
promising. The combination of androgen ablation therapy
and chemotherapy deserves further evaluation.

It seems that early treatment of advanced prostatic
carcinoma with a combination of hormone therapy and
cytotoxic chemotherapy, disappointingly, fails to give
improved results when compared with androgen ablation
alone, when the agents are given separately, though it
appears to work when a combination is used. The approach
remains theoretically promising, but such combination
treatment is still best restricted to a controlled trial
situation.

REFERENCES

Aabo K (1987). Prostate cancer: evaluation of
    response to treatment, response criteria and the need
    for standardisation of the reporting of results.
    Eur J Cancer Clin Oncol 23: 231-236.
Andersson L, Berlin T, Boman J, Collste L, Edsmyr F,
    Esposti P L, Gustafsson H, Hedlund P O, Hultgren L,
    Leander G, Nordle O, Norlen H, Tillegard P (1980).
    Estramustine versus conventional estrogenic hormones in
    the initial treatment of highly or moderately

184 / Richards

differentiated prostatic carcinoma. A randomized study.
Scand J Urol Nephrol, Suppl 55: 143-145.
Beckley S, Wajsman Z, Maeso E, Pontes E, Murphy G
(1981). Estramustine phosphate with multiple cytotoxic
agents in treatment of advanced prostatic cancer.
Urology 18: 592-595.
Benson R C, Gill G M (1986). Estramustine phosphate
compared with diethylstilboestrol - a randomized double
blind, cross-over trial for stage D prostate cancer.
Amer J Clin Oncol 9: 341-350.
Donati R M, Ellis H, Gallagher N I (1966).
Testosterone potentiated 32P therapy in prostatic
carcinoma. Cancer 19: 1088-1091.
Edsmyr F, Andersson L, Konyves I (1982).
Estramustine phosphate (Estracyt): Experimental studies
and clinical experiences. In Jacobi G H, Hohenfellner
R "Prostate Cancer," Baltimore, Williams and Wilkins,
pp253-266.
Fowler J E, Whitmore W F (1982). Considerations
for the use of testosterone with systemic chemotherapy
in prostatic cancer. Cancer 49: 1373-1377.
Gibbons R P, Beckley S, Brady M F, Chu T M,
deKernion J B, Dhabuwala C, Gaeta J F, Loening S A,
Mckiel C F, Mcleod D G, Pontes J E, Prout G R, Scardino
P T, Schlegel J U, Schnidt J D, Scott W W, Slack N H,
Soloway M S, Murphy G P (1983). The addition of
chemotherapy to hormonal therapy for the treatment of
patients with metastatic carcinoma of the prostate.
J Surg Oncol 23: 133-142.
Grossman H B, Kleinart E L, Lesser M L, Herr H W,
Whitmore W F (1981). Androgen stimulated chemotherapy in
the Dunning R 3327 prostatic adenocarcinoma. Urol
Res 9: 237-240.
Isaacs J T, Coffey D S (1981). Adaptation versus
selection as the mechanism responsible for the relapse
of prostatic cancer to ablation therapy as studied in
the Dunning R-3327-H adenocarcinoma. Cancer Res
41: 5070-5075.
Kadia K R, Kellermeyer R W and Persky L (1981).
Hormonal stimulation followed by multiagent chemotherapy
in estrogen unresponsive prostatic adenocarcinoma.
Proceedings of the American Urological Association;
191A.
Konyves I, Muntzing J, Rosencweig M (1984).
Chemotherapy principles in the treatment of prostatic
cancer. The Prostate 5: 55-62.

Lluch J R G, Gaspar E M, Basauri L A, Pousa A L,
  Lopaz J J L (1982). Successful treatment of poor
  prognostic patients with advanced prostatic carcinoma
  with the association of Diethyl Stilboestrol and
  cyclophosphamide. Rev Esp Oncologia 29: 317-324.
Manni A, Santen R J, Boucher A E, Lipton A,
  Harvey H, Simmonds M, White-Hershey D, Gordon R A,
  Rohner T J, Drago J, Wettlaufer J, Glode L M (1986).
  Androgen priming and response to chemotherapy in
  advanced prostatic cancer. J Urol 136:
  1242-1246.
Merrin C E (1980). Treatment of previously
  untreated (by hormonal manipulation) stage D
  adenocarcinoma of prostate with combined orchidectomy,
  estrogens and cisdiamminedichloroplatinum. Urology 15:
  123-126.
Rosenberg C A, Hrushesky W J M, Lamgevin T,
  Kennedy B J (1985). Hormonal and chemotherapeutic
  treatment of prostatic carcinoma; Dunning adenocarcinoma
  of the prostate in Copenhagen-Fischer rats. Oncology
  42: 48-54.
Murphy G P, Beckley S, Brady M F, Chu T M,
  deKernion J B, Dhabuwala C, Gaeta J F, Gibbons R P,
  Loening S A, McKiel C F, McLeod D G, Pontes J E, Prout G
  R, Scardino P T, Shlegel J U, Schmidt J D, Scott W W,
  Slack N H, Soloway M S (1983). Treatment of newly
  diagnosed metastatic prostate cancer patients with
  chemotherapy agents in combination with hormones versus
  hormones alone. Cancer 51: 1264-1272.
Murphy G P, Slack N H, Mittelman A, (1983).
  Experience with estramustine phosphate in prostatic
  cancer. Seminars in Oncology, Volume 10: 3 - 10,
  Supplement 3: 34.
Murphy G P, Huben R P, Priore R, (1986).
  Results of another trial of chemotherapy with and
  without hormones in patients with newly diagnosed
  metastatic prostate cancer. Urology 28; 36-40.
Nickel C J, Morales A (1983). Estramustine
  phosphate versus Stilboestrol as primary treatment for
  metastatic cancer of the prostate. Can J
  Surg 26: 434-438.
Servadio C, Mukamel E, Lurie H, Nissenkorn I
  (1983). Early combined hormonal and chemotherapy for
  metastatic prostatic carcinoma. Urology 21: 493-495.
Smith P H, Suciu S, Robinson M R G, Richards B,
  Bastable J R G, Glashan R W, Bouffioux C, Lardennois B,

Williams R E, de Pauw M Sylvester R, (1986). A comparison of the effects of Diethyl Stilboestrol with low dose estramustine phosphate in the treatment of advanced prostatic cancer: Final analysis of a phase III trial of the European Organisation for Research on Treatment of Cancer. J Urol 136: 619-623.

Suarez A J, Lamm D L, Radwin H M, Sarosdy M, Clark G and Osborne C K (1982). Androgen priming and cytotoxic chemotherapy. Cancer Chemother Pharmacol 8:261-265.

Torti F M, Carter S K (1980). The chemotherapy of prostatic adenocarcinoma. Ann Int Med 92: 681-689.

Valeriote F and Van Putten L (1975). Proliferative-dependent cytotoxicity of anticancer agents; A review. Cancer Res 53: 2619-2630.

EORTC Genitourinary Group Monograph 5: Progress
and Controversies in Oncological Urology II, pages 187-191
© 1988 Alan R. Liss, Inc.

THE MANAGEMENT OF ADVANCED PROSTATIC CANCER

Gerald P. Murphy, M.D., D.Sc.

Urologic Cooperative Oncology Group, Professor
of Urology, University of Buffalo,
Buffalo, New York

In the Session on The Management of Metastatic Prostatic
Cancer, presentations will be appropriately addressing issues
regarding the best endocrine management of prostatic cancer,
as well as a very appropriate and relevant review of Phase II
and Phase III studies. The simultaneous endocrine management
with chemotherapy as an initial treatment will have also been
presented. As a Chairman of the round table, one, however,
wishes to offer some viewpoints anticipating the basis on
which the previous speakers and others will have participated.
Indeed, to reveal one's own subjective prejudice, this is
limited to the current clinical understanding for routine
therapy in the opinion of many studied by the American
College of Surgeons Commission on Cancer in the United States
in a survey (Schmidt et al., 1986; Huben, Murphy, 1986).
At least in the United States, prostatic cancer is generally
managed by most clinicians, urologists or nonurologists, 50%
by bilateral orchiectomy and 50% by some form of exogenous
hormones (Schmidt et al., 1986; Huben, Murphy, 1986).

This Conference deals presumably with evaluation of new
treatments or new points of view. It is important to realize
that what is done by routine practice may well not reflect
such beliefs. Such viewpoints and collection of data in terms
of what is the pattern of care is essential and fundamental
if we are to understand that our proposed treatments, however
complex or innovative they may seem, do not affect the management of the patient and ultimately national figures which are
generally utilized to justify treatment trends, clinical

*Supported in part by the Cancer Fund, University of Buffalo.

trials, and changes in management (Schmidt et al., 1986; Huben, Murphy, 1986). Fundamentally, we proceed from that additional projection and cannot really evaluate new data without also evaluating some of the past (Murphy, 1986). The 14 years of reported experience by the NPCP (National Prostatic Cancer Project) looked forward to evaluating particularly patients with newly diagnosed metastatic disease and those patients with hormone refractory metastatic disease. At the present time, follow-up studies are only being completed on several protocols which may or may not demonstrate that the early use of chemotherapy with a form of hormonal treatment may or may not be of benefit (Murphy, 1986). A recent carefully conducted study failed to show with several chemotherapy agents selected, any measurable improvement in terms of either survival or progression-free interval (Murphy et al., 1986).

We have understood the considerable and perhaps for apparent reasons, our failures in the new management of advanced prostatic cancer beyond that which is considered traditional (Murphy, 1986; Murphy et al., 1986). If one considers the patients who have failed hormonal management, there probably would be no one who would generally disagree that further clinical research is necessary and that a limited amount of information is available (Murphy, 1986; Murphy et al., 1986). Reports have emphasized that a response to chemotherapy must be measured by changes in the size of measurable or two-dimensional soft tissue lesions. However, as seen in our own NPCP series and from Buffalo for the past 33 years, such lesions occur infrequently (Murphy, 1986; Murphy et al., 1986). Moreover, it should not be forgotten that these patients generally die from their disease − a truly complex therapeutic reality (Slack et al., 1986). We are well aware that the bone scan is a sensitive indicator and really is limited in terms of its quantitative evaluation. Acid phosphatase levels are also somewhat variable (Murphy, 1987). As pointed out by the NPCP, we have definitely shown that prostate antigen can be reliable even in some conditions (Murphy, 1987; Killian et al., 1986). Since our data is based on multi-center trials with a central laboratory and quality control, one would only have to emphasize that they should be taken seriously (Murphy, 1987; Killian et al., 1986). Prostate antigen (PA) can be predictive and is predictive − both in terms of time to progression and degree of disease burden based on the level of elevation (Murphy, 1987; Killian et al., 1986). Those who wish to impart that there are other variations in PA that are noneffective have failed to at least in my opinion demonstrate their data; I would like to see such. We have also evaluated multivariant factors at least in 13 potential factors from 1,020 NPCP patients (Emrich et al., 1985). Multivariant analysis revealed that previous hormone response status, degree of analgesics, pain status, elevated acid phosphatase, and anemia were important in independent prognostic factors for response to treatment (Emrich et al., 1985).

In contrast, for the time of survival, the significant prognostic factors were previous hormonal response status, anorexia, elevated acid phosphatase, pain, elevated alkaline phosphatase, obstructive symptoms, tumor grade, performance status, anemia, and age at diagnosis (Emrich et al, 1985). On the basis of these studies, models for newly diagnosed and hormone refractory disease were developed and tested on the actual data. These models work as described and form the basis for the clinical trials that are currently being developed by the new Urologic Cooperative Oncology Group in the United States (Murphy, 1986). Only by the study of the past, in an objective manner, can those who are engaged in the work make any progress in the future. Admittedly, some patients with many bad prognostic factors are going to obviously form a relatively small group of perhaps newly diagnosed patients and obviously the survival for a refractory patient will be limited (Emrich et al., 1985). We are well aware of this factor and have documented this (Murphy, 1986; Emrich et al., 1985). On the other hand, we have also proposed and are evaluating in the Urologic Cooperative Oncology Group (UCOG) other quality of life and subjective response criteria. There are none that are really settled anywhere, but more efforts in any clinical trial must be devoted towards this (Emrich et al., 1985). There probably will be no conclusion as stated what to do beyond the routine. Our current UCOG proposal is that limited Phase II trials comparing a known standard drug that has some effect be undertaken with the understanding that other single agents or combinations can be studied. Such an undertaking would limit the studies to perhaps as few as 15 patients or as many as 25-50 depending upon the observed responses. These types of approaches, along with stratification for disease factors, are in my opinion the only way we can expect to evaluate the possibilities of improvement. Earlier use of other types of biological response modifiers at the present time is unknown, but certainly will be interesting to watch. More recent viewpoints and EORTC studies on hormone therapy also must be rereviewed in view of these viewpoints (Fair, 1986; Smith et al., 1986).

ABSTRACT

The Urologic Cooperative Oncology Group (UCOG) has taken sight of the various disease factors that influence either high risk or low risk evaluation in newly diagnosed or hormonally refractory patients with disseminated prostate cancer. The previous studies of the National Prostatic Cancer Project (NPCP) with regard to the role of prostate antigen and other disease-free interval variations must be at least considered in designing new trials. The recent results of the EORTC Genitourinary Group regarding hormones must also similarly in my opinion, be reviewed for the same factors. If we agree on factors, we perhaps may even agree on the design of trials and our results may indeed in the future be comparable.

REFERENCES

Emrich LJ, Priore RL, Murphy GP, Brady MF, The Investigators of the National Prostatic Cancer Project (1985). Prognostic factors in patients with advanced stage prostate cancer. Cancer Res 45:5173-5179.

Fair WR (1986). Hormonal therapy of advanced prostatic cancer. J Urol 136:653-654.

Huben RP, Murphy GP (1986). Prostate cancer: An update. CA – A Journal for Clinicians 36(5):274-292.

Killian CS, Emrich LJ, Vargas FP, Yang N, Wang MC, Priore RL, Murphy GP, Chu TM (1986). Relative reliability of five serially measured markers for prognosis of progression in prostate cancer. JNCI 76(2):179-185.

Murphy GP (Proceedings in press). To what degree is chemotherapy useful in the treatment of prostatic cancer? Presented at Second International Symposium on Prostatic Cancer, Paris, France, June 16-18, 1986.

Murphy GP, Huben RP, Priore R, members of the National Prostatic Cancer Project (1986). Results of another trial of chemotherapy with and without hormones in newly diagnosed patients with metastatic prostate cancer. Urology 28(1): 36-40.

Murphy GP (in press: 1987). Combinations of hormones and chemotherapy. Actualizaciones Urologicas.

Schmidt JD, Mettlin CJ, Natarajan N, Peace BB, Beart RW, Jr.,

Winchester DP, Murphy GP (1986). Trends in patterns of care for prostatic cancer, 1974–1983: Results of surveys by the American College of Surgeons. J Urol 136:416–421.
Slack NH, Lane WW, Priore RL, Murphy GP (1986). Prostatic cancer: Treated at a categorical center, 1980–1983. Urology 27(3):205–213.
Smith PH, Suciu S, Robinson MRG, Richards B, Bastable JRG, Glashan RW, Bouffioux C, Lardennois B, Williams RE, de Pauw M, Sylvester R (1986). A comparison of the effect of Diethylstilbestrol with low dose Estramustine Phosphate in the treatment of advanced prostatic cancer: Final analysis of a phase III trial of the European Organization for Research on Treatment of Cancer. J Urol 136:619–631.

EORTC Genitourinary Group Monograph 5: Progress
and Controversies in Oncological Urology II, pages 193–198
© 1988 Alan R. Liss, Inc.

ROUND TABLE DISCUSSION: MANAGEMENT OF ADVANCED PROSTATIC
CARCINOMA (Chairmen: G.P. Murphy and J. Shimazaki)

K.H. Kurth

Department of Urology, Erasmus University
Hospital, Rotterdam, The Netherlands

DAHER

I would like you to comment on 2 points. The first
point concerns the time to progression. In my opinion and
maybe I am wrong, there are 2 ways for patients with prostatic cancer to behave. Regardless of the treatment some
patients progress rapidly and die during the first 2 years.
Patients with the second type of prostatic cancer feel well
for 2, 3 or 5 years. Thus, should we not discuss the search
for prognostic factors and propose 2 kinds of treatments? My
second point is the recurrence of the disease. When patients
progress, whatever you give as treatment, most of them will
die within few months. Therefore we must look for new treatment modalities for these patients.

ROBINSON

I think you are absolutely right. What determines the
progression of disease is something within the tumor, and
this is why the prognostic factors are very important. As
far as hormonal therapy is concerned, it is very good as
palliation, there is no doubt about that. Whether it actually delays the time to progression I really cannot tell you.
We need further studies to find this out, as we need further
studies to determine prognostic factors. When we know more
about them we may select patients who should or should not
be treated. I think that is also true for chemotherapy. We
are in a position now that perhaps we can select out a bad
risk group.

JONES

I too would agree with the questioner. The man that is laying in bed with pain and looks anemic and lost some weight is in a different category than the patient that walks into the office just having played 2 rounds of golf. And yet the same patient with the same criteria of evaluability will go into the same study, and of course we get different results. We do need those prognostic factors and we have to use those prognostic factors to stratify prior to randomization into phase-III studies. The idea being that you will have comparable patients in each arm of the study and they will balance out and you will get some idea of how effective one therapy is compared with the other. When the patient eventually relapses and dies within a few months, this is where the nasty scientific oncologist comes in to do his scientific study and he may well have measurable disease and that is what the scientist wants to look at: to develop the new drugs or perhaps to look at the old drugs, so that we can propose them as therapy, rather than as a non-tested drug.

PEELING

I agree with your comment about the prognostic factors, but may I draw your attention to the report, which I think was published in "The Prostate" by Griffith. Looking at the data of the "British Prostate Group" it was noticed that the patients who had high levels of testosterone and low levels of LH pretreatment did well with hormone therapy. Those patients who had low levels of testosterone and high levels of LH - in other words there is some form of failure of the pituitary-testiculary axis - if they have these features pretreatment, these were the ones which in fact recurred very quickly. The concept that we had always felt would be very nice, and Dr. Jones just said the same thing, is to be able to select which patients have the high probability of responding satisfactory to the hormone manipulation before you actually treat them. Thereby you can probably select the patients who in fact will not respond, they probably will go to other forms of treatment, hopefully chemotherapy or something like that in the future.

I have one more comment to complete response. I agree with Bill Jones. I do not think there is actually such a thing, because if you look at the ultrasound appearance of patients who clinically have got no cancer palpable in their prostates after you have treated them, you practically always find out some evidence of heterogeneity and abnormality.

Finally, the third thing I like to mention, patients who relapsed represent the most difficult clinical problem of all. The patients are going to die, we have heard a lot about this. One thing, which has not been mentioned, is whole body irradition as a palliative measure, which is started by Dr. Rider and his colleagues of the Princess Margarete Hospital (Toronto) and which is being continued in our part of the world in Cardiff by Dr. Keen, who worked there originally. We found that whole body irradition for patients who have got pain after the usual hormone manipulations have failed is a very acceptable and very effective palliative measure.

MURPHY

A very important point. There are many different ways of easing prognosis and your findings may supersede our disappointments with receptors.

SCHRÖDER

Could I ask both Dr. Murphy and Dr. Jones, do you think that there is any chemotherapy that is ready for routine use at this moment for the patient that progresses after hormone therapy?

MURPHY

Yes, I think there are, and we do give them agents. The doctor down here in front just got through of expressing his disgust with the urologist hanging on to the patient to the last minute and then expecting him to be saved. This is the difference between trials, scientists investigating a drug and the urge to do something. I don't think that's an unacceptable urge and I think based on the results you can select patients for treatment, even on the rigid criteria that Dr. Jones has selected.

KJAER

We have heard a lot about trials today, but there are
no significant differences between different kinds of treatment. We have also heard about the prognostic factors being
the most important determinators of survival. Is anybody at
all planning a trial, which in my opinion would be the most
important thing to do, namely with no therapy or maximal
supportive care in one arm and some form of therapy in the
other arm. Because if you should conclude what we have heard
today, we have not heard that anything is superior to anything else or to nothing.

MURPHY

You missed the methotrexate plus hormonal deprivation.

ROBINSON

I think ethically we are not prepared to do this at the
moment, but I do think in metastatic disease, a trial of no
treatment or of deferred treatment has to be done.

KJAER

I would like to supplement my question: We could meet
again here in half a year, or in 2 years, and everytime this
topic will come up. Until somebody takes it up rather sooner
than later. So even if we are not prepared - I don't understand the meaning of "prepared" - it should be done, otherwise we will take it up all the time.

PEELING

There is a trial actually at the moment in Britain,
sponsored by the "Medical Research Council" looking at delayed orchiectomy and immediate orchiectomy. This trial is
trying to look at the problem of whether you should treat
non-symptomatic metastatic cancer immediately, or wait. The
recruitment is doing quite well at this moment, so there may
be an answer in 2 or 3 years.

ROBINSON

The real bad prognostic factor is the painful metasta-sis. They progress rapidly. If metastases become symptomatic this is the disease that we have got to treat hard. The other patients we may be overtreating.

KURTH

The question Dr. Schröder asked is still not yet answered. Maybe Dr. Murphy can comment on combination chemo-therapy. We heared from Bill Jones that there is no place for combined chemotherapy and I do not know whether this is also your approach. What is good for routine daily practice, what kind of chemotherapy is just now ready for clinical use?

JONES

To go one step back from there, I would agree that we do need to do studies with a control population. Particu-larly in the far advanced patients who are treated for symptomatic relief, including radiotherapy. As a radiothera-pist I must make this point, that radiotherapy is a very valid aid to treating localized disease and also to treating generalized disease. With hemi-body radiotherapy you can treat one half of the body, and then 3 weeks later you can do the other half. You don't need to use the doses that Rider used in Canada. To come back to the questions of Dr. Schröder and Dr. Kurth: with the risk of advertising for Kyowa from Japan, I would recommend Mitomycin-C. We were very impressed with it in our studies and maybe I am sticking my neck out, but that would be a single agent treatment I would advise in the situation that is described by the doctor down here. Maybe the second drug is Adria-mycin, but I think we have a very limited number of agents that we could use in that situation and I would advocate caution if you would attempt to put drugs together in combi-nation, because my opinion is that combination therapy has not shown any advantage at all.

MURPHY

Whether I do or not, the answers and the expression which you wanted were: the 3 agents I think most frequently

used in the USA as a single agent for patients who failed
are estramustine phosphate, methotrexate in a low dose (20
mg/m2) and similarly in low dose adriamycin. On the other
hand, you can change ideas and the oncologists in the USA
probably more frequently use CMF (cyclophosphamide-metho-
trexate-5-Fu) than anything else. They use it for prostate
and for breast. The results are hard to evaluate. I have not
seen the results. I think that in conferences like this you
have to listen to the disagreements, read the literature a
little more carefully perhaps which might encourage some of
us to publish earlier.

EORTC Genitourinary Group Monograph 5: Progress
and Controversies in Oncological Urology II, pages 199-207
© 1988 Alan R. Liss, Inc.

HISTORY AND PHYSICAL EXAMINATION IN PROSTATIC CANCER -
WHICH INFORMATION IS ESSENTIAL IN DIAGNOSIS AND FOLLOW UP?

Donald W W Newling [1],C. Estrada Arras[2],Aldo Bono[3].

1. Princess Royal Hospital, Hull, U.K.
2. Clinica de Noroeste, Sonora, Mexico.
3. Osp.Di Cicolo e Fundazione E.S.Macchi,Varese,
   Italy.

INTRODUCTION

     The majority of patients with prostatic cancer will
present to their doctor with symptoms and signs of bladder
outflow obstruction. However, up to 10% of patients with
this disease may present with symptoms from metastases as
first evidence that they have prostatic cancer. It would
be very useful to the clinician if, from amongst all those
patients who present with prostatism, most of whom will
have benign prostatic hypertrophy, he was able to identify
the patients most likely to have a malignant aetiology. It
would be of further interest if there were physical signs
which at a very early stage could identify systemic
disease.

     Benign prostatic hypertrophy or adenomatous hyperplasia
of the prostate and prostatic cancer occur in similar age
groups although prostatic cancer has a peak at a slightly
higher age group than benign disease. Nevertheless, the
incidence curves of both conditions overlap substantially.

     There are those patients with prostatic cancer even
with metastases who appear to have benign disease and there
are also a group of patients with benign prostatic
hypertrophy who, for reasons of their age and concomitant
chronic disease, would appear to have a malignant
pathology. The ambition of this study is to identify
features which will help to eliminate the false negative

and false positive cases as shown in Figure 1 and also to separate those patients in the middle ground more clearly into those who probably have malignant disease and those who clearly have not.

FIGURE 1.

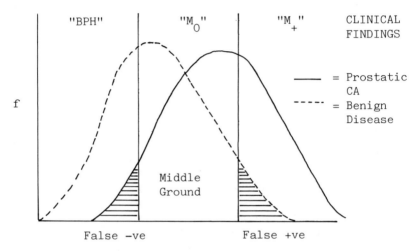

Some features which will help in the identification process will appear in the history the patient gives and others will only be evident on physical examination.

HISTORY OF THE ILLNESS

Important features in the history of the condition include the age of the patient, the duration of his symptoms, any history of persistent pain, loss of weight and/or appetite and symptoms associated with rectal involvement such as constipation or tenesmus.

1. Age of the Patient.

The peak incidence of prostatic cancer is at a slightly higher age than that for benign prostatic hypertrophy. There is, however, a significant incidence of the disease between the ages of 50 and 60 (Bouffioux 1983) and the younger patient presenting with symptoms of prostatism must be viewed with some suspicion. Interestingly, the spread of different stages of prostatic cancer shows that patients presenting with more advanced disease appear to fall into the higher age group. This is probably a reflection of the fact that these patients are more tolerant of their symptoms and attribute many of them to their age and general decrepitude not seeking medical help until the disease is quite advanced.

FIGURE 2.   FIGURE 3.

Incidence of prostatic cancer with the step section technique.

Percentage Distribution of Different stages of Prostatic Cancer by Age.

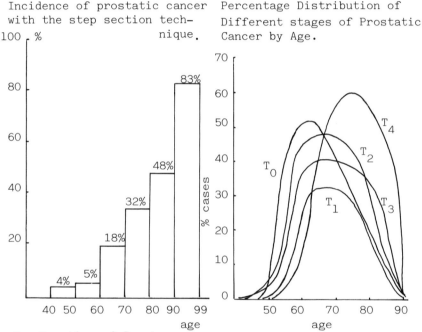

2. Duration of Symptoms.

Patients with prostatic cancer, while having all the same symptoms as those with benign disease, usually admit to these symptoms being inexorably progressive. Frequently they present with crescendo prostatism with retention supervening after perhaps only four or five months of a deteriorating urinary stream. Within the group of patients with prostatic cancer presenting with prostatism those with the shortest history have the most poorly differentiated tumours (Peters 1980, Newling 1983).

TABLE 1.   Duration of Symptoms

        166 patients - AVERAGE DURATION OF SYMPTOMS

                        ALL GRADES   16 months

                            G$_1$ 43 months

                            G$_2$ 9 months

                            G$_3$ 4 months

3. Pain.

        Clearly, back pain, neck pain, pain in the hips, pain
in the femora may indicate metastatic disease (Grayhack
1980) but there are a group of patients who present with
prostatism who have pain of a rather less specific nature
in the perineum or suprapubic region who have no evidence
of infection or retention and who subsequently turn out to
have malignant disease. The majority of these patients are
later found to have significant pelvic node involvement
(Bono 1987). Frequently, patients with pain due to
extensive soft tissue disease in the pelvis complain that
this is worse when they are sitting or standing for long
periods of time. It is also made worse by any concurrent
constipation. One other type of pain is occasionally
present in patients with prostatic cancer. This is the pain
of hydronephrosis due to bladder and/or ureteric
obstruction from the primary tumour. Such a pain is
usually fairly easily differentiated from back pain due to
metastases and is predictably often associated with other
features of uraemia.

4. Rectal Symptoms.

        Patients with large primary carcinomata may well
describe rectal symptoms as well as urological symptoms and
commonly complain that they have a constant urge to
defaecate as well as to urinate. They may be grossly
constipated and suffer from tenesmus. Rarely, prostatic
cancer has presented in a patient with rectal bleeding and
been referred, quite naturally, to a colorectal surgeon.
Larger tumours, ultimately, may cause partial or complete

obstruction of the faecal stream by encircling the rectum.

5. Anorexia and Weight Loss.

In a recent retrospective analysis of 166 personal cases of carcinoma of the prostate this was a very important presenting feature which not only indicated a probable malignant pathology in patients with prostatism but also suggested systemic disease (Newling 1983). Weight gain following the introduction of specific therapy for prostatic cancer is often a good indicator of a response to treatment provided it is not due to the accumulation of oedema following hormonal manipulation.

TABLE 2.

Anorexia and Weight Loss

26/166 (16%) pts. complained of weight loss and anorexia

7/26 (27%) pts. had metastases at presentation

16 other patients subsequently developed metastases

17/26 (66%) died of prostatic cancer within 5 yrs.

Anorexia and weight loss only occurred in pts. with B.P.H. who were uraemic.

(Newling 1983)

6. Rarer Symptoms Due to Metastatic Disease.

Occasionally, patients will present with an abdominal mass due either to hepatomegaly or a large abdominal lymph node mass. Dyspnoea due to pulmonary metastases is rare but has been described (Fergusson 1965) as a presenting symptom of prostatic cancer.

PHYSICAL SIGNS

1. Anaemia.

   Patients with prostatic cancer may be anaemic because
of direct involvement of the bone marrow or, more rarely,
from blood loss per urethram or marrow dysfunction as a
result of uraemia. Patients who have prostatic cancer and
present with a haemoglobin below 11.0 gm have a uniformly
poor prognosis and usually widespread marrow involvement
(Berry 1974).

TABLE 3.

ANAEMIA

   76/166 (46%) WERE ANAEMIC

   25/76 (33%) HAD PROVEN METASTASES

   10/76 (13%) HAD A RAISED S.A.P.*

   31   PTS. WERE ANAEMIC AT PRESENTATION FOR NO
          OBVIOUS REASON

   19/31 (61%) HAVE DIED OF PROSTATIC CANCER

ANAEMIA ONLY OCCURRED IN PTS. WITH B.P.H. WHO HAD MASSIVE
HAEMATURIA OR WERE URAEMIC

(Newling 1983)

2. Palpable Lymph Nodes.

   These must obviously always be looked for and palpable
inguinal nodes are commoner in prostatic cancer than many
clinicians imagine. Not only are they easily palpable but,
of course, they are easily biopsied and, therefore, careful
inspection for them must be made.   Later, lymph node
masses, palpable or imaged, may well be used as
measurements of response.

3. Liver Enlargement.

   This must be discrete and should be shown to be
*S.A.P. = serum acid phosphatase

malignant by ultrasound or CT scanning. Simple enlargement of the liver, particularly once patients are treated for prostatic cancer, is not an indication of progression.
It may be due to metastases but equally can be an indication of fluid retention, possibly due to oestrogen therapy, heart failure, or intercurrent primary biliary disease.

4. Oedema.

    In patients with prostatic cancer oedema may occur either as a result of venous obstruction or, more commonly, lymphatic obstruction. Lymphatic obstruction is frequently unilateral in contra-distinction to venous obstruction, is present around the clock and does not go away when the patient rests. It is often associated with lymphoedema of the inguinal region and the scrotum. There may or may not be associated palpable lymph nodes. Lymphoedema as a result of prostatic cancer is often associated with considerable pain.

5. Rectal Examination.

    This topic is dealt with in detail elsewhere in this publication. At this point it is important to state that the initial rectal examination should be carried out in a properly controlled environment under ideal circumstances and at each follow up examination those circumstances should be the same and preferably the finger also. Another question which will be addressed elsewhere is that of screening by carrying out regular rectal examinations on all patients over the age of 45 (Kimbrough 1956). This might be advocated by those keen to make an early diagnosis of prostatic cancer and to pick up the disease in an extremely early stage. The question as to whether or not prostatic neoplasms at this stage require treatment was not within the remit of this committee.

ESSENTIAL POINTS IN THE FOLLOW UP OF PATIENTS WITH PROSTATIC CANCER

    Prostatic cancer is a very variable disease which may be rapidly progressive or positively indolent with no change occurring with or without treatment for many years. It is essential to establish which sort of disease one is dealing with in an individual patient at an early stage. In order to do this it would seem desirable that the patient should be seen every three months for the first year. At this three monthly appointment a careful history should be taken once more and full clinical examination performed.

The measurement of acid and alkaline phosphatase should be performed at these initial three monthly evaluations (Hovsepian, Byar 1980). Recently, (Siddall et al 1986) evidence has accumulated of the superiority of the measurement of prostatic specific antigen as an indicator of disease activity over acid or alkaline phosphatase. Since its usefulness in predicting is in predicting early invasion of the prostatic capsule and providing first evidence of metastases, it is of particular importance in patients who have apparently localised disease and who are being managed conservatively. In metastatic disease changes on bone scans occur slowly and it is probably only necessary to repeat the bone scan every six months together with a measurement of the primary by rectal ultrasound or CT scan and possibly an ultrasound liver scan.

If the patient is found over the first year to have relatively stable disease with or without treatment, then the follow up intervals may be extended to four months or even six months. If, however, the patient is showing signs of change, be it progression or remission, then the follow up interval should be kept short. In recent EORTC GU Group studies it has been found that many patients who have progressive disease died before objective signs or even subjective signs of progression could be documented.

Many urologists have found that it is extremely useful to have specialised clinics for the follow up of patients with carcinoma of the prostate. Not only does it ensure that the concentration of the staff in the clinic is directed entirely towards this complex disease, but it also enables service facilities, such as radiology, nuclear medicine imaging and biochemistry, to be alerted in advance when they can expect a heavy workload. With prior warning it also ensures that the same clinician has the opportunity to examine individual patients on each successive visit, thereby ensuring the minimum of observer variation in the physical signs of this disease.

REFERENCES

Berry WR, Laszio J, Cox E, Walker A, Paulson D (1974).
  Prognostic factors in metastatic and hormonally
  unresponsive carcinoma of the prostate. Cancer
  44:763-775.
Bono A (1987) (Personal Communication)
Bouffioux C (1983). Prostatic Cancer - epidemiology and
  aetiology. In Pavone Macaluso M and Smith PH, (eds):
  "Cancer of the Prostate and Kidney," New York: Plenum
  Press.
Fergusson JD (1965). The doubtfully malignant prostate.
  Brit J Urol 52:746-750.
Franks LM (1954). Latent carcinoma. Ann R C S (Eng)
  15:236.
Grayhack JT, Lee C, Kolbusz W, Oliver L (1980). Detection
  of carcinoma of the prostate utilising biochemical
  observation. Cancer 45:1986-1901.
Hendry WF, Fergusson JD (1976). Investigation and
  treatment of prostatic cancer. In Hendry WF (Ed) "Recent
  Advances in Urology," London: Churchill Livingstone.
Hovsepian J, Byar D (1980). Pseudo progression and
  regression of bone metastases during endocrine therapy of
  prostatic adenocarcinoma. Proc Am Soc Clin Onc 21:421
  (abstract).
Kimbrough JC (1956). Carcinoma of the prostate - five year
  follow up of patients treated by radical surgery. J Urol
  76:287-291.
Murphy GP (1976). The diagnosis of prostatic cancer.
  Cancer 39:589.
Newling DWW (1983). The presentation and natural history
  of prostatic cancer - paper presented at Symposium on
  Prostatic Cancer - Hull (unpublished).
Peters P (1980). (Personal Communication) quoted in
  Grayhack JT, Lee C, Kolbusz W, Oliver L. Detection of
  carcinoma of the prostate utilising biochemical
  observation. Cancer 45:1896-1901.
Siddall JK, Cooper EH, Newling DWW, Robinson MRG, Whelan P.
  (1986). An Evaluation of the Immunochemical Measurement
  of Prostatic Acid Phosphatase and Prostatic Specific
  Antigen in Carcinoma of the Prostate. Eur Urol
  12:123-130.

EORTC Genitourinary Group Monograph 5: Progress
and Controversies in Oncological Urology II, pages 209–210
© 1988 Alan R. Liss, Inc.

BIOPSY - MINIMAL REQUIREMENTS, PLACE OF CYTOLOGY, TECHNIQUE.

J.H.M. Blom[1], F.K. Mostofi[2], P.J. Spaander[3].
[1]Department of Urology, Erasmus University,
Rotterdam, The Netherlands, [2]Armed Forces
Institute of Pathology, Washington DC, U.S.A.,
[3]Department of Pathology, Rode Kruis Hospital,
The Hague, The Netherlands

Techniques.
   Of the techniques in use to establish the diagnosis
prostatic carcinoma e.g. punch biopsy, aspiration cytology
(which both could be guided by ultrasonography) and T.U.R.P.
it was concluded that T.U.R.P. should not be used to establish the initial diagnosis carcinoma. Of course the
T.U.R.P. material should be screened for the presence of
carcinoma. It was concluded that at least 30% of the
T.U.R.P. material should be examined and if atypia is found
all the material should be examined.
Cytological/histological criteria of malignancy.
   It was emphasized that the criteria of malignancy in
cytological smear preparations are derived only from individual cells and cell groups, while in histological slides
the growth pattern and infiltrative growth are also important criteria of malignancy. In fact infiltrative growth is
the most valid criterium of malignancy.
   Because most experience about the structure of prostatic cancer cell and nucleus has been derived from histological slides it was emphasized that in fact little knowledge is available on the structure of the prostatic cancer
cell.
   Detailed study of prostatic carcinoma cells is essential for better correlation of fine needle aspiration material with behavior.
Grading.
   Grading of malignancy is possible on good aspiration
cytology smear preparations (i.e. sufficient representative
material, well preserved and stained) and correlates with
prognosis. Grading of malignancy is possible on histological

slides of T.U.R.P. and prostatectomy specimens but less
reliable on slides of punch biopsy material.

It is important to realise that grading on aspiration
cytology smear preparations does not always correlate with
the histological grading of the same patient because, by
the method of collecting cytological material, a selection
of less differentiated (-less cohesive cells) can be obtained. This can give a higher grade in the aspiration cytology material than in the T.U.R.P. or prostatectomy material.

Factors relevant to the results of the diagnostic technique.
For accurate diagnosis of malignancy on aspiration
cytology smear preparations the cytological punction procedure should be performed by an experienced person and screened by special trained cyto/histopathologists.

CONSENSUS:

Technique to establish the diagnosis prostatic carcinoma.
- punch biopsy and/or aspiration cytology
  (aspiration cytology alone should only be performed in
  experienced hands),
- punch biopsy preferably transperineal,
- not initially on T.U.R.P.

Grading.
Preferably on: - aspiration cytology smear preparations
                       - T.U.R.P.
                       - prostatectomy
Possible but less reliable on punch biopsy.
N.B. grading of aspiration cytology smear preparations will
not always correlate with grading of histological slides
(technique of collecting material is not comparable).

Additional techniques with possible value for the future.

- D.N.A. measurement
- morphometry
- immunopathology.

EORTC Genitourinary Group Monograph 5: Progress
and Controversies in Oncological Urology II, pages 211–225
© 1988 Alan R. Liss, Inc.

LYMPH NODE STAGING IN POTENTIALLY CURABLE PROSTATIC CARCINOMA

Kenichiro Okada, Osamu Yoshida, David F. Paulson and
Georg Rutishauser

Department of Urology, Faculty of Medicine, Kyoto
University, Kyoto 606, Japan(K.O.and O.Y.), Division
of Urology, Duke University Medical Center, Durham,
NC 27710, U.S.A.(D.F.P.), and Urologische Klinik,
Abteilung fuer Chirurgie der Universitaet, Kanton-
spital Basel, CH-4031, Basel, Switzerland(G.R.)

INTRODUCTION

Nearly 30% of clinically localized prostate cancer is
associated with pelvic lymph node metastasis, which is generally believed to be a systemic extension of the disease.
Non-invasive tests, however, have not been able to predict
the lymph node involvement in accuracy. Biological and
biochemical markers are not conclusive either, although they
are sometimes informative. Accordingly, staging lymphadenectomy commonly is undertaken before any radical treatment of
the primary tumor at present. However, there still remain
several controversial issues on this surgical manoeuvre.

In this session a proposal which seems to be clinically
beneficial will be demonstrated, based on the summary of
recent concepts in pelvic lymph node staging.

Does a Positive Lymph Node Identify a Patient at Increased Risk?

Many investigators have demonstrated that patients
with lymphatic extension relapse much earlier and more frequently than those with intact nodes(Flocks 1973, Bagshaw
1979, Paulson 1980a, Prout et al 1980, Grossman et al 1982)
(Table 1).

Table 1. Impact on prognosis of patients with negative vs. positive pelvic lymph nodes.

Authors	Evaluation	Results	
		Node, neg.	Node, pos.
Flocks (1973)	10-year survival	67% (69)	13% (32)
Bagshaw (1979)	5-year survival	only 1 death (57)	58% (47)
Paulson (1980a)	Median time to first treatment failure	>68 mos. (67)	19.5 mos. (8)
Prout et al. (1980)	5-year progression rate	16% (60)	66% (32)
Grossman et al. (1982)	Survival rate for more than 9 years	N_0, better than N_{1-4} at $p < 0.0001$ (58)	(68)

1) Number in parenthesis indicates number of patients.
2) Treatment modalities widely varied except for the cases with extended radiotherapy in Bagshaw's and with radical prostatectomy in Paulson's series as a single therapy, respectively.

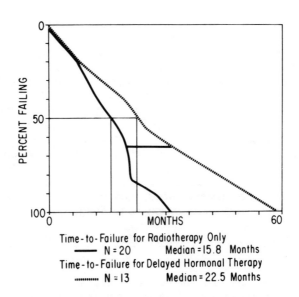

Time-to-Failure for Radiotherapy Only
—— N = 20   Median = 15.8 Months
Time-to-Failure for Delayed Hormonal Therapy
·········· N = 13   Median = 22.5 Months

Fig. 1 Time to treatment failure of delayed hormonal therapy versus radiation therapy.

The early reports from Duke University clearly demonstrated that patients with node positive disease failed at a rate much more rapidly than those who did not have node positive disease(Fig. 1). A subsequent report demonstrated that patients with node positive disease failed at an equivalent rate whether they were treated with radical prostatectomy, external beam radiation, or received no treatment (Fig. 2). The high rate of failure, with over 50% of patients failing within two years, was observed also in the randomized trial which compared extended field radiation therapy to no treatment in patients with node positive disease(Fig. 3).

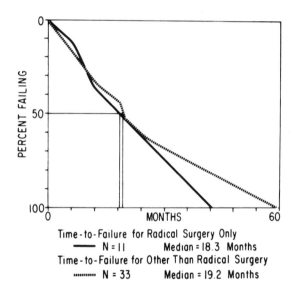

Time-to-Failure for Radical Surgery Only
—— N = 11   Median = 18.3 Months
Time-to-Failure for Other Than Radical Surgery
········· N = 33   Median = 19.2 Months

Fig. 2 Time to first evidence of treatment failure for patients with node positive disease treated by either radical surgery, radiation therapy, or delayed endocrine therapy.

These reports uniformly support the position that patients with node positive disease are at increased risk for early failure. The interpretation has been that patients who have node positive disease have systemic disease and thus should be treated by other than local or regional therapy.

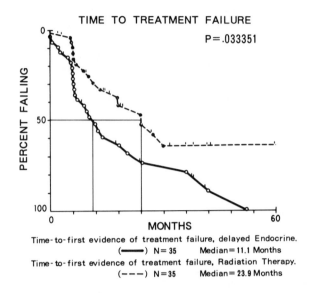

TIME TO TREATMENT FAILURE

P = .033351

Time-to-first evidence of treatment failure, delayed Endocrine.
(———) N = 35   Median = 11.1 Months
Time-to-first evidence of treatment failure, Radiation Therapy.
(– – –) N = 35   Median = 23.9 Months

Fig. 3 Time to treatment failure of delayed endocrine therapy versus radiation therapy.

Is Lymphadenectomy Therapeutic or Diagnostic?

The data would suggest that lymphadenectomy is diagnostic rather than therapeutic. Rutishauser and Hering have demonstrated a marked difference in the disease free survival in pN_0 as opposed to pN_+ patients. There is no suggestion in this data that lymphadenectomy enhances survival, although one is uncertain as to whether patients with pN_1 disease might have done less well had they not had their lymphadenectomy. It is not known whether a single micrometastatic focus might be able to be salvaged by surgical therapy. Rutishauser and co-workers examined the disease free survival of patients who had only a single microscopic focus in a low echelon node. They categorized this level of disease as $pN_{1,1}$. The disease free survival in $pN_{1,1}$ vs. $pN_{1,2}$ ($pN_{1,2}$ being macroscopically detectable unilateral invasion of one lymph node) is given in Figure 4.

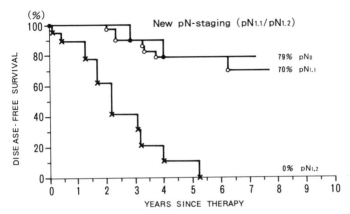

Fig. 4 Different prognosis depending on macroscopic or microscopic pN₁ disease.

(Rutishauser : Personal Communication)

The data generated by the Duke University group would indicate that a patient with a single positive node fails less rapidly than a patient with more than one node, however, one-half of all patients with node positive disease failed within 24 months(Fig. 5).

Prout and associates(1980) reported that in 32 patients with positive nodes progression occurred only in 18 per cent (2/11) of those with a solitary metastatic node compared to 76 per cent (16/21) of those with multiple nodal metastases (p< 0.05) for a similar period. They concluded that a single nodal involvement was not an unfavorable sign and these patients actually survived just as the node-negative patients.

Several other reports also showed that the outcome would be better in those patients with less nodal disease, although a slight difference exists in the terminology (Barzell et al 1977, Prout et al 1980, Schmidt et al 1982, deKernion et al 1985, Smith and Middleton, 1985). These data suggest that lymphadenectomy might be of value in patients with low volume nodal disease, although the longer interval to failure in these patients may occur only as they have less systemic disease. Grossman and co-workers (1982) demonstrated no substantial difference in terms of prognosis among the patients with positive node(s).

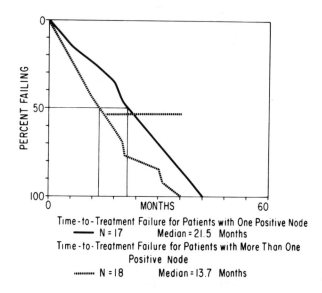

Time-to-Treatment Failure for Patients with One Positive Node
——— N = 17   Median = 21.5 Months
Time-to-Treatment Failure for Patients with More Than One Positive Node
·········· N = 18   Median = 13.7 Months

Fig. 5   Time to first incidence of treatment failure for patients treated by either radical surgery,   radiation therapy, or no treatment as a function of nodal status.

In conclusion lymphadenectomy might be of some therapeutic value in a limited number of cases.   It should be considered as a diagnostic tool only.

What Should be the Limits of Lymph Node Dissection?

If lymph node dissection is diagnostic and not therapeutic, or therapeutic only when a single micrometastatic focus is involved, then it may be reasonable to limit the node dissection to that portion of the anatomy which has a reasonable probability of demonstrating a positive node.

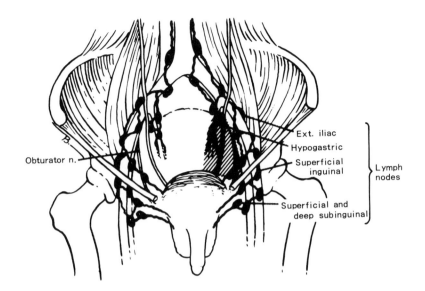

Fig. 6 Shaded area indicate the area of limited pelvic
lymph node dissection for staging of prostatic carcinoma.

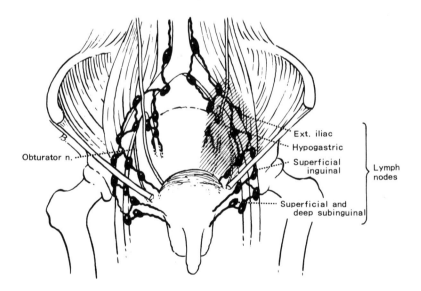

Fig. 7 Area of more extended dissection encompassing the
nodal package around the external iliac vessels. The incidence of nodal involvement by clinical stage is given in
Table 2.

It is well known that morbidity may be higher as the limits of the dissection are increased. As indicated by Paul and associates(1983) the morbidity rate may range between 3.9% to 52.9% in 512 cases. The wide range in morbidity seems to be associated with the extent of dissection.

Paulson(1980a) proposed a limited lymph node dissection, using the external iliac vasculature, the pelvic floor and hypogastric vasculature as the limits of the dissection (Fig. 6). This method has been utilized by many authors (Brendler et al 1980, Lieskovsky 1983, Pilepich et al 1984), and is currently the standard form of dissection. This area of dissection has the probability identifying node positive disease which is equivalent to the more extensive field dissection which includes the nodes surrounding the external iliac vasculature and above the bifurcation of the common iliac(Fig. 7, Table 2).

Table 2. Incidence of positive pelvic lymph nodes as determined by pelvic node dissection

| | | | Lymph Nodes | | | |
| | | | Positive | | Negative | |
	Predissection Stage	No. Patients	No.	(%)	No.	(%)
Series A*	Occult, focal	3	0	(0)	3	(100)
	Occult, diffuse	29	8	(28)	21	(72)
	Localized nodule	52	16	(31)	36	(69)
	Local extension	26	10	(38)	16	(62)
	Any cancer, acid phosphatase elevation, negative bone scan	19	11	(58)	8	(42)
Series B⁻	Occult, focal	27	1	(4)	26	(96)
	Occult, diffuse	24	6	(25)	18	(75)
	Nodule < 1 cm	62	10	(16)	52	(84)
	Nodule > 1 cm	55	14	(25)	41	(75)
	Local extension	32	19	(59)	13	(41)

* Paulson DF and Uro-Oncology Group: The impact of current staging procedures assessing disease extent of prostatic adenocarcinoma. J Urol 121:300, 1979
+ Wilson CS, Dahl DS and Middleton RG: Pelvic lymphadenectomy for the staging of apparently localized prostatic cancer. J Urol 117:197, 1977

A comparison of the incidence of node positive disease by clinical stage would indicate that the probability of identifying positive nodes is equivalent when the distension is either limited or extensive. Morales and co-workers(Golimbu et al 1979, Morales and Golimbu 1980) proposed an extended pelvic lymphadenectomy removing also the presacral and the presciatic nodes. However, their data would indicate the probability of identifying node positive disease in patients who would not have been identified had the nodes within the limited area been removed, is increased by only 7 per cent.

Thus, as the majority of patients who have metastatic disease involving the external or common iliac, or deep pelvic nodes also have hypogastric-obturator nodal involvement, it does not seem appropriate to carry the dissection to the presacral and presciatic nodes.

Can Lymph Node Extension be Identified with Accuracy by Non-invasive Methods?

As yet no alternative for lymphadenectomy that is acceptable for routine use has been established. The efforts accumulated will be reviewed briefly.

1. Biological and biochemical markers

a) Acid phosphatase and other biochemical markers

The VACURG has designated the patient with an elevated acid phosphatase as stage IV in their study, irrelevant to his local finding. The study of Pontes and associates (1981) and others showed that patients with clinically localized tumors and elevated serum enzyme levels have a higher incidence of a lymphatic extension and a poorer prognosis than their counterparts with normal levels. However, high serum acid phosphatase level does not necessarily mean that the disease has already progressed to be systemic. Paulson and associates(1980 a,b) demonstrated only a limited value of serum acid phosphatase in predicting lymph node metastasis.

Nevertheless, elevation in acid phosphatase level in the patients without bone disease by isotope scan indicates node positive disease in 65% of the population. For instance, grade III, stage C carcinoma with an elevated acid phosphatase would have a lymph node metastasis in as much as 92 per cent (Freiha et al, 1979), and vice versa there would be very little chance of node involvement in the very low risk group with normal level.

There have been too few reports on other biochemical parameters to refer to correlation of lymph node metastasis.

b) Tumor grade and other biological parameters

Numerous studies have been done to analyze the correlation between histologic tumor grade and lymphatic extension. These investigators agreed that lymph node metastases increased according to the stage and grade of the primary tumors.

Paulson and co-workers (Paulson et al 1980b, Kramer et al 1980) suggested that a Gleason scale of the primary tumor obtained by a needle biopsy could divide the patients into 3 groups; very low risk (Gleason sum 2 to 4), very high risk (Gleason sum 9 & 10) and the equivocal patients (Gleason sum 5 to 8). They also suggested the possibility that the patients except for an intermediate Gleason scale could avoid staging lymphadenectomy.

Other parameters such as tumor ploidy, DNA histogram or flow cytometry and T-antigenecity of the tumor cells are all in the midst of investigations.

2. Imaging technique

a) Lymphangiography

Lymphangiography is one of the most extensively investigated non-surgical methods to identify node involvement. Numerous reports have been accumulated mostly by using bipedal infusion of oily dye into the lymph channels. Wallace and associates(1977) reported that they could obtain 90 to 95% of sensitivity with a false negative rate of only 15 or 20% in their series of lymphangiograms of various malignant diseases.

However, the following reports especially concerned with pelvic lymph nodes have revealed that lymphangiography is not an acceptable indicator to preclude positive nodes (Loening and associates 1977, Liebner and Stefani 1980, Hoekstra and Schroeder 1981). Apparently several fundamental limitations exist in this examination.

Loening and co-workers(1977) stated that comparative analysis between lymphangiograms and the result of the following lymphadenectomy showed a 59% false positive and a 36% false negative rate in their series of 40 patients. Consequently, Catalona(1984) suggested that accurate diagnosis could be expected in only 50-60% of the cases through a review of the literature. Thus this technique has gradually become devaluated except in the case of lymphangiogram-guided percutaneous aspiration biopsy which will be described below.

b) Computed axial tomography(CAT) and magnetic resonance imaging(MRI)

CAT has routinely been undertaken in clinical management of prostate cancer, mainly for a local staging of cancer or monitoring the grossly involved metastatic lesions. However, it is impossible to identify either a pelvic lymph node smaller than 1 cm in diameter or micro-metastasis, as in other imaging methods. Accordingly CAT is not useful in assessing the status of pelvic lymph nodes in accuracy.

Nothing more can be said about MRI but for the comment above. To our knowledge only 16 articles on MRI appeared up to the end of 1986 focused on prostatic cancer, but chiefly on the local staging. The retrospective study of our series by means of histological sections has revealed that MRI, both T_1 and T_2 imagings, did not give any significant findings distinguishing non-cancer from cancer tissue in the surgically removed prostate gland(Nishimura et al 1987). Therefore, MRI still appears to be of little value in pelvic node staging.

c) Ultrasonography

Numerous studies have been accumulated on local staging of prostate cancer by using different types of scanning methods, none on the staging of the pelvic lymph nodes. A small lymph node or microscopic metastasis is obviously not the target of this examination.

3) Aspiration biopsy

Goethlin(1976), Wallace et al(1977) and others reported that percutaneous aspiration biopsy of the lymph node

guided by lymphangiography and fluoroscopy increased accuracy in detecting metastasis. Encouraged by these reports
several investigators have performed clinical trials(Correa
et al 1981, Wajsman et al 1982). These authors uniformly
agree that this technique will promote histologic proof of
lymphangiographically determined positive nodes and a positive aspiration will eliminate surgical staging. However,
a negative biopsy does not exclude malignancy.

Recognizing this fact, however, one still cannot determine whether the node is truly positive or falsely negative, unless malignancy is proven. In Correa's series of
121 patients, the positive rate of the pelvic lymph nodes
obtained by this technique was 6% for stage A_2, 5% for stage
B, and 24% for stage C, respectively. The frequency of node
positive disease is low compared to the data obtained by
surgical pelvic lymphadenectomy, suggesting that there must
be a high false negative rate.

Thus, the enthusiasm to apply this method now appears
to be diminished.

CONCLUSION

Lymph nodes reflect anatomic distribution of disease in
the host, and positive nodes place a patient at increased
risk. Lymph node extension can be determined accurately
only with surgical staging.

As limited lymph node dissection is the diagnostic and
therapeutic equivalent of extended dissection with fewer
complications, this technique is recommended as a common
manoeuvre.

Whether one could spare the staging surgery in selected
cases, such as a very low(< 4) and a very high(> 8)
Gleason sum in the prostatic primary remains a topical
debate. A patient with an elevated acid phosphatase is
probably not a candidate for surgical staging as the acid
phosphatase elevation predicts metastatic disease, whether
or not it is located in the nodes. Statistical analysis of
accumulated clinical parameters may permit an approximation
of disease risk across a broad patient regulation.

REFERENCES

Bagshaw MA(1979). Perspectives on the radiation treatment
of prostatic cancer: History and current focus. In Murphy
GP(ed): " Prostatic Cancer," Massachusetts: Littleton,
pp 151-174

Barzell W, Bean MA, Hilaris BS, Whitmore WF Jr(1977). Prostatic adenocarcinoma: Relationship of grade and local
extent to the pattern of metastases. J Urol 118:278-282

Brendler CB, Cleeve LK, Anderson EE, Paulson DF (1980).
Staging pelvic lymphadenectomy for carcinoma of the prostate. J Urol 124:849-850

Catalona WJ(1984). "Prostate Cancer," Orlando: Grune and
Stratton, pp 57-83

Correa RJ Jr, Kidd CR, Burnett L, Brannen GE, Gibbons RP,
Cummings KB(1981). Percutaneous pelvic lymph node aspiration
in carcinoma of the prostate. J Urol 126:190-191

deKernion JB, Huang M-Y, Kaufman JJ, Smith RB(1985). Result
of treatment of patients with stage D_1 prostatic carcinoma.
Urology 26:446-451

Flocks RH(1973). The treatment of stage C prostatic cancer
with special reference to combined surgical and radiation
therapy. J Urol 109:461-463

Fowler JE, Whitmore WF Jr(1981). The incidence and extent of
pelvic lymph node metastases in apparently localized prostatic cancer. Cancer 47:2941-2945

Freiha FS, Pistenma DA, Bagshaw MA(1979). Pelvic lymphadenectomy for staging prostatic carcinoma: Is it always
necessary? J Urol 122:176-177

Goethlin JH(1976). Postlymphographic percutaneous fine needle
biopsy of lymph nodes guided by fluoroscopy. Radiology 120:
205-207

Golimbu M, Morales P, Al-Askari S, Brown J(1979). Extended
pelvic lymphadenectomy for prostatic cancer. J Urol 121:
617-620

Grossman HB, Batata M, Hilaris B, Whitmore WF Jr(1982). 125I- implantation for carcinoma of prostate. Further follow-up of first 100 cases. Urology 20:591-596

Hoekstra WJ, Schroeder FH(1981). The role of lymphangiography in the staging of prostatic cancer. Prostate 2:433-440

Kramer SA, Spahr J, Brendler CB, Glenn JF, Paulson DF(1980). Experiences with Gleason's histopathologic grading in prostatic cancer. J Urol 124:223-225

Liebner EJ, Stefani S, Uro-Oncology Research Group(1980). An evaluation of lymphography with nodal biopsy in localized carcinoma of the prostate. Cancer 45:728-734

Lieskovsky G(1983). Pelvic lymphadenectomy. In Glenn JF(ed): "Urologic Surgery," Philadelphia: Lippincott, pp 939-947

Loening SA, Schmidt JD, Brown RC, Hawtrey CE, Fallon B, Culp DA(1977). A comparison between lymphangiography and pelvic node dissection in the staging of prostatic cancer. J Urol 117:752-756

Mclaughlin AP, Saltzstein SL, McCullough DL, Gittes RF (1976). Prostatic carcinoma: Incidence and location of unsuspected lymphatic metastases. J Urol 115:89-94

Morales P, Golimbu M(1980). The therapeutic role of pelvic lymphadenectomy in prostatic cancer. Urol Clin North Am 7:623-629

Nishimura K, Okada Y, Takeuchi H, Miyakawa M, Okada K, Yoshida O, Nishimura K(1987). Differential diagnosis and staging of urological tumor magnetic resonance imaging compared with computed tomography. Acta Urol Jpn 33:210-218

Paul DB, Loening SA, Narayana AS, Culp DA(1983). Morbidity from pelvic lymphadenectomy in staging carcinoma of the prostate. J Urol 129:1141-1144

Paulson DF(1980a). The prognostic role of lymphadenectomy in adenocarcinoma of the prostate. Urol Clin North Am 7:615-622.

Paulson DF, Piserchia PV, Gardner W(1980b). Predictors of lymphatic spread in prostatic adenocarcinoma. J Urol 123: 697-699

Pilepich MV, Asbell SO, Mulholland GS, Pajak T(1984). Surgical staging in carcinoma of the prostate: The RTOG experience. Prostate 5:471-476

Pontes JE, Choe B, Rose NR, Ercole C, Pierce JM Jr(1981). Clinical evaluation of immunological methods for detection of serum prostatic acid phosphatase. J urol 126:363-365

Prout GR Jr, Heaney JA, Griffin PP, Daly JJ, Shipley WU(1980). Nodal involvement as a prognostic indicator in patients with prostatic carcinoma. J Urol 124:226-231

Schmidt JD, Mclaughlin AP III, Saltzstein SL, Garcia-Reyes R (1982). Risk factors for the development of distant metastases in patients undergoing pelvic lymphadenectomy for prostatic cancer. Am J Surg 144:131-135

Smith JA Jr and Middleton RG(1985). Implications of volume of nodal metastasis in patients with adenocarcinoma of the prostate. J Urol 133:617-619

Wajsman Z, Beckley SA, Gamarra M, Pontes JE, Park JJ, Murphy GP(1982). Fine-needle aspiration of metastatic lesions and regional lymph nodes in genitourinary cancer. Urology 14: 356-360

Wallace S. Jing B-S, Zornoza J(1977). Lymphangiography in the determination of the extent of metastatic carcinoma. The potential value of percutaneous lymph node biopsy. Cancer 39:706-718.

EORTC Genitourinary Group Monograph 5: Progress
and Controversies in Oncological Urology II, pages 227–232
© 1988 Alan R. Liss, Inc.

LYMPH NODE STAGING IN POTENTIALLY CURABLE PROSTATIC CARCINOMA

Georg Rutishauser and Franz Hering

Division of Urology, Department of
Surgery University of Basel
Kantonsspital CH-4031 Basel, Switzer-
land

How Often Is Lymph Node Involvement Detected with Modern Imaging Techniques?

At present none of the modern imaging techniques is predictive for lymphatic invasion of prostatic cancer.

In our group of 102 consecutive cases of locali-zed tumors (T_1 or T_2) in which radical prostatec-tomy was planned 43 (42%) turned out to have lymph node invasion (pN_1 or in some cases pN_2) on histo-logic examination. In none of these 43 cases lymph node invasion was seen on CT-scan or lymphangio-graphy. In other words more than 40 % of the pa-tients with localized tumors were understaged pre-operatively (Table 1).

		N neg.	N pos.
pT0	1	1	
pT1	6	4	2
pT2	28	25	3
pT3	66	29	37
pT4	1		1
	102	59	43

Table 1 pT-stage and lymph node invasion

It is interesting to note that of 29 patients
with pT_1 or pT_2 carcinoma 5 (15%) presented already with pN_1 lymph node disease.

Therefore no radical treatment of the primary tumor such as radical prostatectomy or radioactive
seed implantation should be performed without surgical lymph node staging.

Is Lymph Node Involvement a Sign of Systemic Ex-
tension?

There is no question that patients with lymph node invasion relapse much earlier than patients
with pN_0 disease (Fig. 1). This has been observed
by many authors (Paulson 1980, 1986, Prout et al
1980). Our own experience shows after 5 years a
difference of disease free survivors of more than
30%.

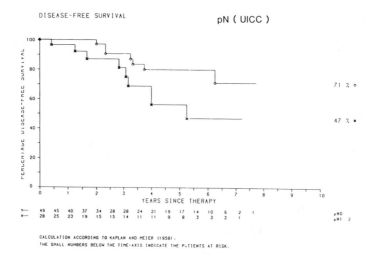

Fig. 1 Disease free survival in pN_0 and pN_1/pN_2
        cases

The lower curve shows patients with lymph node invasion (pN_1/pN_2), the upper patients without lymph

node disease (pN$_0$). It is clearly seen that disease free survival is poor in lymph node positive patients.

Is there a Difference in Prognosis between Micro-scopic and Macroscopic Lymph Node Invasion?

If it is defined that pN 1.1 disease means only
microscopically detectable unilateral invasion of
one lymph node not visible at staging lymphadenectomy and if it is defined that pN 1.2 means macroscopically detectable unilateral invasion of one
lymph node, disease free survival time is much
better in the pN 1.1 group (Fig. 2).
In fact disease free survival time in this group
seems equal to the one of pN$_0$ patients.

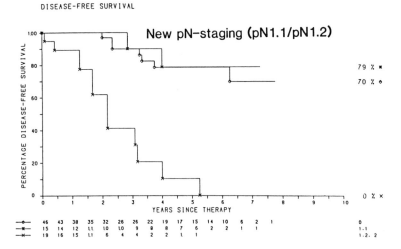

DISEASE-FREE SURVIVAL

Fig. 2 Different prognosis depending on macroscopic or microscopic pN$_1$ disease.

Patients with pN 1.1 disease are in fact the only
(very small) group where staging lymphadenectomy
might be therapeutically efficient (Schmidt
et al, 1982).

Similiar to this observation is the fact that in
patients with pT_3 disease with only micro-invasion
of the prostatic capsule disease free survival is
significantly better than in cases with tumor
spread beyond the capsule and / or invasion of the
seminal vesicles.

How should Lymph Node Staging be done?

We are convinced that lymph node staging is necessary in all patients where treatment of the
primary tumor is planned and we have learned that
it is basically diagnostic - even if it may have
a therapeutic effect in a few patients of the
pN 1.1 subgroup.

Therefore lymph node staging should be an inno-
cuous procedure with low morbiditiy. Extensive radical techniques will not bring better results
and are potentially harmful.

At our institution diagnostic lymphadenectomy is
done from a medial lower abdominal incision as a
limited standard procedure in three portions:

- the external chain beginning over the
  iliac artery in medial direction

- the obturator nodes in the fossa obturato-
  ria. The obturator nerve is spared as well
  as the obturatory artery, if possible.

- the nodes on the internal obturator muscle
  and around the internal iliac artery.

Considering that even macroscopically normal tissue might contain focal (pN 1.1) cancer, all dis-
cernible lymphatic and fatty tissue is resected.
But it is kept in mind that this is not a meticulous therapeutic lymph node dissection as we
are used to do it in the retroperitoneum in selected cases of testicular cancer.

With this concept complications such as infections, lymphoceles, longer lasting lymphatic

drainage occurred only in 9 patients (8.8%).

Are there Alternatives to Lymphadenectomy?

It has already been pointed out that this is not the case.

Imaging techniques such as CT and lymphangiography had a false negative rate of about 40% in our institution.
Fine needle biopsy of lymph nodes which is popular at present, brings only a reliable information if the smear is tumor-positive and it has to be kept in mind that nobody can puncture tumor contaminated lymph nodes which are not visible.

Tumor markers such as prostatic acid phosphatase (PAP) and prostate specific antigen (PSA) are not predictive for lymph node invasion either.
In a recent group of 10 consecutive patients undergoing radical prostatectomy only 2 had elevated acid phosphatase values and - paradoxically - one of these two patients had N_o disease (Table 2).

	PSA	PAP
pT1pN1	+	−
T1pT0pN0	−	−
pT2pN0	+	−
pT2pN1	+	−
pT3pN0	+	−
pT3pN0	+	−
pT3pN1	+	−
pT3.2pN0	+	+
pT3pN2	+	−
pT3pN2	+	+

Table 2 Elevated values for PSA and PAP in relation to pT/pN stage   (- normal   + elevated).

PSA was pathologically elevated in all these 10
cases except in one where the biopsy-proven primary tumor could not be found in the prostatectomy specimen.
It is certainly too early to discuss PSA as an
alternative in this context as elevated values
have been measured in pN_o and pN_+ cases.

In conclusion it can be said that currently diagnostic lymph node dissection is the only reliable
measure to estimate lymph node invasion in
patients with early cancer of the prostate. It is
therefore recommended for all candidates for
treatment of the primary tumor.

REFERENCES

Paulson DF (1980). The prognostic role of lymph-
    adenectomy in adenocarcinoma of the prostate.
    Urol Clin North Am 7: 615-622

Paulson DF (1986). Management of locally advanced
    prostatic carcinoma by surgery: does screening
    for prostatic cancer make sense?
    World J Urol 4: 129-135

Prout GR Jr, Heaney JA, Griffin PP, Daly JJ, Ship-
    ley WU (1980). Nodal involvement as a progno-
    stic indicator in patients with prostatic carci-
    noma.
    J Urol 124: 226-231

Schmidt JD, Mclaughlin AP, Salzstein SL, Garcia-
    Reyes R (1982). Risk factors for the develop-
    ment of distant metastasis in patients under-
    going pelvic lymphadenectomy for prostatic can-
    cer.
    Am J Surg 144: 131-135

EORTC Genitourinary Group Monograph 5: Progress
and Controversies in Oncological Urology II, pages 233–242
© 1988 Alan R. Liss, Inc.

THE STAGING OF M1 DISEASE: THE ROLE OF BONE SCAN, XRAY AND
OTHER IMAGING TECHNIQUES

Brian Richards, Claude Bollack and Christian
Bouffioux

Department of Urology, York District Hospital,
York (B.R.), Service de Chirurgie Urologique,
Hospices Civils, Strasbourg Cedex, France (Cl.B.),
Department of Urology, C.H.U. Sart Tilman, Liege,
Belgium (Chr.B.).

Our purpose is to identify indicators of the presence
of M1 disease - that is of the presence or absence of
distant metastases (UICC, 1978) - which are necessary for
conducting prospective clinical trials in patients with
prostate cancer, considering the investigations needed for
the initial assessment of metastatic disease and also
those required for the assessment of progress at follow
up.

It is assumed that the T and M categories, which are
considered in other chapters, have been fully assessed and
that the diagnosis of the primary prostate cancer has been
confirmed histologically.

THE SITES AT WHICH METASTASES OCCUR

Distant metastases from prostatic cancer have a
great predilection for bone, especially for the pelvis,
vertebral bodies, ribs and skull, and patients who have
disseminated disease generally have bony involvement.
Indicators of deposits in bone are therefore of prime
importance. Metastases to viscera such as the lungs and
the liver are less common, and generally occur late in the
course of the disease. They rarely dominate the clinical
picture. Occasionally, metastases may crop up in unusual
sites such as the testicles, the corpora cavernosa of the

penis or in the brain.

GENERAL INDICATORS OF METASTATIC DISEASE

Secondary deposits in bone must clearly be searched for in every patient, but since there are so many possible sites at which metastases may occur, it seems sensible to consider a general biological survey which may draw attention to the probability that metastases are present somewhere - and which may in addition reveal the presence of significant associated disease. Although they are not imaging techniques, the following are relevant and should be included as part of the initial work-up.

(a) History of weight loss.

(b) History of pain - especially back pain of recent onset.

(c) Performance status.

(d) Hemoglobin. Other hematological variables may be necessary for particular purposes, but are not essential for, and should therefore not be required to assist in, the demonstration of distant metastases.

(e) Liver function tests including bilirubin and liver enzymes. If abnormal these should lead to imaging of the liver by ultrasound. Other biochemical parameters (blood urea, creatinine, albumin, calcium and phospate), can, of course, be measured at the investigator's discretion. But they are not directly relevant to the diagnosis of metastatic disease and are not therefore mandatory.

(f) Acid phosphatase. The serum acid phosphatase has been used to detect metastatic carcinoma of the prostate for 45 years, and the literature provides a lot of contradictory information on its specificity, sensitivity and overall value as a marker of prostatic cancer (Bouffioux, 1979). The situation has not been clarified by the introduction of the more specific radio-immunoassay. Some facts have become clear, however.

(1) Despite early enthusiasm, it is evident that the

prostatic acid phosphatase is of no value as a screening test for localised disease (Watson and Tang, 1980; Vihko et al, 1985).

(2) There are a number of false negatives - patients who have a normal acid phosphatase in the presence of proven metastatic disease, even when radioimmunological measurements are used.

(3) False positives occur in patients with benign disease (Watson and Tang, 1980).

(4) Some patients with elevated pre-operative PAP levels appear to be cured by local therapy (Bruce and Mahan, 1982).

Despite these disadvantages, the presence of an elevated serum prostatic acid phosphatase makes it very likely that there is disseminated malignancy (Byar and Corle, 1984; Whitesel et al, 1984; Killian et al, 1982; de Voogt et al, 1987).

A consistant rise in PAP is a significant indicator of a bad prognosis (Cooper et al, 1983), and estimation of prostatic acid phosphatase is justified both in the initial work-up and in the post treatment monitoring of metastatic prostatic cancer.

(g) Alkaline phosphatase. Alkaline phosphatase has been less closely studied in relation to prostatic cancer than the prostatic acid phosphatase, but it shows at least as good a correlation with the presence of bony metastases, and with response to therapy (Bishop et al, 1985; de Voogt et al, 1987;). It should be included both in the diagnostic screen and as part of the follow-up investigations.

(h) Prostate specific antigen (PSA). Recently there has been growing evidence that serum prostate specific antigen has a distinct advantage in sensitivity and specificity in the monitoring of carcinoma of the prostate compared to standard measurements of serum acid phosphates (Sidall et al, 1986). Nevertheless, PSA measurement is as yet not widely enough available to be adopted as an obligatory investigation in clinical trials.

(i) Other markers such as the urinary hydroxyprolene excretion have no advantage over those already mentioned and should not be included.

SPECIFIC INDICATORS OF METASTATIC DISEASE IN BONE

The Plain Radiograph.

When bony metastases are present, as they are in approximately 40% of newly diagnosed cases of prostatic cancer, they are found in the pelvis in 87% of cases, in the dorso-lumbar spine in 78% and in the ribs in 61%, and they have been considered essential in the primary investigation of all cases (Bouffioux, 1979). This view can no longer be supported.

Plain radiographs may be necessary for the management of individual patients - where symptoms suggest that vertebral collapse is imminent for example, or to help to exclude a false negative scan in patients with diffuse symmetrical bony metastases - but they are not necessary for the generality of patients with metastatic disease and should not be a mandatory requirement.

Bony metastases are not visible on the plain radiograph until about 30% of the bone matrix has been destroyed. The isotope bone scan is a much more sensitive indicator of the presence of skeletal damage (Fitzpatrick et al, 1978). Plain radiographs are still essential, however, to distinguish other causes of increased uptake of the isotope on a scintiscan, such as Pagets disease, degenerative disorders or trauma or even primary bone tumours. A plain film should be taken of at least one hot spot seen on a bone scan, even if the diagnosis of metastatic prostatic cancer appears obvious.

The essential role of the plain Xray, or of tomography if necessary, in the initial work-up prior to a clinical trial is to validate the bone scan by demonstrating the absence of other causes of changes in uptake. Its value as a follow-up investigation is limited by the fact that healing of the 90% of secondaries which are osteoblastic may lead to greater density (Pollen et

al, 1981) and thus be indistinguishable from progression.
There may be doubt whether the appearance of new areas of
sclerosis indicate progression of the disease or merely
healing of a previously unrecognised lesion. Plain Xrays
remain valuable in the direct monitoring of the progress
of metastases only in the 3% of cases where the bone
lesions are lytic. But they are still absolutely
essential in the validation of changes in the appearance
of the bone scan.

The Intravenous Urogram.

This may be useful for investigation of the T
category and possibly for lymph node staging. But it has
no place in the diagnosis of distant metastases.

The Bone Scan

Radio-nuclide bone imaging remains the fundamental
test by which metastases in bone are demonstrated. The
development of technetium-labelled bone-seeking phosphate
complexes has made good quality bone scanning widely
available, although there is still discussion about the
optimal phosphate complex. The methylene diphosphonate is
cleared more rapidly from the blood than the
pyrophosphate, and may be preferable (Pollen et al, 1981).
The bone scan has been shown in many studies to give a
lead time of 3 to 6 months over plain Xrays, and
detectable lesions are seen in 10 to 50% of cases with
negative radiographs. Provided hot spots are Xrayed to
exclude other causes of increased uptake of the isotope,
false positives are rare. False negatives are rare also
and generally occur because of the widespread diffuse
dissemination of metastases which precludes the
development of specific hot spots. The bone scan is
mandatory in the diagnosis of Ml prostatic cancer.

The bone scan has a definite but limited role to play
in the follow-up of patients on treatment. Although
several methods of quantification of the bone scan have
been suggested (Pollen et al, 1981; Grob et al, 1985), the
technique is not sufficiently reproducible to allow
conclusions to be drawn from differences in the density of

hot spots (which may, in any case, get more dense as
initial healing takes place). Follow-up analysis can
detect the presence of new hot spots which need
appropriate checking by plain radiography, and
occasionally repeat bone scans can detect the
disappearance of previously established hot spots. Though
limited objectives, these justify the performance of
repeated bone scan at 6 month intervals during the
follow-up period.

Bone Biopsy

Random iliac biopsies have been considered in patients
with advanced prostatic cancer, but give little additional
information, as they are rarely positive when more
conventional investigations are negative. Biopsy of a
suspected area on scintigraphy may be justifiable when
potentially curative treatment is planned, but it has no
place in the routine monitoring of the clinical trial.

INDICATORS OF METASTATIC DISEASE OTHER THAN IN BONE

The Chest Xray

Chest Xray is mandatory. Pulmonary metastases are rare,
and usually occur as a lymphangitic mottling.
Occasionally they may appear as nodular opacities. Bony
metastases are often seen in the ribs. A chest Xray is at
least as important as an indicator of the common
associated chronic disease or primary lung cancer which
are frequent in elderly patients and may influence their
suitability for treatment.

The value of repeating a normal chest Xray during
follow-up is debatable. Pulmonary abnormalities should be
followed up with 3-monthly chest Xrays. Otherwise the
examination should be repeated annually.

Ultrasound Scan of the Liver

Hepatic metastases are rare except in far advanced
disease. If liver function tests indicate the presence of

liver damage, an ultrasound scan should be performed.

Nuclear magnetic resonance.

This new and very expensive method has not been adequately evaluated and is inappropriate at present in the context of the clinical trial.

CT scanning.

Although CT scan can demonstrate the presence of bone and liver metastases with great clarity, these lesions can be proved by less invasive and less expensive investigations.

Other Investigations

In some specific situations where clinical examination or biochemical investigation suggests the possibility of unusual metastases, other specific investigations may be indicated. These include brain scan, thoracic or abdominal CT scan or bowel radiography. But these are not necessary for routine management, either in diagnosis or in follow-up.

SUMMARY

Patients with newly diagnosed prostatic cancer should be investigated with regard to the presence or absence of distant metastases by

(1) Taking a history especially of weight loss and recent onset backache

(2) Examining them, looking especially for hepatic enlargement or peripheral lymph nodes

(3) Performance status

(4) Hemoglobin, Bilirubin, Liver enzymes, Alkaline and Acid phosphatase

(5) Chest Xray.

(6) Bone scan with specific Xrays directed at hot spots.

(7) Ultrasound scan of liver if liver function tests are abnormal. Ultrasound scan of lymph nodes and kidneys is optional.

(8) Any other tests indicated in special circumstances.

Follow-up, 3-monthly as a rule, should include

(1) The presence of pain and analgesic requirements

(2) Weight

(3) Performance status

(4) Hemoglobin, Alkaline phosphatase, Acid phosphatase

(5) Chest Xray, three monthly if abnormal. Annually otherwise.

(6) Bone scan with Xray of new hot spots, 6-monthly. If there is doubt about the presence of a new hot spot, repeat the bone scan and Xray at 3 months.

REFERENCES

Bishop MC, Hardy JG, Taylor MC, Wastie MC, Lembergar RJ (1985). Bone imaging and serum phosphatases in prostatic carcinoma. Br J Urol 57:317-324.
Bouffioux C (1979). Le cancer de la prostate. Acta Urologica Belgica 47:189-470.
Bruce AW, Mahan DE (1982). The role of prostatic acid phosphates in the investigation and treatment of adenocarcinoma of the prostate. New York Acad Sci 390: 110-121.

Byar D, Corle DK (1984). Analysis of prognostic
  factors for prostatic cancer in the VACURG studies. In
  Denis L, Murphy GP, Prout GR, Schroeder F (eds):
  "Controlled Trials in Urological Oncology" New York:
  Raven Press, pp 147-170.
Cooper EH, Pidcock NB, Daponte D, Glashan RW,
  Rowe E, Robinson MRG (1983).Monitoring of prostatic
  cancer by an enzyme-linked immunosorbent assay of serum
  prostatic acid phosphatase. Eur urol 9: 17-25.
De Voogt HJ, Pavone-Macaluso M, Smith PH,
  Suciu S, Sylvester R, De Pauw M, Members of the EORTC GU
  Group (1987). Prognostic factors in advanced prostatic
  cancer. A statistical analysis of EORTC trials 30761
  and 30762. in press.
EORTC Urological Group Data Centre Report,
  March 1987.
Fitzpatrick JM, Constable AR, Sherwood T,
  Stephenson JJ, Chisholm GD, O'Donohue EPN (1978). Serial
  bone scanning: The assessment of treatment response in
  carcinoma of the prostate. Br J Urol
  50:555-561.
Grob JC, Thiel J, Methlin G, Wolf P, Bollack C
  (1985). Quantitative bone scan and bone metastasis in
  prostatic cancer. Urologia Internationalis 40: 45-47.
Killian CS, Vargas FP, Slack NH, Murphy GP,
  Chu TM (1982). Prostatic specific acid phosphatase
  versus acid phosphatase in monitoring patients with
  prostate cancer. Ann NY Acad Sci 390: 122-132.
Pollen JJ, Gerber K, Ashburn WL, Schmidt JD (1981).
  Nuclear bone imaging in metastatic cancer of the
  prostate. Cancer 47: 2585-2594.
Siddall JK, Cooper EH, Newling DWW, Robinson MRG,
  Whelan P (1986). An evaluation of the immunochemical
  measurement of prostatic acid phosphates and prostatic
  specific antigen in carcinoma of the prostate. Eur
  Urol 12:123-130.
UICC (1978). The TNM classification of
  malignant tumours. UICC, Geneva, 1978.
Vihko F, Kontturi M, Lukkarinen O, Ervasti J,
  Vikho R (1985) . Screening for carcinoma of the
  prostate. Rectal examination, and enzymatic and
  radioimmunologic measurements of serum acid phosphatase
  compared. Cancer 56: 110-121.
Watson RA, Tang DB (1980). The predictive value
  of prostatic acid phosphatase as a screening test for

prostatic cancer. New Engl J Med 303: 497-499.
Whitesel JA, Donohue RE, Mani JH, Edal (1984).
Acid phosphatase: its influence on the management of
carcinoma of the prostate. J Urol 131:70-71.

EORTC Genitourinary Group Monograph 5: Progress
and Controversies in Oncological Urology II, pages 243–260
© 1988 Alan R. Liss, Inc.

OBJECTIVE RESPONSE CRITERIA IN PHASE II AND PHASE III
STUDIES

W G Jones, H Akaza, A T Van Oosterom, T Kotake

University Department of Radiotherapy
Tunbridge Building
Cookridge Hospital
Leeds LS16 6QB UK

The objective measurement of the response to therapy in
patients with carcinoma of the prostate is exceedingly
difficult. There are very few parameters that can be applied
in an objective fashion. Since prostatic cancer is
numerically a great problem, and because over 50% of
patients present clinically with metastatic disease
(predominantly in bone), clinicians exhibit a certain amount
of desperation in trying to identify a systemic therapy that
will bring about a diminution in the amount of disease
present thereby reducing symptoms and hopefully improving
the quality of the patient's remaining survival.
Considerable effort has been expended by many individuals
and co-operative groups in the form of clinical research on
this subject in the last two decades. Unfortunately because
the objective measurement of response is difficult, this has
led to the spawning of a variety of systems using objective,
semi-objective and subjective observations to assess
response. These systems are, on occasions, confounding and
confusing particularly where similar, but not identical,
definitions are used. Unhappily, despite the massive
efforts of research groups there is no real consensus about
treatment response criteria for this disease or how and when
various criteria should be applied.

Prostatic carcinoma presents the clinician with a wide
and fascinating spectrum of clinical problems often related
to a rather variable natural biological history. The
incidence in the population increases with age so that 30%

of men over the age of 50 rising to about 90% of men aged 90 will have carcinomas on histological examination of the prostate gland. Within this population, the tumours exhibit a wide variety of clinical activity from the relatively dormant, indeed almost "benign" tumours which remain localised in the prostate for very many years, to the virulent quickly metastasising tumours which are life threatening and which produce very unpleasant effects in the patient (Kirk, 1985). This paper tries to deal with how the effects of treatment can be assessed in patients with metastatic disease.

In recent years many articles have appeared in the Oncological Press raising very important questions about the objectives of treatment in patients with metastatic solid tumours, particularly when cytotoxic chemotherapy is used. Kearsley (1986) states that "despite the current wave of enthusiasm the vast majority of chemotherapy is given with palliative intent and the decision to use cytotoxic drugs must invariably entail a complex trade-off between likely benefits and expected side effects". He points out that the use of these potentially fatal cytotoxic agents should be questioned unless benefit in terms of cure, long term palliation and improvement of quality of life is obtained. He also says that intensive investigation of patients with advanced cancer may also be detrimental to the patient whilst fulfilling the needs of the clinician to "do something". More specifically Yagoda (1983), and Tannock (1985), considered these and other problems in the management of advanced prostate cancer also raising considerable questions with regard to the ability to define response and thus to answer the all important question as to whether the applied therapy is of benefit to the patient. Eisenberger et al (1985) go further by stating that the palliative role of non-hormonal cytotoxic chemotherapy in the treatment of endocrine resistant prostatic carcinoma has not been established. They also relate the problems in finding effective systemic therapy to the lack of measurable objective parameters to allow for a reliable estimation of anti-tumour effects. Many recent authors have suggested that more objective evidence of response to treatment is required before that treatment can be said to be effective. Some even propose further systems of assessment by which this may be possible (e.g. Aabo, 1987). The response criteria used by the National Prostatic Cancer Project

(NPCP) in the United States are well recognised and the most widely used throughout the world (Murphy and Slack, 1980). The EORTC Genitourinary Group have devised criteria which were initially closely related to the NPCP criteria but which have now gone through phases of development in the direction of much more stringency and objectivity (Schroeder, 1984; Newling, 1985; Robinson et al, 1985) not only in Phase III studies but also in Phase II studies (Jones, 1985).

A properly conducted clinical trial allows an analysis of the relationship between treatment and response. It is a clinical experiment. It has to be accepted that within the limits of clinical variation, the precision of this experiment falls short of that which is achievable in the laboratory. There are those who dislike or reject the notion of this approach involving ill patients, particularly those suffering from a malignant disease, in that a scientific approach implies an unsympathetic disposition. Conversely, because a drug is available and has been shown to be of value in other diseases, it is immediately regarded by some clinicians as being a therapy suitable for use on their patients. It must be accepted however that the drug has to be formally tested in that disease before the conclusion can be reached that it is an applicable therapy and that it might be of benefit to the patient. There are well defined rules for the conduct of clinical trials which must include a consideration of the ethical nature of the study.

Phase II trials are normally performed on patients who have failed standard treatment. In the case of prostatic carcinoma, these are usually patients who have failed prior hormone manipulation(s) or who are considered to be unlikely to respond to such treatment. The selection of patients is on the basis that they have relatively normal physiological and biochemical function and are of reasonable general condition. They should not have other unrelated diseases which prevent the administration of the drug according to the proposed schedule. The patient should also be able to comply with the other requirements of the study. Phase II studies are designed solely to determine whether the drug shows activity in the disease, so the presence of measurable disease is required whereby an objective response can be monitored if it occurs. As a subsidiary to the main aim, further information on the toxicity of the drug can be gathered. Only when a drug is seen to be active at a certain dose level (and a number of Phase II studies of the same drug may be required to determine the latter), should it be released as a proven therapeutic agent into a randomised Phase III study as defined below. Phase II studies usually require only a small number of patients (between 15 and 40). The intention of a Phase II study is to derive an approximate order of activity expressed in percentage terms. A drug is regarded as being active if objective responses (complete and partial remissions only) in excess of 20% are seen, although it is said that drugs with a 30% response rate or higher are the ones most likely to be of real benefit, either as single agents or when used in combination with other proven active drugs.

Randomised Phase II studies are sometimes performed in which new drugs (usually analogues) are compared with known active drugs on a randomised basis. Again only small numbers of patients are required for each arm of the study which is designed to determine the order of response for each drug and to gather valuable data on toxicity.

Phase III studies are much larger randomised trials comparing a standard effective therapy with one or more therapies which have been proved to be or are suggested to be effective from previous studies of a Phase II nature. The aim here is to determine which of the therapies is the more effective resulting in a longer disease free interval or longer survival, or to determine which of two equally potent treatments is less toxic.

The number of patients studied in a Phase III study is determined on a statistical basis depending upon the order of magnitude of difference in effectiveness between the two treatments one wishes to detect. Commonly these studies require hundreds rather than tens of patients in each treatment arm. They may require co-operation between many clinicians, perhaps on a multi-institutional or multi-national basis. Because differences in survival need to be considered the study may take many years to perform, particularly in view of the nature of the disease. In this condition objective end points to Phase III studies are time to progression and overall survival.

In all studies in prostate cancer, the determination of response or progression is obviously time-dependent and frequent evaluation of the patient is necessary (Benson and Gill, 1986). This may require a modification to previous practice where patients may not have been seen at intervals less than three months. Another very important factor with regard to randomised Phase III studies is the presence or absence of useful prognostic factors in the population of patients under study (Berry et al, 1979). Considerable effort is now being expended on identifying such parameters as: previous response to therapy, pain and analgesic usage, elevation of serum alkaline and acid phosphatases, anaemia, age at diagnosis, tumour grade, anorexia, ESR and (perhaps most importantly) performance status of patients at entry into the trial. Such factors are discussed by Emrich et al (1985) using data from patients in the National Prostatic Cancer Project studies. Some of the EORTC Genitourinary Group's data on this subject will be found elsewhere in this volume. Stratification by important prognostic factors before randomisation may well hold the key to some of the problems we presently face.

PHASE II STUDIES

Very few formal Phase II studies have been performed in prostate cancer (Jones et al, 1986a). The EORTC Genitourinary Group embarked on a series of such studies in 1979. Results of the studies of vindesine (Jones et al, 1983) and mitomycin-C (Jones et al, 1986b) have been published. A study of low dose weekly epirubicin has been completed. The present study examines the use of methotrexate, $40mg/m^2$ i.v. every two weeks. During this time, the EORTC Genitourinary Group has developed a philosophy (as described by Jones et al, 1986a) which is very strict, since according to the definitions above, only objectively measurable disease can be used to assess response. Initially lytic bone lesions were accepted but because of difficulties of assessment, this is no longer the case. The only lesions accepted by the Group to assess response are bidimensionally measurable:

a) skin and subcutaneous metastases
b) palpable lymph node masses
c) lung masses as seen on chest X-ray
d) liver metastases measured by CT scan or ultrasound, and

e) lymph node masses in the retroperitoneum or mediastinum as measured by CT scan.

This restriction of criteria by which response is measured is chosen so that only a small group of patients is exposed to potentially dangerous drugs before the application of the therapy to a larger population of patients in a phase III study.

It is accepted that only approximately 10% of patients with metastatic disease will have such soft tissue or visceral metastases (Paulson et al, 1979). It is also accepted that some researchers question whether data obtained from such studies using soft tissue and visceral lesions is applicable to the commoner patient population with bone dominant disease (Citrin et al, 1984), and that this patient population has a much poorer prognosis. However, as stated by Slack et al, (1984) despite the reservations of some researchers, others (Schmidt et al, (1976) and DeWys et al, (1977)) report evidence that response rates are similar in the two types of patient. Both Yagoda (1983) and Tannock (1985) support the approach of studying patients with only measurable soft tissue and visceral disease in these studies. The EORTC Genitourinary Group justifies the continuance of these studies by virtue of there being a clinical need to identify active therapies in this, albeit small, patient population which exhibits such a terribly poor prognosis (Jones et al, 1986a).

Thus in Phase II studies, the EORTC GU Group's philosophy is that only bidimensionally measurable lesions are assessed. Undimensional lesions, such as hepatomegaly, do not allow the requisite accuracy and should therefore be avoided. Indistinct lesions such as lymphangitic changes on chest X-rays, effusions and indefinable lesions such as lymphoedema of limbs, pain etc. should not be accepted. Ideally accessible lesions should be proved to be metastatic cancer by biopsy. All lesions used for the assessment of response must be seen to be progressing prior to the commencement of the study. As many methods as possible are used to document response eg, the use of centimetre rulers and photography to document the size of skin lesions and subcutaneous masses, (after the use of calipers to measure the size), and magnification devices used during plain radiography. Significant changes in the sizes of lesions

Table 1

Lesions for the Objective Assessment of Response
(Bidimensional Measurable Disease)

a) Cutaneous and sub-cutaneous masses:
These should be at least 10mm diameter for skin lesions and 15mm diameter for subcutaneous lesions initially to obtain optimal response measurement (serial photographs with ruler recommended).

b) Lymph nodes :
Single or multiple, measurable by physical examination or CT scan, larger than 25mm initially.

c) Pulmonary metastases:
On chest X-ray these should be at least 10mm diameter. For hilar and mediastinal masses, CT or tomography is essential. Masses should be at least 25mm diameter.

d) Liver metastases :
CT or Ultrasonography only to be used. Masses must be greater than 30mm diameter.

e) Abdominal and Pelvis: lymph node masses
Measured by CT scan and should be at least 25mm diameter.

are required in order to overcome difficulties with regard
to measurement as discussed by Warr et al, (1984) and
Moertel and Henley (1976) and the suggested sizes and
methods of assessment for bidimensionally measurable lesions
as are presented in Table I. A similar and more detailed
discussion of these factors can be found in Van Oosterom et
al, (1986) with regard to the response criteria advocated
for use in the study of patients with bladder cancer.
However we suggest that smaller lesions in skin and
subcutaneous sites are assessable compared to those
advocated by Van Oosterom et al (1986).

     The EORTC Group also believes that the measurement of
response to treatment in bone lesions is at best inaccurate
and therefore should not be attempted in this situation.
The WHO criteria for response assessment of bone lesions are
not acceptable (WHO, 1978). However, Schroeder (1984)
highlights the differences between the subpopulations of
patients with mainly bone and mainly soft tissue/visceral
disease. Similarly the use of biochemical markers cannot be
advocated because of inconsistencies in their behaviour.
Richards et al (1983) reviewed the EORTC group's
experience of acid phosphatase and the current literature
and concluded that changes in acid phosphatase levels were
largely independent of progression of the disease. However,
the search for markers and other parameters which could be
used objectively in the assessment of response must
continue.

     In an attempt to increase recruitment into Phase II
studies, the EORTC Genitourinary group allowed the entry
into two of their studies of patients with non-measurable
metastatic disease but in whom the primary lesion could be
measured by transrectal ultrasound. This group of patients
was shown to have different characteristics to those with
measurable metastatic lesions and it was shown that the
groups were not comparable. It is thus recommended that
this approach should be abandoned (Jones et al, 1986a).
However, evaluation of the prostate by transrectal
ultrasonography may be a valid way of assessing response in
terms of time to progression in Phase III studies
(Schroeder, 1984).

     Our American collegues do not fully accept the very
strict criteria advocated by the EORTC GU group,

particularly with regard to the assessment of response in bone lesions. They consider that this is possible but stress the role of quality assurance and the use of the same facility for repeat examinations. It is accepted that there has been considerable improvement in nuclear medicine imaging in the last decade. Attempts to quantify overall increased uptake using computer technology are in use and hold promise for the future (Citrin et al, 1981). Certainly the total disappearance of increased uptake on isotope scan can be taken as (at least a partial) response, and the appearance of new lesions at different sites to previous ones is accepted as equating with progression.

The Japanese authors of this paper (representing a Japanese prostatic cancer study group supported by the Ministry of Health and Welfare of Japan) also do not fully accept the EORTC group's strict criteria for Phase II studies. The incidence of prostatic cancer in Japan is still very low compared to Europe and the USA, so the numbers of patients with classical bidimensionally measurable lesions is small. In order to increase recruitment into such studies they propose that an assessment of all available parameters should be undertaken including not only bidimensionally measurable lesions, but also the lesion in the prostate (by trans-rectal ultrasonography), bone metastases and the serum levels of prostatic acid phosphatase and possibly other markers. In the situation that there is no established method for the assessment of a lesion, the available methods should be used on a provisional basis. The results obtained should be recorded and reported separately by site and an overall assessment made on the basis of these individual results. Table 2 illustrates this concept showing the results in a small series of patients treated with an L.H./R.H. analogue in the Department of Urology at Tokyo University. Our Japanese colleagues suggest that this method of reporting will allow a much greater degree of analysis of such studies and will facilitate an impartial comparison of the results of studies performed by different groups on an international basis, independent of the individual criteria drawn up by each study group. This is believed as a very important concept for the reporting of results in Phase III as well as Phase II studies.

Table 2. Objective response to treatment of Prostatic Carcinoma by LH.RH Analogues
(Department of Urology, Tokyo University)

Case	Primary Bidi-	Primary Unidi-men	Primary Evals	Bone Bidi-mens	Bone Unidi-mens	Others Bidi-mens	Others Unidi-mens	Others Eval	PAP	Overall Response	Duration of Response (wks)
1) KN	NC				NC				CR	stable	43+
2) YN	PR				PR			PR	PR	PR	18+
3) MO	PR				PD				CR	PD	
4) HM	PR				NC	CR			CR	PR	49+
5) SK	PR								CR	PR	41+
6) ZN	PR				NC				CR	PR	26+
7) SM	NC				PD				PD		
8) KA	PR				NC					PR	12+
9) RS	NC									stable	16+
10) BY	PR									PR	90+
11) TA	NC				NC				CR	stable	44+
12) TA	PR									PR	32+
13) ST	PR		CR(digital exam)						CR	CR	100+
14) SW	PR									PR	80
15) IS	NC									stable	72+
16) HK	PR				NC					PR	28
17) YK	NC				NC					NC	NC	(8)
Response Rate	$\frac{11}{17}=64.7\%$		$\frac{1}{10}=10\%$		$\frac{2}{2}=100\%$	$\frac{6}{8}=75\%$				$\frac{CR+PR}{17}$ $\frac{10}{17}=58.8\%$	

CR+PR+stable $\frac{14}{17}=82.3\%$

Definition of Response Criteria

There appears to be no reason why the standard WHO response criteria (except for bone), (WHO, 1978) should not be used for this disease. A complete response (CR) is defined as the disappearance of all known disease determined by two observations not less than four weeks apart. It is most unlikely that this category of response will be used for patients with metastatic prostate cancer because of the tremendous difficulties in evaluating the presence or absence of disease residual in bone. Partial response (PR) is defined as a 50% or more decrease in the sum of the products of the longest perpendicular diameters of the lesions as determined by two observations not less than four weeks apart. In addition there can be no appearance of new lesions or progression of any one lesion. The no change (NC) category is where a 50% decrease in the total tumour size cannot be established nor has a 25% increase in the size of one or more measurable lesions been demonstrated. Progressive disease is where a 25% or more increase in size of one or more measurable lesions or the appearance of new lesions takes place. The only responses that can be classified as objective responses are those of complete or partial response (CR +PR).

The National Prostatic Cancer Project has defined an identifiable group of patients whose disease "objectively" stabilises (since the disease was progressive at the initiation of the study therapy) rather than exhibiting a no change response. A number of papers have been published regarding the "stable disease" category as being an acceptable objective response state (Slack et al, (1984), Murphy, (1984)). However, the use of this categorisation of response has been questioned by Beynon and Chisholm (1984), Eisenberger et al, (1985), Tannock, (1985) as well as by the EORTC GU Group (Jones et al, 1986a). The NPCP does not now apparently accept the stable category as a response group.

PHASE III STUDIES

Despite a considerable amount of excellent clinical work over the years in attempts to define response criteria, it is suggested that often sight has been lost of the objectives of Phase III studies in terms of determining which of two therapies is better (more effective or less toxic) for the patient.

Because of the difficulties of assessing response in patients with prostate cancer, the major end points of Phase III studies will be time to progression and duration of survival (Schroeder, 1984). Thus the entry criteria do not have to be anywhere near as strict as for Phase II studies.

The patients must have positive histological proof of disease, and good clinical evidence of progression at entry into the study. However, the clinical status of the patient must be fully investigated and an attempt to quantify and document the extent of disease be undertaken as accurately as possible. Only by continued re-assessment and attempting to evaluate response during treatment will better methods of definition of response emerge. Quantification of the extent of disease is seen as a very important step towards achieving a better comparison between the treatments in a Phase III study by facilitating stratification prior to randomisation and the commencement of therapy. Obviously a patient with a locally advanced lesion of the prostate and just two metastases on bone scan has a different prognosis than the patient with multiple bony lesions, weight loss of >10% and lymphangitic changes on chest X-ray. These differences must be taken into consideration by stratification within the study arms, and clinicians designing future studies ought to take this into account, as well as having regard to prognostic factors already identified (see elsewhere in this volume). Because these are numerically fairly large co-operative trials and participating clinicians may have slightly different attitudes to the disease, its assessment and treatment consideration should also be given to the possibility of randomisation by treatment institution so that possible factors of bias introduced into the study by that institution or clinician are distributed randomly, but almost equally, into the study arms.

Considerable efforts have been made to assess response in bone disease with variable success. Serial isotopic bone scans cannot be recommended. Perhaps the most valid conclusion is that arrived at by Condon et al, (1981) in that the determination of progression from changes in uptake in long standing lesions is uncertain and is subsidiary in importance to the detection of new lesions. Care has to be exercised since one previously large area of uptake may appear as two smaller lesions as the disease regresses responding to therapy. Lytic bone deposits can be followed by serial radiographs and it can be inferred that the disease is healing if an osteoblastic rim appears and eventually replaces the radiolucency. On the other hand, pathological fracture through an existing lesion cannot be taken solely as evidence of progression. There would appear to be a considerable degree of agreement on the criteria for the objective determination of progression including objective as well as subjective parameters. These include the appearance of new areas of involvement on bone scan or disease at other sites, increase in symptoms particularly pain, decrease in performance status, weight decrease etc, etc, (Paulson et al, 1985; Beynon and Chisholm, 1984; various publications from the NPCP and the EORTC). Again it must be stated that progression will only be accurately determined by frequent observations. The decision that relapse has occurred may well be a clinical one, perhaps even jointly determined by patient and physician. Determination of progression should not require any special or additional expertise of clinicians who regularly treat this disease. Because of the randomised nature of these studies, similar numbers of patients exhibiting stabilisation of disease showing no, or minimal, response to therapy should be allocated to each arm of the study. Thus the effect of the presence of such sub-populations of patients in each arm will be balanced out allowing a meaningful comparison of the therapies on trial.

Research work attempting to refine response criteria must continue and there are excellent opportunities for this in these larger studies. Evaluation of objective and subjective criteria, the development of "scoring systems", and identification of prognostic factors are important objectives. Obviously the precise definition of an objective response will not be possible in the absence of measurable disease, but imprecise or subjective changes may be helpful here. Measurement of serum acid and alkaline phosphatases, although not useful as objective response criteria because they do not relate directly to the bulk of malignant disease present and do not behave in an exponential manner, may be useful if sharing a trend. Normalisation of serum values usually equates with regression of tumour, and a steady rise in values usually means progression but these have to be considered along with other parameters before a decision on response can be reached. Subjective criteria may also be useful, if taken in conjunction with other factors, but care must be exercised with regard to their interpretation since changes, for example in the severity of the symptom of pain may be relative to other diseases or events or the mental attitude of the patient at the time of interview. Attention must concentrate on those objective and subjective factors which are being shown to be of prognostic value. With pre-randomisation stratifiction by prognostic factors we may well see the better definition of response, but it must be remembered that these are comparative studies of therapy.

With one of the main end points of Phase III studies being length of survival, all patients should be followed to death if possible. The premature reporting of results is to be deprecated, sufficient time must elapse for a meaningful reporting of survival statistics in these studies. An accurate assessment of the cause of death should be made. The cause of death should be defined as being due to: prostate cancer, related to the presence of active cancer (eg general debility leading to a hypostatic pneumonia), deaths due to treatment related causes (eg, vascular accidents due to oestrogen therapy), or death due to intercurrent disease. There should be an increase in the numbers of post-mortem examinations in these patients to precisely define the cause of death.

A most important aspect of a Phase III study is the quality of the patient's survival. It seems nonsensical to apply a therapy which detracts from the quality of survival while causing objective tumour response. The patient only appreciates the toxicity of the therapy unless he is deriving a significant improvement in function as a result of the treatment. In this respect the evaluation of the quality of survival and subjective improvements is important during these studies, but as yet they cannot be used as objective response criteria per se. They are discussed elsewhere in this volume.

CONCLUSION

Among the many concerns of physicians involved in the treatment of prostate cancer is the fact that despite considerable research efforts in recent years there is little evidence of major improvements in therapy. A major concern is that buried in the mounds of paper containing the results of vast numbers of clinical trials is a therapy, or some facet of a therapy, which may have been lost because of the lack of uniformly agreed and easily applied objective response criteria. It is suggested that continued research should be undertaken on a stricter basis. Formal Phase II studies should be performed in which a population of patients with bidimensionally measurable disease should be studied to give an order of response for a therapy applied to this group of patients with a particularly poor prognosis. This rather stringent test is more likely to identify treatments likely to be of benefit to a greater number of patients. If less strict criteria are applied, then response should be reported by site. Only those agents shown to be active in this way should be incorporated into larger randomised Phase III studies, in which larger numbers of patients are required. There will be a need to stratify patients by prognostic factors which are now in the process of being identified. Rather than attempting to assess response on an objective basis, it is easier to determine progression and thereby the time to progression and then to continue to follow the patient until death to see if one of the therapies applied has caused a survival prolongation.

Research into other ways of objectively assessing response must continue in this group of patients but many criteria, as yet, fall far short of the requirements of objectivity. The tasks faced by clinicians throughout the world in this disease are difficult. This has been an attempt to highlight some of the problems. Rather than produce yet another magic formula of response criteria to be followed in clinical trials, we have retracted somewhat to those objective response criteria that are universally agreed and suggest ways by which they can be utilised.

REFERENCES

Aabo K (1987). Prostate Cancer : Evaluation of response to treatment, response criteria, and the need for standardization of the reporting of results. Eur J Cancer Clin Oncol, 23 : 231-236.
Benson RC and Gill GM (1986). Estramustine phosphate compared with diethylstilboestrol. Am J Clin Oncol, 9 : 341-351.

Berry WR, Laszlo J, Cox E, Walker A, Paulson D (1979). Prognostic factors in metastatic and hormonally and unresponsive carcinoma of the prostate. Cancer, 44 : 763-775.

Beynon LL and Chisholm GD (1984). The stable state is not an objective response in hormone - escaped carcinoma of prostate. Brit J Urol, 56 : 702-705

Citrin DL, Cohen AL, Harberg, et al (1981). Systemic treatment of advanced prostatic cancer: Development of a new system for defining response. J Urol, 125: 224-227.

Citrin DL, Elson P, DeWys WD (1984). Treatment of metastatic prostate cancer - an analysis of response criteria in patients with measurable soft tissue disease. Cancer, 54 : 13-17.

Condon BR, Buchanan R, Garvie NW, Ackery DM, Fleming J, Taylor D, Hawkes D, Goddard BA (1981). Assessment of progression of secondary bone lesions following cancer of the breast or prostate using serial radionuclide imaging. Br J Radiol. 54 : 18-23.

DeWys WD, Bauer M, Colsky J, Cooper RA, Creech R, Carbone P (1977). Comparative trial of adriamycin and 5-fluorouracil in advanced prostatic cancer - progress report. Cancer Treat Rep. 61 : 325-328.

Eisenberger MA, Simon R, O'Dwyer PJ, Wittes RE, Friedman MA (1985). A re-evaluation of nonhormonal cytotoxic chemotherapy in the treatment of prostatic carcinoma J Clin Oncol, 3 : 827-841.

Emrich LJ, Priore RL, Murphy GP, Brady MF, (1985). Prognostic factors in patients with advanced stage prostate cancer. Cancer Res, 45 : 5173-5179.

Jones WG, Fossä SD, Denis L, Coninx P, Glashan RW, Akdas A, De Pauw M (1983). An EORTC phase II study of vindesine in advanced prostate cancer. Eur J Cancer Clin Oncol, 19 : 583-588.

Jones WG (1985). EORTC phase II chemotherapy studies in prostate cancer. In : Schroeder FH, Richards B (eds): "Therapeutic principles in metastatic prostatic cancer". New York: Alan R Liss, pp 435-445.

Jones WG, Bono AV, Verbaeys A, De Pauw M, Sylvester R (1986). Can the primary tumour be used as the sole parameter for response in phase II chemotherapy studies in metastatic prostate cancer? An EORTC Genito-urinary Group report. World J Urol, 4 : 176-181.

Jones WG, Fosså SD, Bono AV, Croles JJ, Stoter G, De Pauw M, Sylvester R (1986). Mitomycin-C in the treatment of metastatic prostate cancer: report on an EORTC phase II study. World J Urol, 4 : 182-185.

Kearsley J (1986). Cytotoxic chemotherapy for common adult malignancies : "the emperor's new clothes" revisited? Br Med J, 293 : 871-876.

Kirk D (1985). Prostatic carcinoma. Br Med J, 290 : 875-876

Moertel CG and Henley GA (1976). The effect of measuring error on the results of therapeutic trials in advanced cancer. Cancer, 38 : 388-394.

Murphy GP (1984). Workshop on response criteria and evaluation of the stable disease category in carcinoma of the prostate, breast and large bowel. Oncology, 41 : 64-67.

Murphy GP and Slack NH (1980). Response criteria for the prostate of the USA National Prostatic Cancer Project. The Prostate, 1: 375-382.

Newling DWW (1985). Criteria for response to treatment of metastatic prostatic cancer. In : Schroeder FH, Richards B (eds): "Therapeutic principles in metastatic prostatic cancer". New York : Alan R Liss, pp 205-220.

Paulson DF, Berry WR, Cox EB, Walker A, Laszlo J (1979). Treatment of metastatic endocrine unresponsive carcinoma of the prostate gland with multi-agent chemotherapy: Indicators of response to therapy. J Natl Cancer Inst 63 : 615-622.

Richards B, Sylvester R, De Pauw M (1983). The clinical value of serum acid phosphatase in carcinoma of the prostate. In : Smith PH, Pavone-Macaluso M (eds): "Cancer of the Prostate and Kidney" New York: Plenum Press, pp 167-178.

Robinson MRG, Smith PH, Pavone-Macaluso M, Sylvester R, de Voogt H (1985). The EORTC phase III trials in prostatic cancer. In : Schroeder FH, Richards B: "Therapeutic principles in metastatic prostatic cancer". New York : Alan R Liss, pp 243-249.

Schmidt JD, Scott WW, Gibbons R, Johnson DE, Prout GR, Loening S, Soloway M, de Kernion J, Pontes JE, Slack NH, Murphy GP (1980). Chemotherapy programs of the National Prostatic Cancer Project (NPCP). Cancer, 45 : 1937-1946.

Schroeder FH (1984). Treatment response criteria for prostatic cancer. The Prostate, 5 : 181-191.

Slack NH, Brady MF, Murphy GP (1984). A re-examination of the stable category for evaluating response in patients with advanced prostate cancer. Cancer, 54 : 564-574.

Tannock IF (1985). Is there evidence that chemotherapy is of benefit to patients with carcinoma of the prostate? J Clin Oncol, 3 : 1013-1021.

Van Oosterom AT, Akaza H, Hall R, Hirao Y, Jones WG, Matsumura Y, Raghavan D, Tannock IF, Yagoda A (1986). Response criteria phase II/phase III invasive bladder cancer. In : Denis L, Niijima T, Prout G, Schroeder FH (eds) : "Developments in bladder cancer". New York : Alan R Liss, pp 211-222.

Warr D, McKenney S, Tannock IF (1984). Influence of measurement error on assessment of response to anti-cancer chemotherapy: proposal for new criteria of tumour response. J Clin Oncol, 2 : 1040-1046.

WHO Handbook for Reporting Results of Cancer Treatment (1979). World Health Organisation Offset Publication No 48. Geneva.

Yagoda A (1983). Cytotoxic agents in prostate cancer : An enigma. Semin Urol, 1 : 311-321.

EORTC Genitourinary Group Monograph 5: Progress
and Controversies in Oncological Urology II, pages 261–273
© 1988 Alan R. Liss, Inc.

SUBJECTIVE RESPONSE CRITERIA AND QUALITY OF LIFE

N.K. Aaronson, F. Calais da Silva, H.J. de Voogt

The Netherlands Cancer Institute, Plesmanlaan
121, 1066 CX Amsterdam, the Netherlands; Hopital
Desterro, Praceta Bento Moura 21, Venda Nova
2700 Amadora, Portugal; Academic Hospital, Free
University, de Boelelaan 1117, 1007 MB Amsterdam, the Netherlands

INTRODUCTION

Recent years have witnessed a shifting climate with
regard to the perceived value of incorporating subjective
response criteria and quality of life measures into the
evaluation of cancer therapies. While in earlier years such
evaluation endpoints were, at best, viewed with a good deal
of skepticism, they have more recently received serious
attention from those responsible for planning and carrying
out clinical research.

In general, the increased willingness to consider
subjective outcome measures reflects an awareness that the
traditional evaluation parameters -- tumor response,
disease-free and overall survival, spread of disease, and
control of major physical symptoms -- do not provide a full
picture of the effect of cancer and cancer therapies on the
daily lives of patients. Thus, there is growing concern
with the impact of disease and treatment on a broader set
of health issues related to the physical, functional,
psychological and social well-being of the individual.

A review of the literature suggests that clinical
research in prostatic cancer is only now beginning to
translate this general interest in subjective treatment
effects into protocol designs. While most current studies
routinely employ minimal subjective response criteria

(e.g., measures of performance status and acute toxicities), only a handful of investigations have employed more sophisticated, patient-based evaluations of quality of life or psychosocial outcome (Presant et al., 1985, 1986; Raghavan et al., 1986). To our knowledge, no published data are available from randomized clinical trials in which quality of life outcomes have been evaluated, although two on-going phase III trials of the Genito-Urinary Cancer Cooperative Group of the E.O.R.T.C. are employing patient-based quality of life questionnaires (Denis, 1986; Newling, 1986).

Several arguments can be forwarded for the inclusion of subjective evaluation parameters in prostate cancer clinical trials. Perhaps most important among these is the fact that, in the case of advanced disease, little progress has been achieved in improving survival rates. This lack of progress, coupled with the relatively toxic nature of available treatments, compels us to examine the burden that such therapies place on the patient and his family. Ultimately, we must be able to demonstrate that the physical and psychosocial costs associated with active treatment are justified in the light of expected clinical improvement.

In the expectation that subjective evaluation endpoints will come to play an increasingly important role in future clinical research in prostate cancer, it seems appropriate to attempt to establish basic guidelines for carrying out such assessments. In the following discussions a distinction will be drawn between measures of subjective response and measures of quality of life. The former will refer to subjective evaluations of performance status and treatment toxicity which rely on the judgement of external raters (e.g., physicians, nurses, etc.). In contrast, quality of life assessments will be considered as those measures which rely on direct patient feedback regarding physical, functional, psychological and social health status. While this distinction is somewhat arbitrary, it is useful in organizing the material to be presented.

SUBJECTIVE RESPONSE CRITERIA I: PERFORMANCE STATUS RATINGS

Performance status refers to the ability to carry out a variety of activities that are normal for most people.

Four categories of such activities measured most commonly include: (1) self-care (e.g., feeding, dressing, bathing and using the toilet); (2) mobility (i.e., the ability to move about indoors and outdoors; (3) physical activities (e.g., walking, climbing stairs, etc.); and (4) role activities (i.e., the ability to carry out social roles associated with work, school, family, etc.) (Stewart et al., 1978).

Performance status ratings were first introduced into cancer research in 1949 in the form of an 11 step scale that incorporates global judgements regarding the patient's ability for self-care, ambulation, daily activities, and symptom level (Karnofsky and Burchenall, 1949). This Karnofsky Performance Status Scale (KPS), or alternative, abbreviated assessment approaches such as the 5 step scale developed by the Eastern Cooperative Oncology Group (ECOG) (Zubrod et al., 1960), have gained wide acceptance in clinical cancer research.

While there are a number of factors that have contributed to the adoption of such performance status measures in the design and evaluation of cancer clinical trials, the most important is their demonstrated prognostic value in lung cancer (Aisner and Hansen, 1981; Stanley, 1980), colon cancer (Buroker et al., 1978; Kemeny et al., 1983), prostate cancer (Bery et al., 1979), acute myelogenous leukemia (Kansal et al., 1976) and other tumors (DeConti and Schoenfeld, 1981). Performance status measures are currently used as eligibility criteria for trial patient selection, to stratify patients prior to randomization, to measure the efficacy of treatment or as a proxy measure of quality of life (Orr and Aisner, 1986).

Given the empirical data regarding the prognostic value of performance status measures, there is reason to argue for their routine inclusion in prostatic cancer clinical trials. However, this does not imply that such measures should be viewed with an uncritical eye. For example, while the validity of the KPS appears to be quite good (i.e., it correlates significantly with more sophisticated approaches to assessing patient functional status) (Mor et al., 1984; Schag et al., 1984; Wood et al., 1981), several studies indicate problems with the instrument's reliability. Hutchinson et al. (1979) found that different pairs of physicians reached agreement in KPS ratings in only between 29% and 34% of cases. Yates et al., 1980 reported somewhat higher, but still only moderate levels of inter-observer correlations (r = 0.69) when comparing the KPS ratings of nurses and social workers. Similarly, Schag et al. (1984) found only moderate agreement (i.e, in 59% of cases) between KPS ratings provided by oncologists and mental health professionals.

Orr and Aisner (1986) emphasize that improvement in the reliability of KPS ratings is essential if we intend to employ it as a patient selection criterion or as a stratification variable prior to random assignment to treatment. This, of course, is equally true if it is to be used as a subjective measure of treatment efficacy. A study by Mor and his colleagues (1984) suggests that the reliability of KPS ratings can be improved dramatically (i.e., 97% inter-observer agreement) if raters are provided with training and clear operational definitions of each level of performance status based on activities of daily living.

In contrast to the KPS, the shorter ECOG performance status scale and similar truncated scales developed by other clinical cooperative groups (e.g., the CALGB and SWOG) have yet to be subjected to rigorous validity and reliability testing. Although one can assume that the primary motivation for generating such abbreviated scales is to simplify the rating procedure (and thus improve reliability), no data have yet been published which address this issue. Similarly, no head-to-head comparisons have yet to be made between the KPS and shorter performance status measures, either with regard to their reliability or prognostic value. However, Stanley (1980) reports that, for lung cancer, collapsing the KPS into a more discrete number of categories results in a significant loss of prognostic power. This would suggest that the increased simplicity of the ECOG scale may be achieved at the cost of poorer empirical performance as a subjective measure of response to treatment in prostatic cancer trials.

Thus, at this time it would seem prudent to recommend employing the KPS until sufficient evidence has been amassed to support the use of the ECOG scale as a simpler and equally efficient measure of patients' performance status. Additionally, efforts should be directed toward improving the reliability of the KPS. This may best be accomplished by generating additional operational criteria for placement of patients within the KPS scale continuum.

SUBJECTIVE RESPONSE CRITERIA II: SELECTED TOXICITY SCALES

The systematic evaluation of treatment toxicity is an essential component of any clinical trial. It provides vital information to be considered in establishing the cost-benfit, or therapeutic index, of a given treatment approach. While many of the toxicities associated with anti-neoplastic therapies can be assessed by means of objective laboratory or clinical parameters, there remains a subset of toxic effects that can only be evaluated subjectively (e.g., nausea and vomiting) or are typically evaluated by subjective means due to the invasiveness, inconvenience and cost of more objective procedures (e.g., pulmonary function).

The two major toxicity grading systems employed in oncological clinical trials -- those of the World Health Organization (WHO) and the U.S. National Cancer Institute (NCI) -- both employ a mixture of objective and subjective parameters. It is beyond the scope and mandate of this report to evaluate these systems in a comprehensive manner (see Kisner, 1984 and Vietti, 1980 for overviews). Rather, our focus will be on the adequacy of the subjective elements of these two systems.

The WHO and NCI systems are quite similar with regard to their subjective content. Both include ratings of nausea and vomiting, diarrhea, dyspnea, and state of conscious-ness. Additionally, however, the WHO system includes a rating of treatment-related pain. This would seem to be a serious ommission from the NCI system. Both systems employ a five point rating scale of symptom severity, although the NCI system does not make use of the full scale range for all toxicities (e.g., nausea and vomiting ratings are based on a 4 point scale).

A weakness common to the two systems is their exclusive reliance on severity ratings, without consideration of time of onset or duration. The potential interpretive difficulties resulting from this approach can be illustrated with the nausea and vomiting scales. Within the WHO system, these symptoms are graded as follows: (0) none; (1) nausea; (2) transient vomiting; (3) vomiting requiring therapy; and (4) intractable vomiting. The corresponding NCI gradings are: (0) none; (1) nausea only; (2) controllable; (3) intractable.

Using these grading categories, we would be compelled to rate a patient suffering from continuous, extreme nausea (reflecting a combination of severity and duration) as less symptomatic than a patient who experienced one or two episodes of vomiting on the first day of treatment. It is questionable whether such an a priori rank-ordering reflects accurately the relative burden of such symptoms on the patient's daily life. A possible solution to this problem would be to employ separate gradings for nausea and vomiting, rather than combining them into a single symptom cluster.

A relatively minor, but nevertheless bothersome feature of the NCI system has to do with the occasional use of the same symptom descriptors for several levels of grading. For example, both grades 2 and 3 for diarrhea are described as "watery, 4 times daily". Such redundacy necessitates an abritrary choice between grades, and ultimately results in a collapsing of categories during analysis.

At least with regard to their subjective content, neither of these two toxicity grading systems appears to hold a dramatic edge over the other. The few differences that do exist between the systems (e.g., inclusion of pain, clarity and consistency of grading levels) would seem to favor the WHO appoach. Nevertheless, it would be imprudent to recommend the WHO system on the basis of these considerations alone. Rather, such a decision awaits an integrated evaluation of both the subjective and objective elements of the competing systems. Ideally, this would involve a head-to-head comparison of the validity and reliability of the two systems. Our suspicion is that such an evaluation, rather than uncovering an obvious choice between the two systems, would document the need for refinements in both.

QUALITY OF LIFE ASSESSMENT

While, to a limited degree, observer-based performance status and toxicity ratings represent a form of quality of life assessment, it is often desirable and sometimes obligatory to assess in a more direct fashion the patients' perceptions of the impact of disease and therapy on their daily lives. This is clearly the case where there is interest in assessing such subjective experiences as pain, fatigue or psychological distress. Yet, even in the case of more readily observable symptoms, patient feedback may provide additional insight into their meaning. For example, in assessing alopecia, we are not so much concerned with the amount of hair loss per se, but rather with how the change in physical appearance affects the patient psychologically and socially.

The question that is central to the current discussion is whether there is sufficient consensus regarding the substantive and methodological requirements of quality of life assessment to form the basis for standard reporting procedures in prostatic cancer clinical trials. From a conceptual standpoint, there does appear to be general agreement that quality of life assessment in cancer research should encompass minimally four broad health domains: physical functional status; physical symptom experience; psychological well-being; and social role functioning (Aaronson, 1986; de Haes and van Knippenberg, 1985; Schipper and Levitt, 1985).

This conceptual framework, however, has yet to be translated successfully into an assessment approach that enjoys widespread acceptance by the oncological research community. To the contrary, a review of the literature underscores the diversity of measures employed to assess the quality of life of patients (de Haes and van Knippenberg, 1985). These instruments range from lengthy, omnibus questionnaires intended to assess quality of life among chronic disease patients in general (e.g., the Sickness Impact Profile; Bergner et al., 1981) to more concise questionnaires intended for use among varied cancer populations (e.g., the Functional Living Index – Cancer; Schipper et al., 1984) to ad hoc questionnaires designed with specific clinical trials in mind. None of these instruments have yet to undergo sufficient field testing in oncology settings to justify a recommendation for general use.

In lieu of such a specific recommendation, we prefer to restrict ourselves to some general guidelines for the development and implementation of quality of life studies within prostatic cancer clinical trials. First, we would suggest that a "modular" approach be employed in developing quality of life questionnaires for use in such research. By this we mean the construction of a set of brief, multi-item measures assessing: (1) functional status; (2) common physical symptoms of cancer and cancer treatment (i.e., fatigue and malaise, pain, dyspnea, constipation, diarrhea, sleeplessness, and nausea and vomiting); (3) psychological distress (primarily depression and anxiety); (4) social interaction; and (5) perceived health status and overall quality of life.

These various modules, combined into a "core" or generic questionnaire, could then be supplemented by an additional module focusing on symptoms and side-effects specific to prostatic cancer (e.g., dysuria, diminished urinary flow, hematuria, nocturia, disturbance of libido and sexual function). Adoption of such a measurement strategy would reconcile the two principal requirements in conducting clinical research -- a sufficient degree of generalizability to allow for cross-study comparisons, and a level of specificity adequate for answering those questions of particular relevance in a given clinical trial.

In addition to advocating such a general measurement strategy, there are a number of methodological issues that should be considered carefully in developing a quality of life questionnaire. First, the questionnaire should be designed for patient self-administration, and should minimize the amount of patient burden associated with its completion. While tolerance for answering questions will vary as a function of patient age, education, stage of disease and symptom level, experience within E.O.R.T.C. trials suggests that a questionnaire containing between 30 and 40 items is acceptable to the large majority of patients.

Second, whenever possible, each quality of life domain should be assessed by means of a multiple-item scale, rather than with a single, global question. This strategy will increase the variability of scores, an important requisite for detecting change in health status over time and differences between patient groups. Additionally, if carefully constructed, such multi-item scales will yield substantial gains in reliability and validity over single item measures.

Third, questions should be posed in terms of a specific, and preferably short, time-frame (e.g., the past week). If the time-frame is too long, or is left undefined, patients may be confused as to the relevant period of symptom reporting. This, in turn, can compromise the reliability of the data so obtained.

Fourth, we would recommend the use of Likert-type response scales which provide the patient with a set number of closed-ended possibilities for answering questions (e.g., 'not at all', 'a little', 'quite a bit', 'very much'). This categorical approach is to be contrasted with the linear analog method which presents the patient with a 10 centimeter line anchored at each end with a brief descriptive phrase (e.g., 'no pain' and 'extreme pain'). The patient is then asked to mark the place on the line that best corresponds to his or her experience. While the linear analog approach holds certain formal statistical advantages over the Likert-type, it requires a level of abstract thinking that may be too great for some patients (Aaronson, 1986). Also, preparation of linear analog data for statistical analysis can be quite cumbersome, particularly when collected in large scale trials.

Fifth, it is essential that the requisite psychometric tests be carried out to ensure that the selected quality of life scales are both valid and reliable for use with the population of patients of interest. In an international research context, this implies the need to establish not only statistical validity, but cross-cultural validity as well (via formal 'forward-backward' translation procedures).

A final set of issues concerns the feasibility and practicality of carrying out clinical trial-based quality of life research. Even in those institutions with a strong clinical research tradition, the collection of quality of life data often places novel demands on the research infrastructure. A number of practical steps can be undertaken to maximize the feasibilitiy of such research:

- The quality of life research design should be kept as simple as possible, with the number of required questionnaires reflecting a balance between what is desirable and what is feasible given available data management resources.

- The introduction of practical aids, including study calenders, flow sheets, and 'flagging' of patients' medical records can facilitate timely administration of questionnaires.

- Sufficient time should be allocated for pretesting the questionnaire and for pilot testing the data collection procedures.

- The quality of life component of the trial should be submitted to formal review as an integral part of the protocol review process.

- A key individual in each participating center should be identified who can take responsibility for coordinating the quality of life data collection. In many instances it is preferable that this be someone other than the individual responsible for managing the clinical aspects of the trial.

- In multi-center trials, it may be advisable to limit participation in the quality of life substudy to those centers that have adequate support personnel for such research. Individual centers with extensive resources might be asked to undertake more intensive data collection (e.g., interviews with family members) to supplement the basic quality of life data set.

CONCLUSION

In this paper a number of guidelines have been proposed for the assessment of subjective response criteria and quality of life in prostatic cancer clinical trials. With regard to subjective response criteria, the Karnofsky Performance Status Scale and the subjective components of the WHO Acute and Subacute Toxicity Scales appear, at this moment in time, to be the instruments of choice. As both measures are currently in wide use in cancer research, few difficulties should be expected in calling for their routine inclusion in clinical trials. Despite this recommendation, however, further developmental work is required to improve the precision of these measures.

In the case of quality of life assessment, there does not appear to be a clear choice among available measures. While there are a number of promising instruments, none has yet to be sufficiently tested within the constraints of multi-center clinical trials to justify widespread adoption. This should not be taken to imply that quality of life endpoints can not be introduced successfully into prostatic cancer research. To the contrary, there are several phase III trials currently running in which such assessment is being carried out. Rather, it suggests that the state of the art has yet to develop to a point where a standard method of assessment can be selected. In the hope of facilitating further work in this area, a number of basic recommendations have been proffered regarding quality of life instrument development and research implementation.

REFERENCES

Aaronson NK (1986). Methodological issues in psychosocial oncology with special reference to clinical trials. In Ventafridda V, van Dam FSAM, Yancik R and Tamburin M (eds.): "Assessment of Quality of Life and Cancer Treatment," Amsterdam: Elsevier Science Publishers.

Aisner J and Hansen HH (1981). Commentary: Current status of chemotherapy for non-small cell lung cancer. Cancer Treat Rep 65:979-986.

Bergner M, Bobbitt Ra, Carter WB and Gilson BS (1981): The sickness impact profile: Development and final revision of a health status measure. Med Care 19:787-805.

Berry WR, Laszlo J, Cox E et al. (1979). Prognostic factors in metastatic and hormonally unresponsive carcinoma of the prostate. Cancer 44:763-775.

Buroker T, Kim Pn, Groppe C et al. (1978). 5FU infusion with mitomycin-C versus 5FU with methyl-CCNU in the treatment of advanced colon cancer. Cancer 42:1228-1233.

DeConte RC and Schoenfeld D (1981). A randomized prospective comparison of intermittent methotrexate, methotrexate with leucovorin, and a methotrexate combination in head and neck cancer. Cancer 48:1061-1072.

De Haes JCJM and van Knippenberg FCE (1985). The quality of life of cancer patients: A review of the literature. Soc Sci Med 20:809-817.

Denis, L (1986). E.O.R.T.C. protocol 30853: A randomized
  prospective study of the treatment of patients with metastatic prostatic cancer to compare the therapeutic effect
  of orchidectomy versus lhrh-analogue depot (zoladex)
  preparation supplemented by an anti-androgen (flutamide).
  Brussels: E.O.R.T.C. Data Center.
Hutchinson TA, Boyd NF and Feinstein AR (1979). Scientific problems in clinical scales as demonstrated in the
  Karnofsky index of performance status. J Chronic Dis
  32:661-666.
Kansal V, Omura GA and Soong SJ (1976). Prognosis in
  adult acute myelogenous leukemia related to performance
  status and other factors. Cancer 38:329-334.
Karnofsky DA and Burchenal JH (1949). Clinical evaluation
  of chemotherapeutic agents in cancer. In MacLeod CM
  (ed.): "Evaluation of Chemotherapeutic Agents," New York:
  Columbia University Press.
Kemeny N and Braun DW Jr. (1983). Prognostic factors in
  advanced colorectal carcinoma. Am J Med 74:786-794.
Kisner DL (1984). Reporting treatment toxicities. In
  Buyse ME, Staquet MJ and Sylvester RJ (eds.): "Cancer
  Clinical Trials: Methods and Practice," New York: Oxford
  University Press.
Mor V, Laliberte L, Morris JN et al. (1984). The Karnof-
  sky performance status scale: An examination of its re-
  liability and validity in a research setting. Cancer
  53:2002-2007.
Newling, DWW (1986). EORTC protocol 30865: A randomised
  phase III study comparing estracyt and mitomycin-c in
  hormone escaped advanced prostatic cancer. Brussels:
  E.O.R.T.C. Data Center.
Orr ST and Aisner J (1986). Performance status assessment
  among oncology patients: A review. Cancer Treat Rep 70:
  1423-1429.
Presant CA, Soloway MS, Klioze SS, et al. (1985). Buserelin as primary therapy in advanced prostatic cancer.
  Cancer 56:2416-2419.
Presant CA, Soloway M, Mendex R et al. (1986). Duration
  of response and improved quality of life in buserelin-
  treated prostate carcinoma: Long-term results. Proc Am
  Soc Clin Oncol 5:103.
Raghavan D, Bishop J, Woods R et al. (1986). Mitozantone
  (zan): A non-toxic, moderatetly active agent for hormone-
  resistant prostate cancer. Proc Am Soc Clin Oncol 5:102.
Schag CC, Heinrich RL and Ganz PA (1984). Karnofsky performance status revisited: reliability, validity and

guidelines. J Clin Oncol 2:187-193.

Schipper H, Clinch J, McMurray A and Levitt M (1984). Measuring the quality of life of cancer patients: The functional living index - cancer. J Clin Oncol 2:472-483.

Schipper H and Levitt M (1985). Measuring quality of life: Risks and benefits. Cancer Treat Rep 69:1115-1123.

Stanley KE (1980). Prognostic factors for survival in patients with inoperable lung cancer. JNCI 65:25-32.

Stewart AL, Ware JE and Davies-Avery A (1978). Conceptualizationandmeasurementof health foradultsinthe health insurance study: Vol II: Physical health in terms of functioning. Santa Monica, CA: The Rand Corporation R-1987/2-HEW.

Vietti TJ (1980). Evaluation of toxicity: Clinical issues. Cancer Treat Rep 64:457-461.

Wood CA, Anderson J and Yates JW (1981). Physical function assessment in patients with advanced cancer. Med Pediatr Oncol 9:129-132.

Yates JW, Chalmer B and McKegney FP (1980). Evaluation of patients with advanced cancer using the Karnofsky performance status. Cancer 45:2220-2224.

Zubrod CG, Scheiderman M, Frei E et al. (1960). Cancer - appraisal of methods for the study of chemotherapy of cancer in man: Thiophosphoramide. J Chronic Dis 11:7-33.

EORTC Genitourinary Group Monograph 5: Progress
and Controversies in Oncological Urology II, pages 275-287
© 1988 Alan R. Liss, Inc.

PROGNOSTIC FACTORS FOR RANDOMIZATION AND STRATIFICATION AND ENDPOINTS FOR THE EVALUATION OF TRIALS

Richard J. Sylvester, Stefan Suciu and Hidetoshi
Yamanaka

EORTC Data Center, Brussels, Belgium (R.J.S,
S.S.) and Department of Urology, Gunma University, Gunma, Japan (H.Y.)

INTRODUCTION

The identification of prognostic factors in prostate cancer, as in most diseases, is important because it leads to a better understanding of the natural history of the disease itself and its treatment. It allows a clinician to establish the prognosis of a newly presenting patient based on his disease characteristics, and thus determine the most appropriate treatment.

In carrying out randomized clinical trials, prognostic factors are important for the following reasons:

1. They allow different trials of varying degrees of treatment aggressiveness to be carried out in patients according to whether they have a good or a poor prognosis.

2. Stratification for the most important prognostic factors at entry on study ensures that the distribution of these factors in the various treatment arms will be well balanced. The number of factors that one may stratify for will depend on whether a randomized block design or a dynamic randomization method (Lagakos and Pocock, 1984) is used.

3. Treatment comparisons can be stratified retrospectively at the time of the analysis for those

factors of prognostic importance. In this manner it is possible to adjust for any imbalances of prognostic factors which may exist on the treatments to be compared.

In prostate cancer these last two points are of prime importance since greater differences in survival can be expected based on prognostic factors than for treatments. Thus any imbalance of prognostic factors in the various treatment groups may severely bias the treatment comparisons unless the appropriate adjustments are made.

When discussing prognostic factors, one must necessarily define the endpoints used in determining a variable's prognostic importance. A variable which may be important in predicting whether a patient will respond to treatment may, for example, have little or no value in predicting a patient's survival. Thus in discussing prognostic factors we must always qualify any discussion by specifying the endpoint used in the analysis.

We must likewise qualify any discussion by describing the patient population used to determine a factor's prognostic importance. A variable of prognostic importance in metastatic patients may, for example, be of no importance in non metastatic patients.

The purpose of this paper is to identify, by disease extent, the most appropriate endpoints to use in the comparison of treatments in randomized phase III clinical trials and to present those variables which should be used for stratification at the time of randomization. For this purpose, we shall not attempt an exhaustive review of all possible prognostic factors, but rather limit ourselves to those factors of recognized importance which are both easily and commonly assessed in practice.

One should stratify at randomization only for prognostic factors which can be easily assessed prior to entry on study and which do not require an external review or evaluation. As a general principal one should always stratify by institution and in addition usually by the one or two most important prognostic factors.

STAGING SYSTEMS

Unfortunately there is no universally adopted staging system. The TNM classification (UICC, 1985) is internationally recognized and has been adopted by the EORTC. However the staging system used by the VACURG (Byar, 1977) has also been widely used, especially in the United States. The correspondance between these two classifications is as follows (Schroeder and Van der Werf-Messing, 1982):

Stage I
Incidental carcinoma: $T_0 \ M_0$

Stage II
Palpable intracapsular carcinoma: $T_1\text{-}T_2 \ M_0$

Stage III
Locally extensive carcinoma: $T_3\text{-}T_4 \ M_0$

Stage IV
Metastatic carcinoma: $T_0\text{-}T_4 \ M_1$

It should be noted however that the VACURG included in Stage IV those non metastatic patients who had an elevated acid phosphatase (> 1.1 KAU) although the EORTC did not. Some authors refer to these four categories as stages A to D respectively.

One of the limitations of the above system is that as improved staging techniques have become available, it does not take into consideration the N category.

For the purpose of this paper, we shall follow the initiative of Byar and Corle (1984) and divide patients into two different categories, those with Limited Disease (stage I and II) and those with Extended Disease (stage III and IV) using the above definitions. We shall now consider the endpoints and prognostic factors separately in each of these two groups based on the work of the VACURG and the EORTC.

LIMITED DISEASE

Endpoints

In patients with limited disease, Byar and Corle (1984) found that survival could not be used as an endpoint for treatment comparison since in the VACURG trials only 3% of the stage I patients and 6% of the stage II patients died due to prostate cancer during the course of follow up. For this reason they have taken disease progression as endpoint, defined as an increase in acid phosphatase to > 2.0 KAU, the development of distant metastases, or death from prostatic cancer. However at 5 years they found a progression rate of only 10%.

If randomized clinical trials are to be carried out in this group of patients, and many feel that they should not, it is of interest to widen the definition of progression in order to increase the number of events which are observed during follow up. With more widespread use of imaging techniques such as ultrasound and CT scan, one could also take into account objective progression of the primary lesion and also assess its response to therapy. However until such techniques become common practice and a standardized set of response criteria agreed upon, it is recommended that the main endpoint for use in clinical trials in this group of patients be time to disease progression as defined by Byar and Corle.

Prognostic Factors

Using disease progression as defined above as endpoint, Byar and Corle (1984) found three variables to be of prognostic importance in a multivariate analysis:

1. Gleason sum (Gleason, 1966).
2. Size of the primary tumor (cm^2).
3. Acid phosphatase.

The Gleason sum was by far the most important factor. All three of these variables are recognized to be of prognostic importance in prostatic cancer, despite the fact that different methods for their measurement or assessment are available. Based on these variables a small subgroup of patients was identified in which one third progressed within 5 years. Although tumor size was measured, no data on the T or N categories were available.

Other authors (Prout et al, 1981) have reported a high rate of progression in patients with pelvic lymph node "metastases" in apparently locally confined disease.

Discussion

Because of the small percentage of progressions or deaths due to prostate cancer and the large percentage of these patients that can be expected to die of cardiovascular or other associated chronic diseases, it is very difficult to carry out randomized clinical trials in this patient group. In practice, for trials in limited disease it is recommended to stratify at entry on study for the T category (or tumor size). It is not practical to stratify by tumor grade or Gleason sum since an external review will not generally be available at the time of entry on study. Variables such as grading, acid phosphatase and N category should be taken into account by stratification at the time of the analysis. Further work is needed however to better define really high risk patients in this group and one step in this direction would be through the routine assessment and evaluation of the N category.

EXTENDED DISEASE

Endpoints

The choice of endpoints in patients with extended disease is by no means an easy one. There is no universally accepted method or criteria for objectively measuring the response of the primary lesion and assessment of the response of bone metastases is not without difficulties (Schroeder, 1984; Newling, 1985). In addition the work involved in extramural review of xrays and bone scans is considerable (Lund et al, 1984). Due to the nature of the disease, a large number of patients can be expected to remain stable during the initial treatment assessment period. While response to treatment may be assessed as a secondary endpoint, it is thus not recommended as the primary endpoint in randomized phase III trials.

In stage III patients, perhaps the most appealing endpoint is the time to the appearance of distant metastases. However in EORTC trials 30761 and 30762 only 25% of the stage III patients developed distant metastases during the course of follow up (Pavone-Macaluso et al, 1986; Smith et al, 1986). Thus large sample sizes would be required to carry out randomized clinical trials using this endpoint.

In stage IV patients the EORTC has more recently adopted in trial 30805 time to objective progression as its main endpoint, with progression being defined as an increase in size > 50% of the primary lesion or the appearance of new metastases. However the use of disease progression as defined here has not been totally satisfactory because:

1. patients may die of malignant disease (or associated chronic disease) prior to confirmation of objective progression.

2. patients may go off study due to subjective disease progression or drop out of the trial before objective signs of progression can be established.

Consequently in its most recent trials (30843, 30853) the EORTC has defined an additional category of subjective or nonspecific progression as an endpoint, based on changes in acid or alkaline phosphatase, pain or performance status. In this way patients without signs of objective progression, but for whom it is no longer ethical to leave them in the protocol due to a subjective worsening, will not be inevaluable for this endpoint.

Due to problems in assessing response to treatment and time to progression, duration of survival would appear to be the endpoint of choice, especially since there is no effective second line treatment for patients with hormone resistant disease. However as we are dealing with an old patient population, many patients will die due to (treatment related?) cardiovascular disease or due to other associated chronic diseases.

Among patients entered in EORTC trials 30761 and 30762, approximately 50% (30%) of the stage III patients and 70% (50%) of the stage IV patients died during follow up due to any cause (due to malignant disease). It was estimated that approximately two thirds of the deaths were due to malignant disease. Since it is not always possible to establish the cause of death with certainty and because deaths due to reasons other than malignant disease may be treatment related, it is preferable to base duration of survival calculations on all deaths.

For patients with extended disease it is thus recommended to take duration of survival as the primary endpoint. In addition the time to progression should also be assessed, making a distinction as to the type of progression (local, distant, or subjective).

Prognostic Factors

In Stage III or Stage IV disease, a list of 18 factors found to be of prognostic importance for duration of survival by the EORTC and/or the VACURG are listed in Table 1.

Table 1. EORTC/VACURG Prognostic Factors For Survival in Extended Disease

Variable:

Metastatic Status
T Category
Size of Primary
Histology: G Category, Gleason Sum
Extent of Bone and Lung Metastases
Ureteral Dilatation
Acid Phosphatase
Alkaline Phosphatase
Performance Status
Pain
Electrocardiogram
Chronic/Cardiovascular Disease
Hemoglobin
Age
Weight
Fibrinogen
Haptoglobin
17-OH Corticoids

This list is not meant to be exhaustive and does not include all factors of possible importance. For example, variables such as the erythrocyte sedimentation rate and the serum testosterone have not been listed.

The identification of such variables by means of univariate analyses does not take into account however the correlation between the various variables. For example, once performance status is determined, the relative importance of the other variables remains unknown. Thus multivariate analyses that allow all the variables to act together simultaneously are required so that the relative importance of the variables can be determined and a small subset of factors for stratification purposes identified.

Multivariate analyses of prognostic factors for Stage III/IV disease have been performed by both the EORTC (De Voogt et al, 1987) and the VACURG (Byar and Corle, 1984).

The EORTC found the following factors to be of greatest prognostic importance with regard to duration of survival (any cause of death) in trials 30761 and 30762:

Table 2. EORTC Prognostic Factors in Stage III and Stage IV

Stage III

Univariate Analysis	Multivariate Analysis
1. Performance Status	1. Performance Status
2. Pain	2. Acid Phosphatase
3. Age	3. Pain
4. T Category	4. Age
5. Hemoglobin	5. T Category
6. G Grade	

Stage IV

Univariate Analysis

1. Performance Status
2. Hemoglobin
3. Size of Primary Tumor
4. Pain
5. T Category
6. G Grade
7. Acid/Alkaline Phosphatase
8. Chron/Card Disease

Multivariate Analysis

1. Performance Status
2. Alkaline Phosphatase
3. T Category
4. Chronic/Cardiovascular Disease

Not only is the prognosis different in Stage III and Stage IV patients (Pavone-Macaluso et al, 1986; Smith et al, 1986), but except for performance status, which was the most important factor in both groups, the relative importance of the prognostic factors is also different. Combining Stage III and Stage IV patients together, the following prognostic factors were obtained:

Table 3. EORTC Prognostic Factors in Stage III+IV

Stage III + IV (Combined)

Univariate Analysis

1. Performance Status
2. Hemoglobin
3. Pain
4. Metastatic Status
5. Acid/Alk. Phosphatase
6. T Category
7. G Grade
8. Age
9. Chron/Card Disease

Multivariate Analysis

1. Performance Status
2. T Category
3. Chronic/Cardiovascular Disease
4. M Category
5. Acid/Alk. Phosphatase
6. Age

In all these analyses the performance status proved to be the most important prognostic factor.

Byar and Corle (1984), in a multivariate analysis of the Stage III + IV (combined) VACURG patients, found the duration of survival (all causes of death) to be correlated with the following factors:

Table 4. VACURG Prognostic Factors in Stage III+IV

VACURG Multivariate Analysis

1. Age/Acid Phosphatase
2. Performance Status
3. Gleason Sum
4. Weight
5. M Category
6. Size of Primary
7. Hemoglobin

Acid phosphatase for patients < 70 years and the performance status were the two most important prognostic factors.

Discussion

As metastatic patients have a worse prognosis than non metastatic patients, it is generally agreed that separate trials should be carried out for Stage III and Stage IV patients. If not, then patients should be stratified at entry on study by their metastatic status.

All Stage III and Stage IV patients should be stratified at randomization by the most important prognostic factor, performance status, and also by the T category. Stratification for other factors such as acid and alkaline phosphatase, histology and N category should be done at the time of analysis. In trials with drugs of known or potentially important cardiovascular side effects, patients should also be stratified according to their cardiovascular status.

Instead of stratifying for individual factors, patients could also be stratified based on a prognostic index used to divide patients into risk groups. Such an index would be composed of the most important prognostic factors, the weights of which would be determined by a multivariate model. Before such an index is used in practice however, it should be validated using an independent data set.

In Stage III patients the EORTC found that 10/197 (5%) patients with pain and 13/197 (7%) patients with an acid phosphatase more than twice the upper normal limit had a poor prognosis and may thus have had undetected metastases at entry on study. Such patients should probably be excluded from future Stage III trials and included in Stage IV studies. The EORTC has also recently adopted the policy of including N4 patients in Stage IV trials.

There is also increasing evidence that <u>Stage IV</u> patients with soft tissue or visceral metastases have a worse prognosis than patients with only bone metastases (Yagoda et al, 1979; EORTC, 1986). The percentage of such patients is relatively small, approximately 10-15% of all metastatic patients, however their actual number may increase through more extensive patient staging procedures.

CONCLUSIONS

It is thus recommended to stratify limited disease patients at entry on study by the T category or tumor size and take time to disease progression as the main endpoint. Extended disease patients should be stratified by performance status and T category with the primary endpoint being duration of survival, death due to any cause.

A plea is also made for the more routine assessment of the N category and lymph node metastases outside of the pelvis (mediastinal nodes, supraclavicular nodes) in all disease stages in order to more fully determine their prognostic importance, both individually and also relative to other established prognostic factors.

REFERENCES

Byar DP (1977). VACURG Studies on prostatic cancer and its treatment. In Tannenbaum M (ed): "Urologic Pathology: The Prostate", New York: Lea and Febiger, pp 241-267.

Byar DP, Corle DK (1984). Analysis of prognostic factors for prostatic cancer in the VACURG studies. In Denis L, Murphy GP, Prout GR, Schroeder F (eds): "Controlled Clinical Trials in Urologic Oncology", New York: Raven Press, pp 147-169.

De Voogt HJ, Pavone-Macaluso M, Smith PH, Suciu S, Sylvester R and De Pauw M (1987) Prognostic Factors in Advanced Prostatic Cancer: a statistical analysis of EORTC trials 30761 and 30762. In preparation.

EORTC (1986). Interim analysis, trial 30805.

Gleason DF (1966). Classification of prostatic carcinomas. Cancer Chemotherapy Reports 50,3:125-128.

Lagakos SW, Pocock SJ (1984). Randomization and stratification in cancer clinical trials: an international survey. In Buyse ME, Staquet MJ, Sylvester RJ (eds): "Cancer Clinical Trials: Methods and Practice",

Oxford: Oxford University Press, pp 276-286.

Lund F, Smith PH, Suciu S (1984). Do bone scans predict prognosis in prostatic cancer? A report of the EORTC protocol 30762. British Journal of Urology 56:58-63.

Newling DW (1985). Criteria for response to treatment of metastatic prostatic cancer. In Schroeder FH, Richards B (eds): "Therapeutic Principles in Metastatic Prostatic Cancer", New York: Alan R Liss, pp 205-220.

Pavone-Macaluso M, De Voogt HJ, Viggiano G, Barasolo E, Lardennois B, De Pauw M, Sylvester R (1986) Comparison of diethylstilbestrol, cyproterone acetate and medroxyprogesterone acetate in the treatment of advanced prostatic cancer: final analysis of a randomized phase III trial of the European Organization for Research on Treatment of Cancer Urological Group. The Journal of Urology 136:624-631.

Prout GR, Griffin PP, Daly JJ, Shipley WU (1981). Nodal involvement as prognostic indicator in prostatic carcinoma. The Journal of Urology (Suppl.) 17:72.

Schroeder FH (1984). Treatment response criteria for prostatic cancer. The Prostate 5:181-191.

Schroeder FH, Van der Werf-Messing B (1982). Prostate. In Halnan KE (ed): "Treatment of Cancer", London: Chapman and Hall, pp 475-493.

Smith PH, Suciu S, Robinson MRG, Richards B, Bastable JRG, Glashan RW, Bouffioux C, Lardennois B, Williams RE, De Pauw M, Sylvester R (1986). A comparison of the effect of diethylstilbestrol with low dose estramustine phosphate in the treatment of advanced prostatic cancer: final analysis of a phase III trial of the European Organization for Research on Treatment of Cancer. The Journal of Urology 136:619-623.

UICC (1985). "TNM-Atlas", Berlin: Springer-Verlag, pp 180-188.

Yagoda A, Watson RC, Natala RB, Barzell W, Sogani P, Grabstald H, Whitmore W (1979). A critical analysis of response criteria in patients with prostatic cancer treated with cis-diamminedichloride platinum II. Cancer 44:1553-1562.

EORTC Genitourinary Group Monograph 5: Progress
and Controversies in Oncological Urology II, pages 289–311
© 1988 Alan R. Liss, Inc.

IMMUNODIAGNOSIS AND IMMUNOIMAGING

William R. Fair, M.D.
Urology Service, Memorial
Sloan-Kettering Cancer Center
New York, New York 10021

The title of the afternoon's discussion could appropriately be expanded to include the topic of Immunoprognosis since much of the promise of the application of immunologic techniques to clinical medicine lies in the _potential_ of using these methods to establish the heterogeneous nature of neoplastic growth in the hope that the delineation of various immunophenotypic subsets of malignant tumors will identify malignant cells with very different biologic potentials and varying response to treatment. While the potential benefits of immunodiagnosis and immunotherapy are great, in actual fact the position of clinical immunology in the current practice of urologic oncology is "on the cusp", if you will, being poised between the limited demonstrable practical benefits achieved thus far and the unlimited potential for future application in diagnosis and therapy of genitourinary disease, including, but not limited to those in the domain of the urologic oncologist.

In the following discussion, We will attempt to review the current use of immunodiagnostic techniques in clinical practice, elaborate briefly on how this approach has furthered our understanding of the histochemistry of the normal nephron and urinary collecting system and confirmed the origin of renal cell carcinoma. I will also share with you some preliminary data on the use of monoclonal antibodies to detect serum antigens which appear to predict prognosis in patients with renal carcinoma. We will then move on to a discussion of the role of immunohistochemistry in determining the malignant or aggressive potential of urothelial cancers and the techniques of combining monoclonal antibody and flow cytometry technology in clinical application to predict biologic potential and treatment response in bladder cancer. This will be followed by a consideration of the current status of immunophenotyping as an indication of heterogenity in the cellular composition of urothelial tumors and the influence of the expression of blood group antigens in the normal and malignant cell. We will conclude our discussion of this complex and rapidly evolving subject with an update on the clinical and experimental results of immunotargeting - the attempt to image or treat malignancies utilizing modern immunologic techniques in an effort to develop a specific diagnostic or therapeutic probe.

I:

IMMUNODIAGNOSTIC TECHNIQUES CURRENTLY USEFUL IN UROLOGIC ONCOLOGY

1) Testes Cancer: Assays of serum alpha-fetoprotein (AFP) and beta-human chorionic gonadontrophrin (BHCG) are of vital importance in the management of patients with germ cell testicular tumors. Serum AFP, a product of mononuclear embryonal cells is elevated in as many as 75% of patients with non-seminomatous germ cell tumors, (NSGCT) but is not elevated in patients with seminomas except those relatively rare patients with liver regeneration as a result of metastatic disease (Javadpour, 1980). AFP is useful in detecting NSGCT even in patients with no clinically detectable evidence of embryonal cell carcinoma. BHCG is produced by syncytiotrophoblastic cells in embryonal cell carcinomas, seminomas, endodermal sinus tumors and choriocarcinomas. Although serum BHCG levels may be elevated in 20-60% of patients with NSGCT and 10% of patients with seminomas, high levels of BHCG are seen only in the presence of choriocarcinoma (Grossman, 1985; Javadpour, 1980).

In addition to their usefulness in detection and staging, the serum tumor markers also serve as prognostic indicators in testicular tumor patients; high levels of BHCG or AFP correlated with a poor therapeutic response (Vugrin, 1982) and the amount of metastatic disease present. (Vugrin, 1982)

At Memorial Sloan-Kettering Cancer Center (MSKCC), the serum lactic dehydrogenase has proved to be the most useful marker in determining the extent and progression in testicular cancer patients. A high LDH level indicates extensive metastatic disease and the LDH value, considered in conjunction with the numbers of metastatic lesions, has been utilized to construct a highly accurate mathematical formula to predict response to therapy. (Bosl, 1983)

Despite the indisputable value of serum markers in patients with advanced testicular cancers, they are, unfortunately of much less value in detecting patients with low stage disease - the very patients in whom serum markers are most needed. The current controversy over retroperitoneal lymph node dissection versus surveillance in clinical Stage I patients would be largely obviated by highly accurate serum markers to identify micro-metastatic disease in patients with no clinically obvious metastatic disease.

2) Prostatic Cancer: Serum acid phosphatase levels are useful in following patients with prostatic carcinoma. However, elevations of serum acid phosphatase (SAP) occur in a variety of conditions other than prostatic carcinoma and may be normal even with obvious metastatic disease.

In 1980, the report by Foti and Cooper (Foti, 1977) published in the New England Journal of Medicine created a great deal of excitement with the observation that 33% of Stage I patients and 79% of Stage II patients had an elevated serum acid phosphatase when measured by an radioimmunoassay technique. In patients with Stage C disease the marker was elevated in 71%; in

Stage D disease 92% of patients had an elevated acid phosphatase. In benign prostatic hyperplasia (BPH) only 6% had a false positive result. In an attempt to confirm this study a number of authors did similar studies. Table 1 gives our results in comparing the acid phosphatase level measured by both enzymatic and radioimmunoassay methods on the same sample. (Fair, 1982) Overall, only 29.7% of patients with documented carcinoma of the prostate had an increased serum acid phosphatase; one of sixteen (6.2%) Stage A patients had positive results. In Stage D disease, almost 35% of the patients had a normal acid phosphatase in the presence of widespread metastases.

We also considered the accuracy of the serum acid phosphatase as a diagnostic test. When the upper limit of normal was set to exclude 92.5% of patients with BPH, thereby accepting a false positive rate of 7.5%, only 31 of 113 patients (27.4%) in whom the enzymatic method was used to measure acid phosphatase had an elevation of the enzyme in the serum. Of 118 patients in whom the radioimmunoassay was used to measure acid phosphatase, the results were virtually identical with 35% of 118 (29.7%) having an elevated value.

In an effort to assess the utility of acid phosphatase in detecting advanced disease, various subsets of patients were examined. It appeared that acid phosphatase was more valuable in detecting advanced stage disease (Stages C and D) in black males compared with white. Sixteen of 20 blacks (80%) with Stage C or higher carcinoma of the prostate had an elevated acid phophatase, compared to only 14 of 41 (34%) Caucasian males. Thus, it may be that acid phosphatase is of slightly greater value in the black population in assessing the extent of the disease.

In those patients with the highest degrees of clinical suspicion, that is, those admitted to the hospital for a prostatic biopsy, the serum acid phophatase value was minimally helpful in predicting the biopsy results. Of 203 patients hospitalized for a prostatic biopsy, serum acid

TABLE 1

ACID PHOSPHATASE IN UNTREATED PATIENTS

| STAGE | # ELEVATED ASSAYS (%) | |
	ENZYMATIC	RIA-PAP
A	1/16 (6.2)	1/16 (6.2)
B	1/32 (3.7)	3/35 (8.6)
C	10/36 (27.8)	13/37 (35.1)
D	17/25 (68.0)	17/26 (65.4)
UNSTAGED	2/4 (50.0)	1/4 (25.0)
TOTALS	31/113 (27.4%)	35/118 (29.7%)

*Adapted from Fair et al, J Urol 128:735, 1982.

phosphatase was elevated in only 24 of 61 in whom the biopsy was positive (39.3%). False positive elevations were detected in 11 of 142 men in whom the biopsy was negative (7%). Overall the positive predictive value was 69% and the negative predictive value 75%; the test was of little value as a screen for carcinoma of the prostate.

A number of other studies were done with the radioimmunoassay measurement of acid phosphatase in an attempt to confirm the early results . The work of Bruce et al (Bruce, 1981; Griffiths, 1980) and our own data, failed to document that the radioimmunoassay of prostatic acid phosphatase was of significant benefit in the diagnosis of prostatic cancer.
Although acid phosphatase is of little value as a screening test in the general population, a persistently elevated acid phosphatase may provide significant clinical information in the individual patient. In a study by Whitsel, Donohue, and colleagues (Whitesel, 1982) the results of acid phosphatase determination in patients with carcinoma of the prostate undergoing pelvic lymph node dissection were assessed. Of the 343 patients, 318 had a negative pre-operative acid phosphatase. Of these, 70 (22%) were found to have positive lymph nodes. Of the 25 patients with a elevated acid phosphatase pre-operatively, 15 were found to have positive lymph nodes; in 10 of these, the lymph node dissection was negative for metastatic disease. When these 25 patients were followed for 2 years, 10 of 12 patients with positive lymph nodes had evidence of distant metastatic disease. Therefore, 83% of patients with elevated acid phosphatase, even in the presence of negative lymph nodes on pelvic node dissection, can be expected to develop metastatic disease within 2 years. The authors stressed that the presence of a persistently elevated acid phosphatase is strong evidence of metastatic disease and radical attempts at local cure in this population should be discouraged.

Recently, prostatic specific antigen (PSA or PA), a chemically and immunobiologically well defined glycoprotein distinct from PAP has been found to be more valuable than PAP in monitoring patients for disease recurrence; the absolute level of PA also correlated with the positive predictive value of the tests. (Papsidero, 1981)

While prostate specific antigen may indeed be prostate specific, it is not specific for prostate carcinoma, with more than 60% of patients with BPH having elevations in PSA.

A more recent study has indicated that prostate specific antigen may be of some value in the biochemical staging of prostatic disease. In a study from Roswell Park (Killian, 1985) the probable predictive value of PSA in detecting metastatic disease was correlated with the prostatic antigen level in the serum. When the PSA level was in the normal range, only 2/26 patients were found to have metastatic disease. However, when the prostatic antigen level was elevated more than 20 times above the normal level, 22/25 patients (88%) were found to have metastatic disease. A similar correlation was noted in patients followed for clinical recurrence.

In the group remaining in remission, the prostatic antigen level stayed in the normal range in approximately 80% of patients. However, in those patients with a clinically detectable recurrence, prostatic specific antigen was elevated in more than 90% ; in many cases the PSA rose well in advance of the clinically detected relapse. Even more recently, Stamey and colleagues (Stamey, 1987) have shown an excellent correlation between PSA levels and prognosis.

    3)   **Renal Cancer:** Several recent communications have reported a variety of candidate substances for monitoring patients with various renal disorders. Serum levels of urokinase - Type plasminogen activator were found to be increased in renal cancer by Kircheimer and colleagues (Kirchheimer, 1985) Tolkoff-Rubin and associates. (Tolkoff-Rubin, 1986) noted increased urinary excretion of brush border protein in patients with benign nephropathy and have utilized this observation successfully to monitor rejection in renal transplant recipients. The preliminary report by Klotz and associates of the relationship of The Uro-4 antigen to the eventual fate of patients operated on for renal carcinoma is particularly interesting. Increased levels of Uro-4 antigen were found in patients with higher stage renal cell carcinomas and appeared to be directly related to prognosis. (Klotz, 1985) At present the clinical relevance of these tests in urologic oncology is limited since all may be elevated in other common non-neoplastic conditions.

In summary then, with the exception of testicular and prostatic cancer, there is little or no widely accepted clinical applicability of immunodiagnostic techniques in other urologic malignancies although, as discussed below, monoclonal antibody (mAb) technology promises to unfold additional applications in the future.

The Promise of Monoclonal Antibodies:

Over the past decade, exciting advances in technology have occurred following the seminal observations of Kohler and Milstein (Kohler, 1975) which led to the wide scale production of monoclonal antibodies directed at a single antigen. This technique allows maximum utilization of the sensitivity and specificity of the immune system. Unlike conventional anti-serum which consists of a heterogeneous mixture of antibody against a multitude of different antigens, the hybridoma technology provides the opportunity to produce huge amounts of antibody in a purified state and holds great promise for major advances in immunodiagnosis and immunotherapy. To date, at least 20 different monoclonal antibodies have been raised against various parts of the human nephron. The differentiation antigens detected by these monoclonal antibodies constitute a series of glycoproteins characteristic of different cell types. The antigens recognized by these monoclonal antibodies represent an immunohistologic dissection of the human nephron and have a broad range of potential applications in studying embryogenesis and pathogenesis of a variety of kidney diseases, both neoplastic and non-neoplastic. Figure 1 illustrates the immuno-anatomy of the human urinary system defined by 5 mouse monoclonal antibodies. (Cordon-Cardo, 1984) The intensity of the staining pattern is indicated by the broadness of the band. These antibodies are specific for a single differentiation antigen, that is, an antigen expressed only by cells of a particular lineage or during a particular phase of development. Thus, Uro-1 (J 143) detects antigens found only in the human glomerulus and urothelium. In contrast, Uro-2 expresses a strong staining pattern in the glomerulus and stains cells of the proximal tubule less intensely. Uro-2 (S 4) is not found in the urothelium. Uro-3 (F 23) is restricted to proximal tubular cells. Thus, by differential staining patterns, it is possible to determine the origin of cells in specimens that may not be readily identifiable by standard histologic means. As a result of similar studies, the observation that renal cell carcinoma arises from the proximal convoluted tubual has been confirmed. (Bander, 1987)

By studying the phenotypic expression of renal cancers, Bander and associates (Bander, 1986) have found the expression of the gp160/gp120r phenotype to correlate with disease progression. Whether additional experience will allow an accurate delineation of tumor subsets into those requiring more aggressive therapy and those in whom less radical therapy, such as partial nephrectomy may be considered, awaits further experience.

IMMUNOPATHOLOGY AS AN INDICATOR OF TUMOR HETEROGENEITY OR TREATMENT RESPONSE

Table 2 lists the bladder monoclonal antibodies (mAbs) currently useful at Memorial Sloan-Kettering Cancer Center. (Fradet, 1986) T-16 which recognizes a 42,000-48,000 glycoprotein is

FIGURE 1:

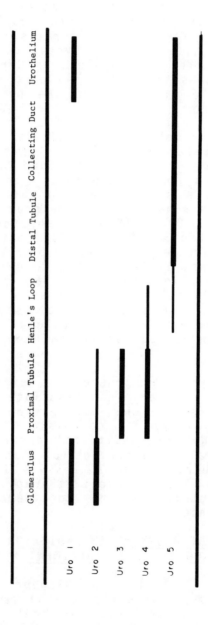

With permission: Cordon-Cardo, C. et al
J Histochem CytoChem 32:1035, 1984

TABLE 2:

ANTIBODIES DETECTING CELL SURFACE ANTIGENS OF TRANSITIONAL CELL EPITHELIUM (22,23)

ANTIBODY	Ig CLASS	IMMUNOGEN	ANTIGEN CHARACTERISTICS	EXPRESSION		
				KIDNEY	NORMAL UROTHELIUM	OTHER CELLS
OM-5	IgG$_1$	Fresh papilloma	Not Known	Neg.	50-60%	Neg.
T-43	IgG$_1$	T24	85gp	Neg.	Neg.	Yes
T-138	Igm	T24	25 gp	Neg.	Neg.	Yes
T-23	Igm	Normal kidney	Not known	Neg.	Neg.	Yes
T-16	IgG$_{2b}$	T24	48,42 gp	distal & collecting tubules	Yes	Yes
T-87	IgG$_1$	T24	60 gp	distal & collecting tubules	Yes	Yes
J-143	IgG$_1$	253-J	140,30 gp	glomerulus	Yes	Yes

expressed on normal urothelial cells. In contrast T-43 has no expression on normal transitional cells but does appear on some invasive urothelial cancers. The OM-5 antibody is particularly interesting in that it is positively expressed in specimens of superficial bladder cancer and 50-60% of normal urothelial specimens. Thus, differential expression of OM-5 and T-43 antigen may have prognostic implications; if further experience bears out this hypothesis, it may be prudent to initiate early aggressive treatment in tumors expressing antigens to these antibodies rather than waiting for conventional indicators of invasion to appear.

Fradet and colleagues (Fradet, 1986a), have combined DNA flow cytometry (FCM) and monoclonal antibody technology to refine the predictions of FCM. In these studies, diploid tumors with low levels of T138 did not progress. In contrast, lesions with high T138 levels usually progressed to an invasive tumor, metastases, or death, regardless of whether the tumor was diploid or aneuploid. Chopin et al (Chopin, 1985) utilized mAbs to identify malignant and premalignant exfoliated cells from human bladder wash specimens. Using an immunoperoxidase staining technique, the diagnostic accuracy of mAbs was similiar to Papanicolaou staining, in controls and patients with higher grade transitional cell carcinomas, and provided specific morphologic criteria not possible by conventional cytology studies. One-third of cases of superficial low grade transitional cell carcinomas also reacted with the G4 and E7 mAbs which may indicate a distinct subpopulation of these tumors. At present, the prognostic or therapeutic implications of these observations are unknown. Ramaekers and colleagues in the Netherlands (Ramaekers, 1983) have utilized similar FCM - monoclonal antibody studies to gate DNA analysis, utilizing monoclonal antibodies to cytokeratins and intermediate filaments. These authors have shown that mAbs to cytokeratin can provide an indication of the processes involved in neoplastic changes in bladder and renal tumors and as a means of studying the relationship of tumor cells to their normal counterparts.

A particularly appealing potential use of mAb technology is in predicting response to therapy. Huffman and colleagues (Huffman, 1985) utilized mAbs to detect a urothelial differentiation antigen in exfoliated bladder cells of patients receiving intravesical Bacillus Calmette-Guerin (BCG). Prior to BCG treatment, exfoliated cells reacted with OM-5 , a highly restricted differentiation antigen found in approximately 50% of samples of normal urothelium, and frequently and predominantly expressed on the cells of superficial bladder cancers, in 13 of 15 cases. Following BCG treatment 4 patients whose urothelial cells were OM-5 positive before treatment reverted to negative. Five of 9 patients showing persistence of OM-5 positive cells after therapy had recurrent tumor on biopsy and 2 of the remaining 4 had a positive cytology, but no obvious tumor, during the median follow up of 13 months. The 4 patients without detectable antigen positive cells remained free of disease. (median follow-up period was 12 months).

BLOOD GROUP ANTIGENS:

In recent years, interest in the ABH and Lewis antigen expression in normal tissues and tumors has increased as a result of several clinicopathologic observations:

1) Deletion of the antigens of the ABH system in human urinary bladder tumor. (Emmott, 1979; Coon, 1985; Coon, 1981)
2) Evidence that loss of the ABH antigen in cells of the urinary bladder and larynx may be an early event in malignant transformation (Lin, 1977).
3) Elevated levels of Lewis antigen have been reported in the serum of patients with certain epithelial tumors such as colon carcinoma (Koprowski, 1981)
4) The observation that certain of these antigens appear to act as oncofetal and developmental

markers (Cooper, 1980; Ghazizade, 1985; Gooi, 1981).
5) Incompatible blood group expression in some neoplasms. (Hattori, 1981)

Blood group antigens are carbohydrate structures formed by the sequential addition of saccharides to the carbohydrate side chains of both lipids and proteins. (Fig. 2) The genetic control of the expression of these structures is related to genes controlling antigen synthesis and another gene locus controlling expression in bodily secretions and cells other than red blood cells. As a result of the variance in antigen expression, the term "secretor" and "non-secretor" indicate the ability of an individual to secrete these substances in the saliva. (Race, 1975) Secretor individuals are categorized by ABH, Lewis b and Lewis y antigens in their saliva; non-secretors produce Lewis a and Lewis x. (Sakamoto, 1984) The Lewis antigens are not synthesized by the red cells but are absorbed onto the erythrocytes from the plasma. Lewis antigens are, in general, found in plasma, secretions and secretor epithelial cells. (Sakamoto, 1984; Cartron, 1980) Cordon-Cordo et al (Cordon-Cardo, 1986) found that individuals could be subdivided into 2 categories according to the immunostaining patterns observed. Secretors generally express precursor type 1, H, Le^b and Le^y antigens on the epithelial cells of the thin loop of Henle and collecting ducts in the deep medulla, as well as on the urothelium. Non-secretor individuals either minimally express or totally lack expression of H, Le^b and Le^y in the epithelial cells of the collecting ducts and urothelium. Due to the variable expression of the H antigen and Lewis determinants depending on secretor status, reports of observations of antigenetic loss should be re-evaluated correlating secretors status of the individual to antigenic determinants.

Monoclonal antibodies to cell surface antigens have dramatically illustrated the heterogeneous nature of most urothelial tumors.

If this tumor heterogenity is reflected in a similiar variability in biologic behavior and response to therapy among tumors that appear histologically identical the potential for more accurate estimation of prognosis and assessment of treatment is obvious. Figures 3A and 3B represents bladder tumors from 2 different patients. Both tumors were poorly differentiated and deelply invasive. Both patients were treated with MVAC chemotherapy prior to cystectomy. Patient 86-95-10 (FIgure 3A) had a complete response to the chemotherapeutic agents while patient 85-22-114 had absolutely no response noted. Although clinically and histologically virtually indentical a comparision of the immunophenotype is particularly revealing and indicates a differences not appreciated by histologic parameters only the tumor in FIgure 3A had a positive reaction to Le^b and Le^x; both of these antigens were not observed on the tumor of the patient in Figure 3B. Additionally, a difference in the reativity to A and B suface antigens was also noted.

Whether these immunophenotypic changes are related to the differential response to chemotherapy is not possible to state with certainty but the difference in therapeutic response is reflected in the variance in immunohistology and reveals the variability of histologically similar tumors in a manner not formerly possible.

Indeed, one can envision that in the not too distant future, the current tumor grading systems based previously on histologic pattern recognition will yield to a more precise mapping of the immunophenotype of a given tumor.

In contrast to the large number of mAbs against urothelial cell surface antigens, similiar antibodies against prostatic tissue or prostatic carcinoma are relatively few. Wright and colleagues have described a series of characterized incompletely mAbs directed against both benign and malignant prostatic epithelial cells.(Starling, 1984) Webb et al (Webb, 1986) and Ware et al (Ware, 1982) generated a series of mAbs by immunizing mice with the prostatic carcinoma cell lines PC-3, DU-I45, and LnCAP. These authors also described a unique approach to prostatic tumor targeting by producing a hybrid monoclonal immunotoxin (HT) linking immune spleen cells secreting antibody to ricin A chain (RAC) to a hybridoma secreting prostate directed mAb, alpha Pro-15 - resulting in a hybrid monoclonal with dual specificity linked by a conventional antigen-antibody reaction and not by a chemical linkage. The investigators felt that the resulting HIT-RAC conjugate would not interfere with the biological function of either the antibody or the toxin. This intriguing idea has yet to be tested clinically.

M. Bazinet and co-workers at Memorial Sloan-Kettering Cancer Center have generated 2 mAbs utilizing human prostatic cancer tissue as the immunogen. P25.91, an IgG_2a class antibody and p25.48 an IgG_3 class antibody appear, on the basis of preliminary testing, to be expressed only on maligant prostatic epithelial cells and not on epithelial cells in samples of benign prostatic hyperplasia or other non-prostatic tissue, although much more extensive specificity testing is currently underway. (Bazinet, 1986)

IMMUNOTARGETING:

The clinical application of labeled monoclonal antibodies in attempts to label and/or treat tumors utilizing immunologic techniques has been primarily focused on the area of renal cancer. This is not surprising since metastatic renal cell carcinoma is essentially resistant to all current therapy and has been the subject of intense investigational efforts utilizing various immunotherapeutic approaches. Also, a relatively large number of renal mAbs are available which recognize proximal tubular cell surface antigens and have facilitated research in this area.

Early efforts at developing mAbs for therapy were fueled by the hope that a **"tumor specific"** mAb might be found which would be directed against antigens found only on the tumor cell surface and would not recognize normal cells of the same or other histologic types. To date, no **"tumor specific"** antigens, found exclusively on malignant tissue, have been shown to exist. However, as discussed above, a number of "tumor associated" antigens in renal carcinoma have been identified. Those tumor associated antigens are not unique to malignant cells and are also found on normal renal proximal tubules. In addition, there is considerable heterogenity within tumors and not every cell of the tumor expresses the same antigen. Differential expression of antigens between the primary tumor and metastatic deposits have been observed. This heterogeneity makes it extremely unlikely that any single mAb will be of universal benefit in immunoimaging or immunotherapy, although mixtures of mAbs or polyclonal antibodies may be considered for use.

Chiou, Lange and associates (Chiou, 1985; Lightner, 1986) reported consistent imaging of renal cell carcinoma (RCCa) xenografts in nude mice usings an IgG_1 mAb (AGH) reactive against most RCCa's, the proximal tubules of normal and fetal kidneys and some breast and colon cancers. In these studies, the implanted RCCa was imaged without background subtraction when AGH was coupled to ^{125}I, ^{121}I or ^{111}IN. On the basis of the results obtained within the immunoimaging studies, the Minnesota group explored immunotherapy utilizing ^{131}I labeled AGH mAb.(Lightner, 1986) Dosimetry calculations revealed good localization of the radiation with a greater than 20:1 uptake of radioactive iodine found in the tumor as compared to other tissues. In a small number of animals treated, significant reduction in tumor size (60%) was observed.

However, it is not surprising than the excellent results utilizing mAbs directed against human tissues implanted into the mouse have not been confirmed in metastatic RCCa in situ. Since a human xenograft in the animal is the only tissue likely to take up a mAb directed against an antigen found only on human tissue, one might expect little or no competition from other mouse tissue. Obviously such an "exclusive uptake" would not exist in human tumors.

Preliminary studies utilizing mAbs to treat metastatic renal cell cancer in humans at both Minnesota and MSKCC are underway. In New York, the Phase I trial of mAb therapy in RCCa has enrolled 17 patients on an escalating dosage schedule. To date, 3 of 17 have had significant partial remissions of disease in metastatic (Ueda, 1981) sites. In these studies 1 of 3 mAbs (S4, S22, F23) was selected for therapy based on the results of preliminary tissue typing to determine which of the mAbs bind to cellular antigens expressed by the tumor.

CONCLUSION:

While the potential for the development of new diagnostic and therapeutic strategies utilizing immunologic techniques appears unlimited, much arduous work remains to be done before clinical immunoimaging and immunotherapy of genito-urinary malignancies becomes a reality. However, tremendous studies have occurred in expanding our knowledge of monoclonal antibody technology and in utilizing this advance to understand the basic biologic behavior of normal and malignant cells.

We are now able to demonstrate, by immunophenotyping, the heterogenity that exists within tumors that appear histologically identical. The prospects are indeed exciting to contemplate that such phenotypic differences will identify biologic tumor subsets of different biologic potential and may predict therapeutic response. Clearly a new era appears to be at hand and the already exciting advances in immunodiagnosis and immunotargeting will prove to be only the first steps along the road.

REFERENCES

Bander NH. Monoclonal antibodies. State of the Art April (1987). J Urol 137:603-612.

Bander NH (1986). Personal communication.

Blaszczyk M, Cote RJ, Daly ME, Old LJ (1986). Specificity analysis of mouse monoclonal antibodies reactive with prostatic cancer. J Urol 135:111a-abstract 32.

Bosl GJ, Geller NL, Cirrincione C, Vogelzang NJ, Kennedy BJ, Whitmore WF, Jr, Vugrin D, Scher H, Nisselbaum J, Golbey RB, (1983). Multivariate analyses of prognostic variables in patients with metastatic testicular cancer. Cancer Res: 3403-3407.

Bruce AW, Mahan DE, Sullivan LD, Goldenberg L (1981). The significance of prostatic acid phosphatase in adenocarcinoma of the prostate. J Urol 125:357-360.

Cartron JP, Mulet C, Bauvois B, Rahuel C, Salmon C (1980). ABH and Lewis glycosyltransferases in human red cells, lymphocytes and platelets. Blood trans immuno hematol 23:271-xxx.

Chiou RK, Vessela RL, Elson MK, Clayman RV, Gonzalez-Campoy JM, Klicka MJ, Shafer RV, Lange PH (1985). Localization of human renal cell carcinoma xenografts with a tumor preferential monoclonal antibody. Cancer Res 45:6140-6146.

Chopin DK, deKernion JB, Rosenthal DL, Fahey JL (1985). Monoclonal antibodies against transitional cell carcinoma for detection of malignant urothelial cells and bladder washing. J Urol 134:260-265.

Coon JS, McCall A, Miller AW III, Farrow GM, Weinstein RS (1985). Expression of blood group related antigens in carcinoma in situ of the urinary bladder. Cancer 797-804.

Coon JS, Weinstein RS (1981). Detection of ABH tissue isoantigens by immunoperoxidase methods in normal and neoplastic urothelium: Comparison with the erythrocyte adherance method. Amer J Clin Path 76:163-171.

Cooper HS, Cox J, Patchef AS (1980). Immunohistologic study of blood group substancies in
polyps of the distal colon: Expression of a fetal
antigen. Amer J Clin Path 73:345-350.

Cordon-Cardo C, Bander NH, Fradet Y, Finstadt CL,
Whitmore WF, Jr, Lloyd KO, Oettgen HF, Melamed
MR, Old LJ (1984). Immunoanatomic dissection of
the human urinary tract on monoclonal antibodies.
J Histochem and Cytochem 32:1035-1040.

Cordon-Cardo C, Lloyd KO, Finstadt CL, McGroarty
ME, Reuter VE, Bander NH, Old LJ, Melamed MR
(1986). Immunoanatomic distribution of blood
group antigens in the human urinary tract-
influence of secretor status. Laboratory
Investigation 55:444-454.

Emmott RC, Javadpour N, Bergman SM, Soares T
(1979). Correlation of the cell surface
antigens with stage and grade in cancer of the
bladder. J Urol 121:37-39.

Ernst C, Atkinson B, Wysocka M, Blaszczyk M, Herlyn
M, Sears H, Steplewski Z, Koprowski H (1984).
Monoclonal antibody localization of Lewis
antigens in fixed tissue. Lab Invest 50:394-400.

Fair WR, Heston WDW, Kadmon D, Crane DB, Catalona
WJ, Ladenson JH, McDonald JM, Noll BW, Harvey G
(1982) Prostatic cancer, acid phosphatase,
creatinine kinase-BB and race: A prospective
study. J Urol 128:735-738.

Foti AG, Cooper GF, Herschman H, Malvaez RR (1977).
Detection of prostatic cancer by solid phase
radioimmunoassay of serum prostatic acid
phosphatase. N Eng J Med 297:11357-1361

Fradet Y, Cordon-Cardo C, Thompson T, Daly ME,
Whitmore WF, Jr, Lloyd KO, Melamed MR, Old LJ
(1986). Cell surface antigens of human bladder
cancer defined by mouse monoclonal antibodies.
Proceedings Natl Acad Sci USA 81:224-228.

Fradet Y, Cordon-Cardo C, Whitmore WF, Jr, Melamed
MR, Old LJ (1986). Cell surface antigens of
human bladder tumors: Definition of tumor
subsets by monoclonal antibodies in correlation
of growth characteristics. Cancer Res
46:5183-5188.

Ghazizadeh M, Kagawa S, Kurokawa K (1985).
Immunohistochemical studies of human renal cell
carcinomas for ABO(H) blood group antigens, T
antigen-like substance and carcinoembryonic
antigen. J of Urol 133:762-766.

Gooi H, Feizi T, Kapadia A, Knowles BB, Solter D,
Evans MJ (1981). Stage specific embryonic
antigen involves alpha 1 3 fucosylated type 2
blood group change. Nature (London) 292:156-158.

Griffiths JC (1980). Prostate specific acid
phosphatase: Re-evaluation of radioimmunoassay
in diagnosing prostatic disease. Clin Chem
26:433-435.

Grossman HB (1985). Tumor Markers in Urology.
Sem Urol 3, pp 10-17 .

Hattori H, Uemura K, Taketomi T (1981). Glycolipids of gastric cancer, the presence of blood
group A-active glycolipids in cancer tissues
from blood group O patients. Biochem Biophys
Acta 666:361-369.

Huffman JL, Fradet Y, Cordon-Cardo C, Herr HW,
Pinsky CN, Oettgen HF, Old LJ, Whitmore WF, Jr,
Melamed MR (1985). Effect of intravesical
Bacillus Calmette-Guerin on detection of a
urothelial differentiation antigen in exfoliated
cells of carcinoma in situ of the human urinary
bladder. Cancer Res 45:5201-5204.

Javadpour N (1980). Management of seminoma based
on tumor markers. Urology Clinic North America
7:773-780.

Javadpour N (1980). Significance of elevated
serum Alpha Feto Protein (AFP) in seminoma.
Cancer 45:2166-2168.

Killian CS, Yang N, Emrich Lj, Vargas FP, Kuriyama
M, Wang MC, Slack, NH, Papsidero LD, Murphy GP,
Chu TM and Investigators of the National
Prostatic Cancer Project (1985). Prognostic
importance of prostate specific antigen for
monitoring patients with stages B_2 to D_1
prostate cancer. Cancer Res 45:886-891.

Kirchheimer JC, Pfluger H, Hienert G, Binder BR
(1985). Increased urokinase activity ratio in
human renal cell carcinoma. Int J Cancer
35:737-741.

Klotz LH, Bander NH, Thompson RE, Rubin RR, Whitmore WF, Jr, Old LJ (1985). Staging and monitoring of renal cell carcinoma (RCC) by serum assay for proximal tubular antigen. J Urol 133:155a-abstract 165.

Kohler G, Milstein C (1975). Continuous cultures of fused cells secreting antibody of predefined specificity. Nature 256:495-497.

Koprowski H, Herlyn N, Steplewski Z, Sears HF (1981). Specific antigen and serum of patients with colon carcinoma. Science 212:53-54.

Lightner DJ, Vesseala Rl, Chiou RK, Palme DF, Lange PH (1986). Immunotherapy for renal cell carcinoma: Recent results. World J Urol 4:222-227.

Lin F, Lin PI, McGregor DH (1977). Isoantigens a, b, and h in morphologically normal mucosa and in carcinoma of the larynx. Amer J Clin Path 68:372.

Papsidero LD, Kuriyama M, Wang MC, Horoszewicz J, Leong SS, Valenzuela L, Murphy GP, Chu TM (1981). Prostate Antigen: A marker for human prostate epithelial cells. J Natl Cancer Inst 66:37-42.

Race RR, Sanger R, (1975). Blood group antigens in man (6th edition): Oxford, Blackwell Scientific Publications.

Ramaekers FCS, Puts JJG, Moesker O, Kant A, Huysnans A, Haag D, Jap PHK, Herman CJ, Vooijs GP (1983). Antibodies to intermediate phylum proteins in the immunohistochemical identification of human tumors: An overview. Histo Chem J 15:691-713.

Sakamoto J, Yin BT, Lloyd KO (1984). Analysis of the expression of H Lewis, X, Y, and precursor blood group determinants in saliva and red cells using a panel of mouse monoclonal antibodies. Mol Immunol 21:1093-1098.

Stamey TA, Yang N, Hay AR, McNeal JE, Freiha FS, Redwine E (1987). Prostate-specific antigen as a serum marker for adenocarcinoma of the prostate. N Eng J Med 317:909-916.

Starling JJ, Beckett ML, Wright DL, Jr, (1984). In monoclonal antibodies in cancer edited by Wright DL, Jr p253-286 New York Marcel Dekker Inc.

Tolkoff-Rubin NE, Cosimi AB, Delmonico FL, Russell PS, Thompson RE, Piper DJ, Hansen WP, Bander NH, Finstad CL, Cordon-Cardo C, Klotz LH, Old LJ, Rubin LH. (1986). Diagnosis of tubular injury in renal transplant patients by a urinary assay for a proximal tubular antigen, the adenosine-deaminase-binding protein. Transplantation 41:593-597.

Ueda R Ogata SI, Morrissey DM, Finstaldt CL, Szkudlarek J, Whitmore WF, Jr, Oettgen HF, Lloyd KO, Old LJ (1981). Cell surface antigens of human renal cancer defined by mouse monoclonal antibodies: Identification of tissue specific kidney glycoproteins. Proceedings National Academy of Science USA 78:5122-5126

Vugrin D, Friedman A, Whitmore WF, Jr (1984). Correlation of serum tumor markers in advanced germ cell tumors with responses to chemotherapy and surgery. Cancer 53:1440-1445.

Vugrin D, Whitmore WF, Jr, Nisselbaum J et.al. (1982). Correlation of serum tumor markers and lymphangiography degrees of nodal involvement and surgical stage II testis cancer. J Urol 127:683-684.

Ware JL, Paulson DF, Parks SF, Webb KS (1982). Production of monoclonal antibody alpha Pro3 recognizing a human prostatic carcinomic antigen. Cancer Res. 42-1215-1222.

Webb K, Ware JL, Paulson DF (1986). A review: Prostate monoclonal antibodies-the magic bullet. World J Urol 4:193-199.

Whitesel JA, Donohue RE, Mani JH, Fauver HE, Augspurger RR, Biber RJ, Scanavino DJ, Pfister RR, May (1982). Acid phosphatase. Its influence on pelvic lymph node dissection. Abstract 236 American Urological Association, Kansas City, MO.

EORTC Genitourinary Group Monograph 5: Progress
and Controversies in Oncological Urology II, pages 313-326
© 1988 Alan R. Liss, Inc.

BIOLOGICAL RESPONSE MODIFIERS IN RENAL CANCER

R. Ackermann

Department of Urology, University of Düsseldorf,
D-4000 Düsseldorf, Federal Republic of Germany

Biological response modifiers are a heterogeneous group of agents which differ from each other in many ways. Isolation, purification and characterization, and eventually mass production of many of these substances are the result of enormous advances in the field of molecular biology. Nucleic acid sequencing, protein sequencing and synthesis, and cloning of individual genes required to obtain a sufficient amount of highly purified products of the mammalian genome for analysis, are areas which should be mentioned in this context. The development of mass cell culture techniques, and the hybridoma technology, which allows the production of monoclonal antibodies, were basic requirements for the isolation and purification of these agents and for the definition of their chemical, physical, and biological properties. The progress in many of these areas is closely related to advances in computer technology.

The application of biological response modifiers in cancer treatment intends to interfere with the complex bilateral interactions between host and tumor in order to enable the host to control the disease. Several approaches are conceivable (Oldham, 1986).
1. Augmentation of the host defense by administering cells, natural biological or synthetic derivates as effectors or mediators of an antitumor response.
2. Increase of antitumor response through the restauration of effector mechanisms and/or decrease of deleterious host reactions.
3. Augmentation of antitumor response with modified tumor cells or vaccines, or increase of tumor cell sensitivity to an existing response.

4. Decrease of malignant transformation and/or increase of differentiation of tumor cells.
5. Increase of host tolerance to cytotoxic treatment modalities.

It is obvious that the concept of biological response modification comprises more than the conventional approaches of immunotherapy. Biotherapy is probably the term which may describe the various aspects more properly.

Biological response modifiers have been used in the treatment of metastatic renal cell carcinoma for two reasons. Due to the observation that spontaneous regression of metastases following tumor nephrectomy occurs in a small number of patients it is believed that renal cell carcinoma is particularly susceptible to biological treatment modalities. Clinical studies with biological response modifiers have been further stimulated by the fact that conventional therapy is usually ineffective in metastatic renal cell carcinoma. Earlier studies with BCG, Corynebacterium parvum, transfer factor and levamisole should be mentioned although no beneficial effects on patients have been observed. More recent approaches are listed in Table 1.

Table 1. Recent Approaches of Biological Response Modification in Renal Cancer

---

- Immune RNA
- Interleukin-2 (IL-2) and lymphokine-activated killer cells (LAK)
- Modified tumor cells and vaccines
- Tumor necrosis factor (TNF)
- Thymosin Fraction 5

The application of immune RNA is based on the experimental observation that RNA extracted from lymphocytes which have been exposed to specific antigens is capable of transferring specific immunological activity into non-immune lymphocytes (Mannick and Egdahl, 1962). Furthermore, there is experimental evidence that immune RNA may magnify a tumor directe immune response (Ramming and Pilch, 1971). In addition to that it has also been reported that extracted xenogeneic immune RNA still contains the injected antigen resembling an antigen RNA complex which may be highly immunogenic in comparison to the antigen alone. Basically, tumor cell suspensions or tumor extracts have been injected into animals. Following sensitization, RNA was extracted from the stimulated lymphocytes and administered repeatedly by intracutaneous injection over many weeks. DeKernion and Ramming (1976) reported minor responses in 8 out of 23 patients. The lack of any detectable, efficient antitumor response in this study has been attributed to a possible inactivation of the injected xenogeneic immune RNA by the patient's enzymes. The possible interference was eliminated in the study reported by Richie and coworkers (1984), who treated in vitro autologous lymphocytes obtained by leucophoresis with the extracted xenogeneic immune RNA. One complete response and one partial response with a duration of 18 and 8 months respectively, were observed in this small series. This approach has not been adopted in spite of the significant antitumoral response in 2 patients.

Particular interest has been focused on the administration of interferons (IFN) as treatment of metastatic renal cell carcinoma. Interferons are considered to be the prototype of a biological response modifier. According to their biological chemical and antigeneic properties, interferons can be devided in 3 distinct types: alpha-, beta- and gamma-interferons. It is well known that all 3 types of interferons have antiviral, immunomodulating and antiproliferative properties. This has been clearly shown in many experimental and clinical investigations. The antiproliferative activity requires the expression of IFN-receptors on the tumor cell surface which are necessary for the binding of IFN-molecules, and subsequent internalization of the complex. This is followed by the induction of several intracellular enzyme systems which effect macromolecular activities and protein synthesis. Alpha- and beta-interferons share the same receptor whereas the receptor for gamma-interferons is different.

In most of the clinical studies either natural or recombinant alpha-interferons were tested. The number of evaluable patients in each series is usually small except for the studies reported by Kimura (1984) and by deKernion (1983) respectively (Table 2). A summarizing evaluation of the reported studies is almost impossible as many of the trials have been updated with the time. Some of the publications do not include cases which have been reported earlier while those are included in other reports although this is not specifically mentioned. The analysis of treatment results of more than 350 patients with metastatic renal cell carcinoma treated with various types of alpha-interferon, demonstrates that a complete regression of metastatic lesions is a rare event occurring in only 4 patients (Kimura, 1984; deKernion et al, 1983; Kempf et al, 1986; Kirkwood et al, 1983; Krown et al, 1983; Marumo et al, 1984; Muss et al, 1984; Neidhart, 1984; Otto et al, 1985; Queseda et al, 1983; Vugrin et al, 1984).

Table 2. Interferon Therapy in Renal Cell Cancer

Author (year)	Interferon (type)	No. of pts. (evaluable)	Remission CR/PR
deKernion et al (1983)	HuIFN (Le)	47 (43)	1/6
Kempf et al (1984)	rIFN-a2	9	0/1
		26	0/2
Kimura (1984)	HuIFN (Ly)	56	0/11
Kirkwood et al (1985)	HuIFN (Le)	14	1/2
		16	0/0
Krown et al (1983)	rIFN-a (A)	27 (19)	0/2
Marumo et al (1984)	HuIFN (Ly)	18	0/1
Muss et al (1984)	rIFN-a	10 (7)	0/0
Neidhart et al (1984)	HuIFN (Ly)	33	0/5
		23	0/4
		11	0/2
Otto et al (1987)	rIFN-a2	33	1/8
Quesada et al (1985)	rIFN-a (A)	15	0/0
		15	0/4
		26	1/7
Vugrin et al (1985)	HuIFN (Ly)	22 (21)	0/3

The rate of partial regression appears to be variable within the range of 0-20% of the cases. Apart from the fact that in the various studies different interferons have been administered the evaluation of clinical experience is further complicated by important differences in the route of administration and the schedule of the protocol (single and total doses of IFN).

In addition, studies with alpha-interferons, natural and recombinant beta-interferons have also been tested. Again, partial regressions were achieved in about 10% of the patients. Recently, various gamma-interferons have been studied with respect to their efficacy in metastatic renal cell carcinoma. In our own protocol, recombinant gamma-interferon is administered subcutaneously at a daily dosage of 0.15 mg/m2 between day 1 and 13. This is followed by a dose of 0.2 mg/m2 between day 14 and day 20, and a further increase in dosage to a maximum of 0.25 mg/m2 thereafter. IFN therapy is continued if the first follow-up evaluation after 6 weeks shows either stable disease or signs of remission. In case of progressive disease, treatment was discontinued. Twelve patients with metastatic renal cell carcinoma have entered this protocol. Eleven patients are evaluable with a follow-up of at least 3 months. One patient is free of disease 8 months following the beginning of IFN therapy. One patient developed a partial remission for 6 months, while another patient has a stable disease since 13 months. Eight patients developed progressive disease within 5 months following initiation of treatment and 7 patients died within half a month to 9 months. The toxicity encountered during therapy was variable. Apart from flu-like symptoms, such as fever, malaise, fatigue and nausea, cardiovascular, gastrointestinal, hematologic and hepatic disorders have been observed. Side effects in the renal or nervous system, which have been reported in the literature, did not occur. One partial regression of a patient who underwent tumor nephrectomy for renal cell carcinoma stage pT3 N+ M+ is demonstrated in Fig. 1. Although a significant response was noted during treatment, IFN therapy had to be discontinued due to severe side effects. This was followed by the rapid development of local recurrence and growth of the remaining lesions of the lung.

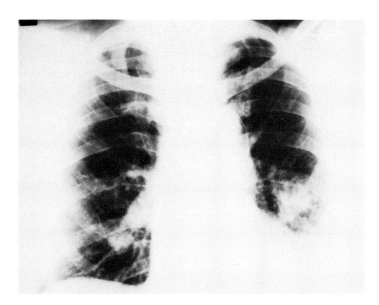

Figure 1a: Chest X-ray of a patient with metastasized renal cell carcinoma (E.M. 70 years) prior to nephrectomy (09.30.1985).

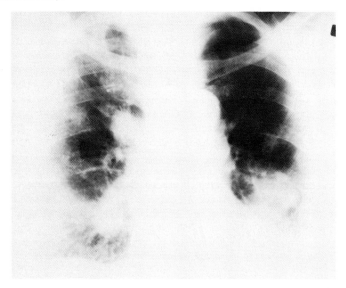

Figure 1b. Chest X-ray of a patient with metastasized renal cell carcinoma (E.M. 70 years) prior to therapy with recombinant IFN-gamma (03.17.1986)

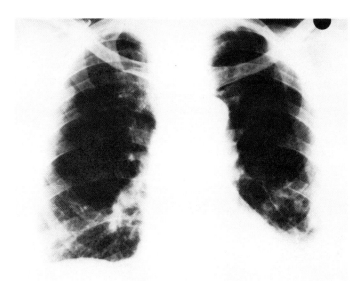

Figure 1c. Chest X-ray of a patient with metastasized renal cell carcinoma (E.M. 70 years) 3 months following the initiation of IFN therapy (06.24.1986)

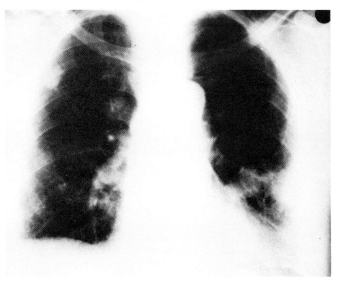

Figure 1d. Chest X-ray of a patient with metastasized renal cell carcinoma (E.M. 70 years) 5 months following the end of IFN therapy.

Cummings and coworkers (1986) have shown in in vitro experiments that the antiproliferative activity of interferons can be increased by additive hyperthermia or by additional treatment with vinblastin. In clinical studies, combinations of alpha-interferon with vinblastin and recombinant alpha-2 interferon with doxorubicin have failed to achieve any improvement in comparison to IFN monotherapy (Figlin et al, 1985). However, a significant increase in toxicity has been noted. It is obvious from this analysis that the various treatment concepts with interferons do not seem to be of any significant benefit to patients with metastatic renal cell carcinoma. However, it is important to realize that antitumor responses have been observed in many cases. The limiting factors remain a matter of speculation. In this context one aspect seems to be of particular interest. It is quite conceivable that the limited clinical response is related to an insufficient antiproliferative activity of the various types of interferons. It is currently attempted to hybridize interferons in order to produce hybrids with increased antiproliferative activity. In in vitro experiments it has been shown that the presence and number of B-domains in the molecule augment the cytotoxic activity of interferons. When tested on a metastatic variant of human renal cell carcinoma kept as xenograft and in cell culture, the appropriate interferon hybrid exhibits a 100% increased cytostatic activity. Taking into consideration that more than 100 different hybrids are conceivable, many more clinical studies with interferons are yet to be carried out.

Until recently 4 types of effector cells have been identified which possess the ability to lyse human tumor cells in vitro. Using experimentally induced tumors it can be demonstrated by in vivo experiments that these effector cells, i.e. cytotoxic T-cells, natural killer cells, macrophages and K-cells are under certain circumstances capable of mediating immunological antitumoral host reactions. Studies on the regulatory mechanisms of the various systems have shown that the activity and proliferative capacity of cytotoxic T-cells and natural killer cells are mediated by a T cell derived cytokine designated as T-cell growth factor and renamed interleukin-2. Apart from these functions, interleukin-2 stimulates the production of other cytokines such as B-cell growth factor and interferons. During the process of defining the functional abilities of interleukin-

2, it became evident that this lymphokine generates a sub-population of the mononuclear cells which is not identical to the 4 well known effector cells. This subpopulation designated as lymphokine-activated killer cells (LAK) or LAK-cells was found to lyse in vitro fresh tumor cells which were resistent to natural killer cells. The generation of LAK-cells following incubation with interleukin-2 occurs withing 2-3 days. The kinetics differ from that of the generation of cytotoxic T-cells by a specific antigen. Interferon is not the primary stimulus for the production of lymphokine activated killer cells. The cells do not adhere to plastic surface or nylon wool as do macrophages and B-cells. They are not present in mononuclear cell populations obtained from the thoracic duct which do not contain natural killer cells. The generation of LAK-cells is radiosensitive. Although the kinetics of the formation of LAK-cells are different from that of cytotoxic T-cells, LAK-cells express surface markers such as OKT3 and Leu-1, which are also expressed on T-cells. There is further evidence that LAK-cells do not belong to the T-cell lineage as their cytotoxic activity is not HL-A restricted. Taking into consideration the biological properties of lymphokine activated killer cells two aspects are of importance. Firstly LAK-cells do not require the expression of a tumor specific or related antigen which has not been identified for renal cell carcinoma. Secondary, LAK-cells are able to lyse solid tumor cells which are unaccessible to natural killer cells.

Rosenberg and coworkers (1987) were the first who used LAK-cells in the therapy of malignant disease. LAK-cells were generated from peripheral mononuclear cells obtained from the patients by lymphocytophoresis. Following purification of the cells, activation was obtained by in vitro incubation with interleukin-2 for 3-4 days. This was followed by reinfusion of the isolated cell fractions in combination with recombinant interleukin-2 (IL-2) by infusion on day 5, 6 and 8.

According to a recent update of the experiences with this mode of treatment, 36 patients with metastatic renal cell carcinoma received combination therapy with LAK-cells and IL-2. Twenty-one patients received IL-2 monotherapy (Rosenberg et al, 1987). In the group of patients with combination therapy, 4 complete responses, 8 partial responses and 7 minor responses were observed. In the monotherapy group, only 1 complete regression was detected. Although this mode of treatment has certain limitations mainly due to technical difficulties and severe side effects, further randomized studies in qualified centers should be carried out to confirm these results. These studies should also clarify the question, whether additional administration of LAK-cells is mandatory for the efficacy of this concept.

Apart from this approach, preparation of modified tumor cells in combination with various adjuvants have been tested for their antitumoral activity in patients with metastatic renal cell carcinoma. This concept is based on the assumption that tumor cells of renal cell carcinomas express specific antigens which can be used to augment a specific immune response, which in turn might be efficient to control the disease. Tallberg and Tykkä (1985) have administered insoluble antigenic polymer particles prepared from the patient's own tumor tissue in combination with tuberculin and/or candida albicans antigens as adjuvants. The autologous tumor material is insolubilized by polymerization using ethylchlorformiate. In a summarized update of their experiences including 71 patients who received active specific immunotherapy, and 56 non-randomized patients with conventional therapy, the overall survival was significantly better in the immunotherapy group. In this study 14 complete remissions and 5 partial regressions of pulmonary metastases in a total of 21 patients were observed. These results contradict observations reported by Neidhart and coworkers (1980) and by Fowler (1986). Using the same method for the preparation of the vaccine as Tallberg, Fowler observed 3 minor responses in a total of 23 patients. Although the selection of patients in these 2 studies might have been different with regard to the tumor load and patients performance status, thus not allowing a comparison of the results, the value of this treatment modality remains controversial. Schärfe and coworkers (1986) used single cell suspensions obtained by mechanical dissection of the tumor which were then inactivated by radiation and given in combination with candida antigen as adjuvant. Complete responses of metastatic lesions in 3 out of 53 patients and partial regression in 6 out of 53 patients have been achieved. These results are in the range of those reported by Fowler (1986) and Tallberg and coworkers (1985), respectively. It is evident that active specific immunotherapy is still in a stage of clinical investigation. Controlled clinical trials are needed in order to establish the true value of this biological therapeutic approach.

Two biological response modifiers, tumor necrosis factor (TNF) and thymosin fraction-5 (TF-5) though still under experimental investigation, have been tested for their therapeutic potential in renal cell carcinoma. Tumor necrosis factor is a molecule closely related to lymphotoxin and is produced by a variety of cell lines of the hematopoetic system, in particular by one lymphoblastoid cell line designated as Luk-II. TNF is characterized by its strong necrotizing and cytotoxic activity. There is a strong synergistic cytotoxic activity with various types of interferons. When tested against various cell lines derived from human renal cell carcinoma with different metastatic propensities it became evident that tumor cells derived from a single human renal cell carcinoma exhibit a heterogeneic response to the cytotoxic effects of recombinant TNF (Heicappell et al, 1987). TNF is currently being clinically tested with and without interferons.

The biological activity of thymus extracts on the immune system has been well documented in a variety of experiments. Apart from the synthetic alpha-1 fraction, thymosin fraction -5 has received the most attention. Stimulated by promising results of phase II trials with TF-5, Dimitrov and coworkers (1985) administered this biological response modifier in 19 patients with metastatic renal cell carcinoma. TF-5 was given at a dose of 100 mg/m2 subcutaneously on days 1 through 5 for 3 weeks during the period of induction, followed by maintenance therapy with the same dose twice weekly until evidence of disease. Fifteen out of 19 patients were evaluable. None of the patients developed tumor regression. Only 2 of the patients remained stable for 32 and 44 weeks of treatment, respectively.

CONCLUSION

For those who are interested in the area of biotherapy it is not surprising that results obtained with various biological response modifiers are not as impressive as one would like them to be. This is not unexpected considering that tumors do not consist of homogenous cell populations with identical biological properties that the microenvironment is extremely variable, and that the complex system responsible for the defense reactions is not fully understood. However, the presence of antitumoral responses confirms the assumption that host/tumor interactions are essential for the pathogenesis of clinical manifestations of malignant disease. This in turn implicates that research in this field remains the most promising aspect for the future.

REFERENCES

Cummings KB, Schmid SM, Bryan GT, Borden EC (1986). Antiproliferative activity of recombinant interferon alpha and beta for human renal carcinoma cells: Supra-additive activity with elevated temperature or vinblastine. World J Urol 3:230-233.

deKernion JB, Ramming KP (1976). Treatment of hypernephroma with xenogeneic immune RNA. In Bonney WW (ed): "Genito-urinary Cancer Immunology", National Cancer Institute Monographs, pp 347-350.

deKernion JB, Sarna G, Figlin R, Lindner A, Smith RB (1983). The treatment of renal cell carcinoma with human leukocyte alpha-interferon. J Urol 130:1063-1066.

Dimitrov NV, Arnold D, Munson J, Singh T, Borst J, Stott P (1985). Phase II study of thymosin fraction 5 in the treatment of metastatic renal cell carcinoma. Cancer Treat Rep 69:137-138.

Figlin RA, deKernion JB, Maldazys J, Sarna G (1985). Treatment of renal cell carcinoma with alpha (human leukocyte) interferon and vinblastine in combination: a phase I-II trial. Cancer Treat Rep 69:263-267.

Fowler JE (1986). Failure of immunotherapy for metastatic renal cell carcinoma. J Urol 135:22-25.

Heicappell R, Grütter MG, Fidler IJ (1987). Cytostatic and cytolytic effects of human recombinant tumor necrosis factor on human renal cell carcinoma cell lines derived from a single surgical specimen. J Immunol 138:1634-1640.

Kempf RA, Grunberg SM, Daniels JR, Skinner DG, Venturi CL, Spiegel R, Neri R, Greiner GM, Rudnick S, Mitchell MS (1986). Recombinant interferon alpha-2 (Intron A) in a phase II study of renal cell carcinoma. J Biol Resp Modif 5:27-35.

Kimura K (1984). A cooperative Phase I-II study of HLBI in patients with malignant tumors. Jpn J Cancer Chemother 11:1326-1331.

Kirkwood JM, Harris JE, Vera R, Sandler S, Fischer DS, Khandekar J, Emstoff MS, Gordon L, Lutes R, Bonomi P, Lytton B, Cobleigh M, Taylor SJ (1983). A randomized study of low and high doses of leukocyte alpha-interferon in metastatic renal cell carcinoma: The American Cancer Society Collaborative Trial. Cancer Res 45:863-871.

Krown SE, Einzig AI, Abramson JD, Oettgen HF (1983). Treatment of advanced renal cell cancer (RCC) with recombinant leukocyte A interferon (rIFN-alpha A). Proc Am Soc Clin Oncol 2:58.

Mannick JA, Egdahl RH (1962). Ribonucleic acid in "transformation" of lymphoid cells. Science 137:976-978.

Marumo K, Murai M, Hayakawa M (1984). Human lymphoblastoid interferon therapy for advanced renal cell carcinoma. Urology 24:567-571.

Muss HB, Caponera M, Cooper MR (1984). A phase II trial of recombinant alpha-2 interferon in renal cell carcinoma. Proc Am Assoc Cancer Res 25:231.

Neidhart JA, Murphy SG, Henic LA, Wise HA (1980). Active specific immunotherapy of stage IV renal carcinoma with aggregated tumor antigen adjuvant. Cancer 46:1128-1134.

Neidhart JA (1984). Interferon-alpha therapy of renal cancer. Cancer Res 44:4140-4143.

Oldham RK (1986). Immunotherapy: old concepts and new approaches. In Klippel K-F, Macher E (eds): "Present Status of Non-Toxic Concepts in Cancer", Karger Verlag, Basel, pp 1-18.

Otto U, Huland H, Denkhaus H, Klosterhalfen H (1985). Therapie mit rekombinantem Alpha-2 oder rekombinantem Gamma-Interferon bei Patienten mit metastasierendem Nierenkarzinom. Verhandlungsbericht der Deutschen Gesellschaft für Urologie, 1986, pp 152-153.

Queseda JR, Swanson DA, Trinodade A, Gutterman JK (1983). Renal cell carcinoma: antitumor effects of leucocyte interferon. Cancer Res 43:940-947.

Ramming KP, Pilch YH (1971). Transfer of tumor-specific immunity with RNA: inhibition of growth of murine tumor isografts. J Natl Cancer Inst 46:735.

Richie JP, Steele GD, Wilson RE, Ervin T, Wang BS, Mannick JA (1984). Current treatment of metastatic renal cell carcinoma with xenogeneic immune ribonucleic acid. J Urol 131:236-238.

Rosenberg SA, Lotze MT, Muul LM, Chang AE, Avis FP, Leitman S, Linehan WM, Robertson CN, Lee RE, Rubin JT, Seipp CA, Simpson CG, White DE (1987). A progress report on the treatment of 157 patients with advanced cancer using lymphokine-activated killer cells and interleukin-2 or high-dose interleukin-2 alone. New Engl J Med 316:889-897.

Schärfe T, Becht E, Klippel KF, Jacobi GH, Hohenfellner R (1986). Active immunotherapy of stage IV renal cell cancer using autologous tumor cells. World J Urol 3:245-248.

Tallberg T, Tykkä H, Mahlberg K, Halttunen P, Lehtonen T, Kalima T, Sarna S (1985). Active specific immunotherapy with supportive measures in the treatment of palliatively nephrectomized renal adenocarcinoma patients. A thirteen-year follow-up study. Eur Urol 11:233-243.

Vugrin D, Hood L, Taylor W, Laszlo J (1984). Two trials of lymphoblastoid alpha-interferon (IFN) in patients with advanced renal carcinoma. Proc Am Soc Clin Oncol 3:153.

EORTC Genitourinary Group Monograph 5: Progress
and Controversies in Oncological Urology II, pages 327–328
© 1988 Alan R. Liss, Inc.

Discussion: Biological Response Modifiers in Renal Cancer

Jan G.M. Klijn, Rotterdam, The Netherlands

N.N.: I do not think that increasing the antiproliferative
activity of interferons will be beneficial for the patients,
because so far nobody has demonstrated that the direct
antiproliferative effect at the level of the tumor target
cell is really the way interferons exert their antitumor
effects. Neither is there a clear dose-response relationship
in the clinic.

Ackermann: Well, I agree that it has not been demonstrated.
As I mentioned, there are several mechanisms which operate
the immune modulating system and antiproliferative activities. I agree that there is no close dose-effect relation in
the studies so far, but it has been clearly shown that tumor
cells can be attacked and can be inhibited in their proliferation. What this means is not understood, but it is clearly
shown that interferons interfere with the protein synthesis
of these cells and what we have seen is that the antiproliferative effect is present as long as the cells are exposed
to interferons. As soon as you withdraw the interferons, the
cells will start to proliferate again. This is one major
disadvantage. One aspect which seems to be promising is that
one tries to increase the cytotoxic activity of these mole-
cules in order to damage the cell metabolism more effectively than it has been achieved with the natural and recombinant interferons, which are currently available.

N.N.: Could you explain to me how the antitumor mechanism of
immune RNA is.

Ackermann: Well, there are three hypotheses. One is that,
and this is based on experimental findings, the exogenous
immune RNA can transfer immunity into non-immune lymphocytes. Furthermore, as Kona has demonstrated in his experiments, immune RNA acts as what he calls a superantigen. It
binds to an antigen and behaves like a superantigen
increasing an antitumor response which is already present.

And the third aspect is that exogenous immune RNA may work as adjuvant rather than as a specific immune stimulating agent.

Fosså: I want to ask you Dr. Ackermann, if you had a metastatic renal cell carcinoma with lung metastases, would you choose not to be treated at all, or would you choose a cytostatic drug as vinblastine, or would you choose a biological response modifier and if so, what type?

Ackermann: Well, I would suggest that you can try either a treatment with interferons or a combination of IL-2 with LAK cells. Then evaluate your patients within a short period of time, let us say 4-6 weeks. If you get stable disease continue the treatment and if you get progression discontinue. I think that is one aspect which should be followed.

Pinedo: But the question was lung metastasis and I think you should remove it.

Ackermann: No, I did not consider the particular situation of removable lung metastases, I was speaking about a patient with metastases in general.

EORTC Genitourinary Group Monograph 5: Progress
and Controversies in Oncological Urology II, pages 329–344
© 1988 Alan R. Liss, Inc.

BENIGN TUMORS OF THE KIDNEY

F. K. Mostofi, M. D., I. A. Sesterhenn, M.D.,
and C. J. Davis, Jr., COL, MC, USA

Armed Forces Institute of Pathology
Washington, D. C. 20306

INTRODUCTION
Considerable controversy has existed in pathological diagnoses and criteria of both epithelial and non epithelial
tumors of the kidney. In this presentation we intend to
present the controversies and clarify the confusion.

1. Epithelial Tumors of Renal Parenchyma

One of the enduring controversies in oncopathology has been
the existence of renal adenoma and the criteria for its
diagnosis. One school of thought has maintained that renal
adenomas do not exist and that all renal adenomas are, in
fact, small adenocarcinomas (Bennington & Beckwith, 1975).
Another group,   quoting Bell (1950), has claimed that
tumors less than 3 cm are adenomas, those over 3 cm are
carcinomas. We believe that renal adenomas do exist, that
size is not a reliable criterion for distinguishing adenomas
from carcinoma and that a reliable diagnosis of adenoma can
be made on histological basis (Mostofi,1979). This position
has been endorsed by the World Health Organization (Mostofi,
Sesterhenn & Sobin, 1981).

2. Criteria for Diagnosis of Adenoma

Renal adenomas are for the most part incidental findings
mostly at autopsies but occasionally in kidneys surgically
removed for other causes. Grossly, they are usually small
but may attain large size. Histologically, they are defined
as epithelial tumors composed of uniform cells with regular
nuclei seldom exhibiting mitotic activity. The cells have
scant cytoplasm, the nuclei are small, round and regular.

The cells form uniform glandular structures which may be
compact, tubular, cystic, with or without papillation (Mostofi, Sesterhenn & Sobin, 1981). Generally speaking, adenomas merge imperceptibly with the surrounding tissue.

Size, as a criterion for distinguishing adenomas from carcinoma, has long been considered unreliable. While observing
that renal tumors which were less than 3 cm in diameter
rarely metastasized, Bell (1950) himself reported 2 tumors
less than 2 cm in diameter that had metastasized. Murphy
and Mostofi (1970) studied 180 renal adenomas. About half
were found at autopsy, the other half surgically removed
but none had been clinically diagnosed; thirty-seven were
over 3 cms in diameter.

3. Categories of adenomas

We recognize 3 categories of renal adenomas: the tubulo
papillary, the metanephric and the oncocytic.

A. The tubulo papillary type is characterized by the presence of tubules lined by small cuboidal cells with small
regular fairly uniform nuclei. (Fig. 1) The papillae are
usually small and covered by small cuboidal cells with uniform nuclei. These adenomas are usually found in autopsy
kidneys, the frequency ranging from 7 to 22% (Olsen, 1984).
in those over 40, the frequency increasing with age and care
with which the lesion is searched for. Significant association has been demonstrated between these adenomas and smok-
ing and with arteriolar nephrosclerosis. In the last few
years we have encountered the lesion in kidneys of patients
on dialysis. Sometimes the distinction between these adenomas and carcinoma may be difficult.

B. In recent years we have recognized another category of
adenoma - metanephric adenomas. While studying Wilms tumors
in adults we were impressed by a group of purely epithelial
tumors which showed adenomatous differentiation. Histologically, the cells were uniform, very small and formed small
tubulo-papillary structures. (Fig. 2) The close resemblance
of these tumors to metanephric hamartomas of the nephroblas-
tomatosis complex has led us to label the lesion as metanephric adenomas. These lesions occur mostly in female
patients in their second to sixth decade.

C. The most interesting and again pathologically controver-

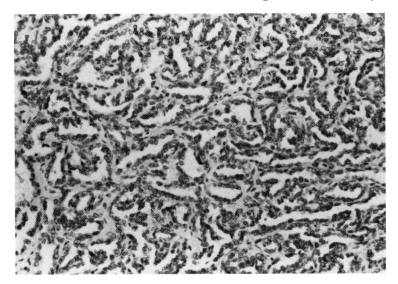

Fig. 1. Renal adenoma. Papillary tubulo-acinar structures lined by uniform small epithelial cells. AFIP Neg. 87-6236 X 100.

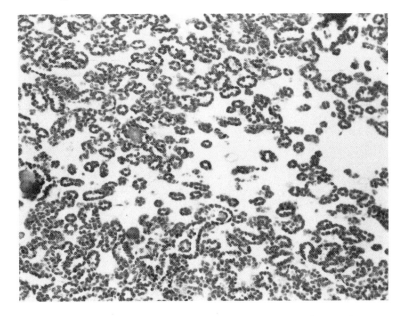

Fig. 2. Metanephric adenoma. Tiny tubules lined by small cuboidal cells. AFIP Neg. 87-6237 X 100.

sial epithelial tumor of the kidney is renal oncocytoma or
renal adenoma oncocytic type. Originally recognized by
Zippel (1941), subsequently reported by Apitz (1944), Hamperl
(1962), Zollinger (1966), Blessing and Weinert (1973). Their
existence escaped American attention until the report by
Klein and Valensi (1976) who designated the lesion as adenoma of proximal convoluted tubules. Oncocytomas have a
fairly distinct radiological and pathological appearance.
(Quinn et al, 1984).

Computed tomography demonstrates a large homogeneous well
defined mass with or without a central low density linear
scar which is usually large but without evidence of hemorrhage and necrosis in contrast to renal cell carcinomas
which are non homogeneous and show areas of hemorrhage and
necrosis. If CT is equivocal angiography may be helpful as
it often shows spoke wheel arterial distribution or a homogeneous tumor blush but this appearance is not always present.

Grossly, the tumors are usually large, ranging in size from
2 to 25 cms with a mean of 5-8 cm. They are round or oval,
well circumscribed. They are usually single and unilateral
but we have seen multiple tumors in the same kidney and bi-
laterally. The larger tumors often expand into perinephric
fat but there, too, they are well circumscribed. The cut
surface is smooth, bulging, uniform, mahogany brown, usually
with a central grayish white scar.(Fig. 3)

Microscopically, the cells are uniformly small and cuboidal.
The cytoplasm is intensely granular and eosinophilic. The
granules represent abundant mitochondria. The nuclei are
uniform, small and vesicular with 1 or 2 delicate nucleoli.
(Fig. 4) Mitoses are rare. Moderate nuclear and cellular
pleomorphism may be present focally. Binucleated cells and
giant cells are not infrequent.

Olsen (1984) has described the ultrastructure in detail.

In most cases the cells are closely packed into rounded or
ovoid aggregates. At the periphery of the tumor the cell
aggregates are tightly packed together with little or no
stroma. Toward the center they become progressively separated from each other by edematous or acellular hyalinized
stroma constituting the central scar. Less frequently the
cells may form tubules or microcysts.

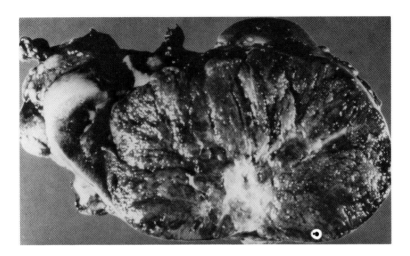

Fig. 3. Renal Oncocytoma. The tumor is circumscribed and homogeneous throughout except for a white scar near center. AFIP Neg. 85-7528. Reproduced by permission of Year Book Medical Publishers, Inc. Current Problems In Cancer, Vol. X #2, 1986.

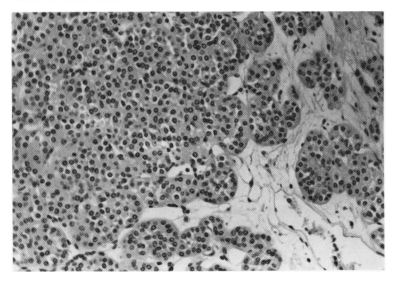

Fig. 4. Renal Oncocytoma. The cells are uniform, have small regular nuclei, form compact nests at periphery, and separated by edematous stroma in center. AFIP Neg. 87-6239 X 100.

The differential diagnosis is between oncocytoma and granular cell carcinoma. Aside from the different appearance in CT scan and angiography renal cell carcinomas have a variegated cut surface with areas of hemorrhage and necrosis. The cells are larger, less regular and granular, the nuclei are larger and more hyperchromatic. There are usually associated clear cell areas. The cells form tubular structures surrounded by a delicate vascular network. No condensation of cell masses is seen at the periphery, areas of hemorrhage and necroses are frequent. However, it should be emphasized that no sharp distinction exists between the small granular cells of oncocytoma and the large granular cells of renal cell carcinoma and there are definitely many gray areas.

In larger tumors hemorrhagic foci may be present but hemorrhage and necrosis are uncommon. We have seen several instances in which tumor cells are present in vascular spaces. These are designated as borderline cases requiring long term follow-up.

Oncocytomas are usually discovered accidentally but about 10% of patients have vague abdominal pain and about the same number have gross or microscopic hematuria. In our group the age range is 26 to 87 years with a mean age of 56. The male to female ratio is 1.6 to 1 and white to black ratio 8.5-1.

While recognizing borderline cases and the need for long term follow-up, we believe that oncocytomas as described are benign. We do not grade our oncocytomas as has been proposed by Lieber et al (1981).

Oncocytomas may coexist in the same kidney with renal cell carcinoma either separately or closely related. Gross and microscopic are quite dissimilar. Oncocytomas should be widely sampled.

II. Non Epithelial Tumors

Benign mesenchymal tumors of the kidney are quite common and the frequency increases with the age of the patient but they are usually small and of no clinical significance. One group of mesenchymal tumors, renal angiomyolipomas, however, are of clinical significance and source of considerable controversy.

Are they tumors or hamartomas? Are they benign or malignant? Are they invariably associated with tuberous sclerosis complex?

Although we recognize the lesion as a hamartoma this term is rather indefinite and ambiguous and we believe angiomyolipoma is better. In our experience it is the most frequently misdiagnosed renal mass - often diagnosed as liposarcoma, leiomyosarcoma or carcinoma.

Eighty percent of patients with tuberous sclerosis have multiple renal angiomyolipoma but a large majority of these have no renal symptoms. Only 15-20% of patients with symptomatic angiomyolipoma have tuberous sclerosis complex. In this group symptoms appear by the age of 25 and since there may be associated bilateral cysts the lesion is confused with polycystic disease but manifestation of polycystic disease is rare in this age group.

Symptomatic angiomyolipomas occur in all ages, the youngest in our material is 12, the oldest 70, with a mean age of 40 for males and 42 for females. The female to male ratio is 4:1. The symptoms may be indolent or intermittent consisting of abdominal pain or mass but most often they are abrupt, resulting from massive hemorrhage with severe abdominal or flank pain and shock. In younger patients there may be renal failure.

Radiological studies may or may not be helpful depending on the recognition of fat on plain abdominal film. Ultrasound may be more valuable in clinical diagnosis demonstrating a well defined mass as echogenic as the central echo complex (Hartman et al, 1981). Unfortunately, if fat cells are not abundant, ultrasound is not diagnostic.

Computed tomography is most helpful in the diagnosis. Detecting density differences of one percent it recognizes the fat component as well as hemorrhage and extra renal extension (Sherman et al, 1981).

Oftentimes the severe abdominal symptoms lead the patients to a general surgeon who, encountering a massive hemorrhagic fatty tumor involving the kidney and perinephric tissue, is inclined to diagnose liposarcoma which diagnosis may be carried over to pathology.

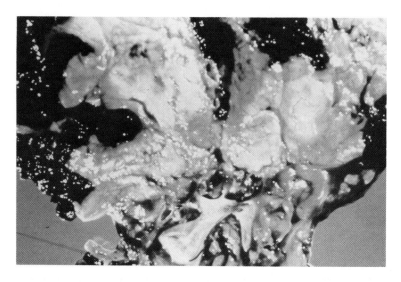

Fig. 5. Angiomyolipoma. Masses of fatty tissue with hemorrhage. AFIP Neg. 79-15082.

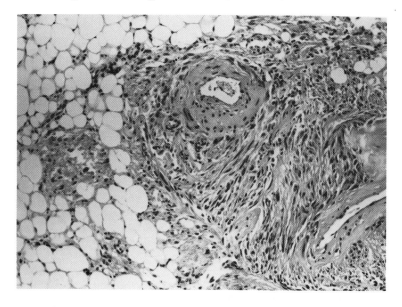

Fig. 6. Angiomyolipoma. The tumor consists of islands of fat cells, spindle shaped cells and thick walled, hyalinized blood vessels. AFIP Neg. 87-6240 X 70.

The tumors are usually unilateral but a few may be bilateral. They range from 3 to 20 cms in diameter with a mean of 9.4 cms. The color depends on the proportion of fat ranging from yellowish to grayish. Necrosis, cyst formation and calcification are occasionally present. Extensive hemorrhage may be seen. (Fig. 5)

Histologically, the tumors are composed of 3 distinct elements: adipose tissue, thick walled, tortuous blood vessels and sheets of smooth muscle cells. (Fig. 6) However, the proportions may vary from tumor to tumor or from area to area.

The adipose tissue consists of fat cells which may vary in size but show no anaplasia. The smooth muscle elements may show considerable variation in size, shape and staining. They range from elongated cells with typical cigar shaped nuclei and longitudinal cytoplasmic myofibrils to large plump cells or darker bizarre shaped cells. The smooth muscle cells may form small bands in between adipose tissue or form perivascular cuffs or large sheets resembling leiomyoma. Rarely the cells may have an epithelioid appearance. Not infrequently the origin of smooth muscle elements from the vessel walls is obvious. The vascular components present one of several pictures. Usually they consist of large thick-walled arterial type of vessel which are tortuous. The vascular lumens vary greatly in diameter and are often eccentric. While the endothelial cells are normal, the subintimal connective tissue and the media often show variable thickness and structure. Sometimes they consist of hyalinized collagenous connective tissue, sometimes of smooth muscle cells alone and sometimes of admixture of the two. Little or no elastic tissue is seen in vascular walls. The vessels tend to aggregate. The small arteries and arterioles lack elastic tissue but consist of closely packed immature appearing smooth muscle cells arranged circumferentially around a lumen.

This histological picture is typical of angiomyolipoma. As mentioned earlier, the tumor may not only involve the kidney it may be extra renal as well. In 315 cases that we have studied, 21 showed regional lymph node involvement which we have attributed to multicentricity rather than metastases.

Despite the large size, the absence of encapsulation, the presence of hemorrhage and necrosis, the described variations in size, shape and staining of the smooth muscle cells and the presence of the lesion in the regional lymph node, we believe the lesion is benign as todate we have seen no metastases in any of our cases.

III. Nephroblastic Tumors

Nephroblastoma or Wilms' tumor is, of course, the most common nephroblastic tumor of childhood. Two related lesions: congenital mesoblastic nephroma and multilocular cystic nephroma have been a source of much controversy and confusion.

A. Congenital mesoblastic nephroma

The lesion was variously referred to as leiomyoma, fetal renal hamartoma, and leiomyomatous hamartoma. (Mostofi,1979). Congenital mesoblastic nephroma, introduced by Bolande et al (1967), has now been generally accepted.

This is the most common solid renal mass in the neonates, but we have seen them in a 0-1/2 year old girl and in a 10 year old girl. The main symptom is a large abdominal mass.

Hartman et al (1981) have described the radiographic findings. Ultra sound is the most frequent initial radiological procedure.

The tumor is often evenly echogenic with low level echoes. The tumor may be detected in utero on maternal sonogram, as a solid abdominal mass in the infant.

If sonogram is equivocal plain film of the abdomen shows a large noncalcified soft tissue mass that may cross the midline. Excretory urogram outlines a renal mass 2 to 7 times the size of the kidney with marked distortion of calyceal system. Computed tomography reveals a fairly uniform solid intrarenal mass. Angiography, if necessary, shows a moderately vascular tumor with irregular bizarre vessels. The nephrogram is often nonhomogeneous with small laking or blush (Hartman et al, 1981b).

The size varies from 0.8 to 14 cm in diameter with a mean of 6.2 cm in diameter. Most lesions are solid but an occasional one may have cysts or even cartilage. The tumors are spherical and fairly well circumscribed. Grossly, they resemble uterine fibroids. (Fig. 7) Microscopically, the tumors con-

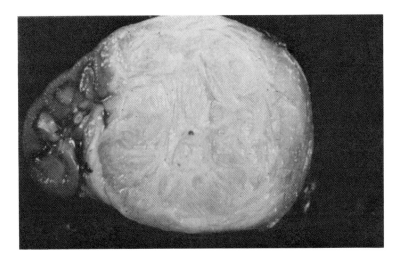

Fig. 7. Mesoblastic nephroma. The tumor is made up of lobules of fibrous tissue resembling a uterine fibroid. AFIP Neg. 54-1465.

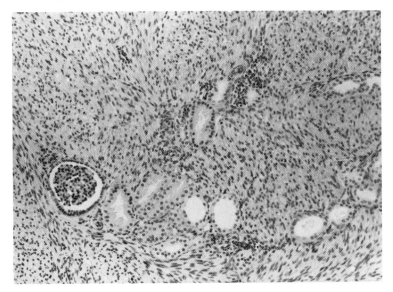

Fig. 8. Mesoblastic nephroma. Fascicles of spindle cells interdigitate with nephrons. AFIP Neg. 87-6241 X 76.

sist of interlacing bundles and whorls of spindle shaped
cells with cigar-shaped nuclei intermingled with various
amounts of fibrous tissue and primitive mesenchymal cells.
(Fig. 8) Mitotic figures may be quite frequent. The cells
are fairly uniform with little or no pleomorphism. Thin
walled blood vessels and sinusoids course the tumor. Islands
of cartilage may be present. Hemorrhage and necrosis may
be present.

The distinguishing feature of the lesion is the unusual
growth pattern in which the smooth muscle elements interdigitate with groups of nephrons consisting of glomeruli
and tubules. The nephrons may be immature, mature or both,
depending on the age of the patient.

The lesion as described is benign but it may recur if incompletely removed. Occasionally clones of darker, mitotically
active anaplastic cells may be seen with the loss of fasci-
cular pattern. These have been referred to as atypical cellular mesoblastic nephroma (Joshi et al, 1986). They are
in fact undifferentiated sarcomatous areas and the category
could more accurately be called malignant mesoblastic nephroma to distinguish them from typical lesions.

It is currently held that these focal anaplastic features
as well as hemorrhage and necrosis may be disregarded if the
infant is less than 3 months of age. In older infants consideration may be given for a low stage nephroblastoma type
regimen to forestall possible recurrence and metastasis
(Beckwith & Weeks, 1986).

The controversy relative to the relationship of the lesion
to nephroblastoma is beyond the scope of this presentation
but has been discussed elsewhere (Mostofi, 1979).

B. Multilocular cystic nephroma.

Designated also as multilocular cyst, the lesion is often
misdiagnosed as cystic renal cell carcinoma and segmental
multicystic kidney and occasionally as lymphangioma. The
lesion has been a source of considerable controversy. Is
it congenital or acquired? Is it benign or malignant? Is
it related to Wilms?

The lesion is seen in boys from 2 months to 4 years. Usually
manifested as a mass but hematuria may also be present. A

similar tumor is seen in adult females over 30 years of age. Whether the histogenesis of the 2 are the same or not,there is sufficient similarity to have the same designation for them and described together.

Madewell et al (1983) have described the radiological findings. Plain films and excretory urogram shows a well defined intra renal mass in a normally functioning kidney. The sonographic findings depend on the size of the locules, their content, and the amount of the stroma. If the cysts are large the sonogram will demonstrate a cluster of echo free masses separated by intense echo. If locules are small a non specific complex intrarenal mass is seen. On computerized tomography the lesion appears as a well defined mass in the kidney, usually surrounded by a thick capsule with no external lobulations.

The size of the lesion may vary from 3 to 30 cms or more but most are in the range of 8-10 cm. It invariably has a thick capsule as the growth is entirely expansile. The cut surface shows multiple non-communicating spherical locules separated by thin septae. (Fig. 9) As they enlarge, they often protrude into perinephric fibroadipose tissue or more frequently into the renal pelvis and upper ureter. Hematuria may ensue as a result of pelvic herniation, but no hemorrhage or necrosis as seen in the cyst, a feature that distinguishes it from cystic renal cell carcinoma.

Histologically, the lesion is composed of 2 components:Eosinophilic cuboidal, hobnail or flat epithelium lining the cysts which are supported by small cells. In infants the stroma is edematous while in adults it is very cellular, simulating ovarian stroma. (Fig. 10).

The tumors are benign but two facts should be remembered. In infants elements of nephroblastoma may be seen in the stroma. Designated as cystic partially differentiated nephroblastoma (Joshi et al 1977), these lesions require only nephrectomy. In adults, rarely, the stroma may be sarcomatous and metastasize (Madewell et al, 1983).

CONCLUSION: We have described a number of benign epithelial, mesenchymal and nephroblastic tumors of the kidney. Before such a diagnosis is made it is essential to examine the tumor thoroughly to rule out the presence of any malignant elements.

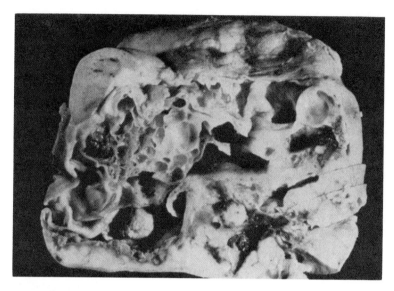

Fig. 9. Multilocular cystic nephroma. The tumor consists of multiple non communicating locules. AFIP Neg. 60-228.

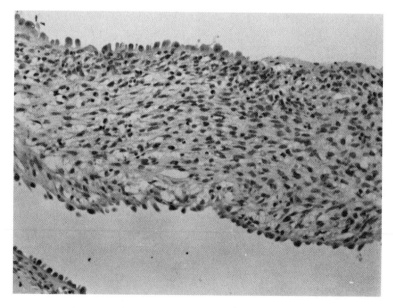

Fig. 10. Multilocular cystic nephroma. Fibrous stroma is covered by tear-drop cells. AFIP Neg. 87-6242 X 100.

REFERENCES

Apitz K (1943). Die Geschwulste und Gewebsmissbildungen der Nierenrinde; die intrarenalen Nebenniereninsein. Virchow Arch Pathol Anat 311:285-305.

Beckwith JB and Weeks DA (1986). Congenital mesoblastic nephroma. Arch Pathol Lab Med 110:98-99.

Bell ET (1950). Renal diseases. 2nd Ed. Philadelphia, Lea & Febiger, p 435.

Bennington JL and Beckwith JB (1975). Tumors of the kidney, renal pelvis and ureter. Fascicle 12, Atlas of Tumor Pathology, 2nd Series, Washington, DC, Armed Forces Institute of Pathology.

Blessing MH, Wienert G (1973). Onkozytom der Niere. Klinische und pathologisch-anatomische Befunde. Zentralbl Allg Pathol 117:227-234.

Bolande RP, Brough AJ, Izant RJJ (1967). Congenital mesoblastic nephroma of infancy. A report of eight cases and the relationship to Wilms tumor. Pediatrics 40:272-278.

Hamperl H (1962). Onkozyten und Onkozytom. Virchow Arch Pathol Anat 335:452-483.

Hartman DS, Goldman SM, Friedman AC et al (1981a). Angiomyolipoma: ultrasonic-pathologic correlation. Radiology 139:451-458.

Hartman DS, Lesar MSL, Madewell JE, Davis CJ (1981b). Mesoblastic nephroma: radiologic-pathologic correlation of 20 cases. AJR 136:69-74.

Joshi VV, Banerzie AK, Pathakic (1977). Cystic partially differentiated nephroblastoma. Cancer 40:789-795.

Joshi VV, Kasynics J, Walters TR (1986). Atypical mesoblastic nephroma. Arch Pathol Lab Med 110:100-106.

Klein MJ and Valensi QJ (1976). Proximal tubular adenomas of kidney with so-called oncocytic features. Cancer 38:906-914.

Lieber MM, Tomera KM, Farrow GM (1981). Renal oncocytoma. J Urol 125:481-485.

Madewell JE, Goldman SM, Davis CJ et al (1983). Multilocular cystic nephroma. A radiologic-pathologic correlation of 58 patients. Radiology 146:309-321.

Mostofi FK (1979). Tumors of renal parenchyma in kidney disease, present status. In Churg J, Spargo BH, Mostofi FK, Abell MR (eds.), Baltimore, Williams and Wilkins Co.

Mostofi FK, Sesterhenn IA, Sobin LH (1981). Histological typing of kidney tumors. Int Histol Classification of Tumors, no 25, Geneva, World Health Org.

Murphy GP and Mostofi FK (1970). Histologic assessment and clinical prognosis of renal adenoma. J Urol 103:31-36.

Olsen S (1984) Tumors of the kidney and urinary tract. Copen-
hagen, Munksgaard, pp 23-25.
Quinn MJ, Hartman DS, Friedman AC et al (1984). Renal oncocy-
toma, new observations. Radiology 153:49-53.
Sherman JL, Hartman DS, Friedman AC, Davis CJ, Goldman SM
(1981). Angiomyolipoma: computed tomographic pathologic
correlation of 17 cases. AJR 137:1221-1226.
Zippel L (1941). Zur Kenntnis der Onkocyten. Virchow Arch
Pathol Anat 308:360-380.
Zollinger HU (1966). Niere und ableitende Harnwege. In Doerr
W and Uhlinger E (eds): "Spezielle Pathologische Anatomie,
Vol 3," Springer Verlag, pp 676-677.

The opinions or assertions are the private views of the
authors and are not to be construed as official or as reflecting the views of the Departments of the Army or Defense.

EORTC Genitourinary Group Monograph 5: Progress
and Controversies in Oncological Urology II, pages 345-346
© 1988 Alan R. Liss, Inc.

Discussion: Benign Tumors of the Kidney

Jan G.M. Klijn, Rotterdam, The Netherlands

Fair: Dr. Mostofi, I think either the pathologists are
confused or the clinicians are confused by oncocytoma. Recently there was a disturbing report from Farrow and his
group, which shows that about 15% of oncocytomas had an
aneuploid peak on DNA flowcytometry which raises the possibility that at least 15% might be in fact malignant. So does
this mean that the pathologists are actually reading, in
some cases, renal cells with oncocytic features or does it
mean that we clinicians are not paying enough attention to
oncocytomas as far as their malignant potential goes?

Mostofi: I think your first conclusion was correct.

Schröder: I am very worried about those 21 patients with
angiomyolipoma and lymph node involvement and I would like
to know on what you base your conclusion that this is not a
malignant disease. I have never heard about any disease
spreading to the lymph nodes that is not called malignant by
the pathologist.

Mostofi: Well, they are present in the lymph nodes but we
have not seen a single case of metastasis elsewhere. Many
years ago there has been a report of an angiomyolipoma that
was malignant from Great Britain but it was not an
angiomyolipoma after all.

N.N.: Mr. Mostofi, would you advocate follow-up for patients
with oncocytoma and for how long?

Mostofi: I think that any patient with a renal cell
epithelial tumor should be followed over a long period.
Precisely how often and so on, I have to ask my urologist
friends this because they have more experience in this than
I do.

Huland: The same group as Dr. Fair mentioned, divided oncocytoma in grade 1 and grade 2, is that your experience too?

Mostofi: We think that typical oncocytoma should not be confused with renal cell carcinoma. And, as Dr. Fair mentioned, sometimes renal cell carcinoma may have the features that we see in oncocytoma namely that they occurred in solid cell masses and that they do not have the vascularity which you see in renal cell carcinoma. But nevertheless, if you examine carefully, you will find typical renal granular cell carcinoma elsewhere.

EORTC Genitourinary Group Monograph 5: Progress
and Controversies in Oncological Urology II, pages 347–356
© 1988 Alan R. Liss, Inc.

INCIDENTAL RENAL NEOPLASMS: INCIDENCE IN LOS ANGELES COUNTY,
TREATMENT AND PROGNOSIS

Alastair W.S. Ritchie and Jean B. deKernion

Department of Surgery, Division of Urology,
UCLA School of Medicine, Los Angeles, California
90024

ABSTRACT

    The proportion of 3232 malignant renal parenchymal
tumors diagnosed at an asymptomatic stage in Los Angeles
County over a 13 year period was 15%. A comparison of the
proportion of tumors that were asymptomatic at diagnosis
over two four year periods, showed no significant change.
Asymptomatic tumors were localized to the kidney in 77.5%
of cases and had produced metastases in 9.4%. Conversely,
symptomatic tumors were localized in only 43.9% and had
metastases in 28%. These data are compared with recent
literature concerning the incidence, diagnosis, pathology,
prognosis and treatment of incidental renal neoplasms.

INTRODUCTION

    The reported incidence of renal tumors discovered by
chance depends on the source of data. Careful post mortem
studies on hospital in-patients have shown that a significant
number of cases are not diagnosed during life (Hellsten et
al., 1981 a,b, Hajdu and Thomas, 1967). A series of 16,294
autopsies performed in Malmo, Sweden, revealed 350 cases of
renal cell carcinoma, 235 of which were unrecognized during
life (Hellsten et al., 1981 a,b). Most large clinical series
contain a proportion of tumors, varying from 3.6 to 8.4%,
which were diagnosed by chance (Table 1).

    The present study is based on data from the Cancer
Surveillance Program, University of Southern California.
This program obtains information from hospital pathology

reports for Los Angeles County, a population of approximately
7.5 million. Benign and malignant renal parenchymal tumors
were separately identified using ICD-O codes and analyzed
according to presenting symptoms, sex and extent of disease
at presentation. Cases of Wilms' tumor were excluded from
analysis.

PROPORTION OF TUMORS THAT ARE INCIDENTAL FINDINGS

From the literature it would appear that the proportion of tumors discovered incidentally is increasing
(Table 1).

Table 1 Incidental Renal Carcinoma

Date	Total No.	% Incidental	Reference
1951	1746	3.6	Riches, 1951
1971	309	6.5	Skinner et al, 1971
1982	311	8.4	Haertig & Kuss, 1982
1972-84	3232	15.1	Present study

In Los Angeles County, the proportion of incidentally
diagnosed cases was unchanged in two four year periods:
16% in 1976-9 and 14% in 1980-3. In a small series,
Konnak and Grossman (1986) reported that 7 of 56 (13%) of
their tumors were discovered incidentally during the period
1961 to 1973, whereas 22 of 46 (48%) were incidental
findings during the four years from 1980.

The trend towards an increase in diagnosis of renal
neoplasms at an asymptomatic stage, since the 1950s, may be
related to the advent of computer assisted tomography and
ultrasound. Small lesions can easily be missed or are not
imaged by excretory urography. Of nine small neoplasms
less than 3 cm in diameter when first imaged, three were
not visible on the IVU, even in retrospect and a further 3
were overlooked (Curry et al 1986). Lang (1986) has
reported that CT will establish the diagnosis for an asymptomatic renal mass in 79% of cases, compared with only 7%
for IVU.

PATHOLOGY OF THE INCIDENTALLY DIAGNOSED RENAL MASS

Asymptomatic renal masses are found in up to 20% of

elderly patients (Lang, 1986). Accurate diagnosis by non-invasive means depends heavily on CT and ultrasound imaging. To place the proportion that prove malignant in perspective, Table 2 shows the final pathology in a large series reported by Lang (1986).

Table 2   Final diagnosis in 1594 asymptomatic renal masses (adapted from Lang 1986)

Pathology	Number	%
Simple cysts	1055	66.2
Benign cystic lesions	228	14.3
Inflammatory lesions	125	7.8
Pseudotumors	93	5.8
Malignant neoplasms	72	4.5
Benign neoplasms	13	0.8
Vascular lesions	8	0.5

Benign tumors: Unequivocally benign lesions such as lipomas, angiomyolipomas and fibromas are rare and are usually grouped with small clear cell tumors classified as benign adenomas. In Los Angeles County only 38 benign tumors were registered, compared with 3232 malignant tumors, over a 13 year period.

Historically, the term adenoma has been bestowed on well differentiated renal cortical glandular tumors less than 3 cm in maximum diameter. Bell (1950) reported a direct relationship between size and the frequency of distant metastases. He did however note metastases in 3 of 65 (4.6%) tumors of diameter less than 3 cm. Further justification for the distinction of benign from malignant, was the greater frequency with which the adenomas were reported in autopsy series, compared to carcinomas. The shared cell of origin, the absence of histological differentiating features, the shared male predominance and age range and the occurrence of metastases from small lesions, have led some pathologists to express the view that adenomas are simply small carcinomas (Bennington 1973, Petersen 1986). Conversely, Mostofi and Davis (1986) have stated that they believe in the existence of adenomas but use both clinical aspects of the lesions behavior and histology to distinguish the two. For the clinician, however, there is no reliable method to identify which lesions will produce metastases. Size alone is not a good criterion, since widespread metastases have been reported

from 10 tumors less than 3 cm in diameter (Petersen, 1986)
and histology of nine renal neoplasms first visible when
less than 3 cm in diameter, showed that only one lesion was
benign (oncocytoma). The remainder were all classified as
carcinomas and two produced metastases (Curry et al., 1986).

The term adenoma has also been applied to tumors
containing cells with oncocytic features, devoid of mitoses
and with no evidence of local extension, metastases or
hemorrhage and necrosis (Kline and Valensi, 1976). The
"adenomas" with oncocytic elements have been renamed oncocytomas (Lieber et al., 1981). Renal oncocytomas comprise
about 4% of all parenchymal tumors previously labelled
together as renal cell carcinoma. These lesions are incidental
findings in approximately 70% of cases and have a low but not
absent potential for local penetration and metastases. Many
renal carcinomas have oncocytic features in certain areas but
may have aggressive clinical behavior. Thus the term oncocytoma has to be reserved for a tumor composed solely of
oncocytes (Lieber and Tsukamoto, 1986).

Malignant tumors: Incidentally diagnosed malignant
lesions may be primary or secondary. In the current study,
analysis of cell type in asymptomatic, primary, malignant
tumors, revealed no significant differences from that in
patients with symptoms. Metastases to the kidney are usually
silent (Table 3).

Table 3 Proportion of patients with renal metastases having
no symptoms, normal urinalysis and normal renal
function

#Pts.	No symptoms	Normal Urinalysis	Normal Renal Function	Reference
27	23(85)	9(33)	25(93)	Choyke et al (1987)
116	115/142* (81)	43(37)	96(83)	Klinger, 1951
10	8(80)	NS	NS	Bhatt et al (1983)

*115/142 patients with metastases to the urinary tract: the
proportion of 116 with renal metastases was not specified.
NS - not stated.

Although it is not possible to differentiate an incidental renal carcinoma from a metastasis to the kidney, the
factors favoring the diagnosis of renal metastases are small,
multifocal, avascular renal masses in association with wide-

spread metastases elsewhere in the body. Renal metastases do not tend to enhance with contrast CT studies and do not usually involve the renal venous sytem (Pagani, 1983). When both kidneys are involved the commonest primary is a lymphoma, whereas if one kidney is involved the commonest primary is the lung (Klinger, 1951).

CLINICAL BEHAVIOR AND PROGNOSIS OF ASYMPTOMATIC, SOLID RENAL LESIONS

Overall the outcome of a small, asymptomatic lesion will depend on the histology and stage at diagnosis. It would however be helpful to have more precise prognostic indicators as guidelines for management.

DNA content of the primary tumor has emerged as a useful prognostic indicator in metastatic renal carcinoma (Ljunberg et al., 1986) and has been applied to "adenomas" and onco-cytomas. Bennington and Mayall (1983) reported on 21 renal cortical glandular neoplasms (15 adenocarcinomas and 6 adenomas) studied using the azure A Feulgen reaction for DNA. The cytometric features showed no significant difference between adenomas and grade 1 adenocarcinomas. These data were interpreted as evidence that renal adenomas are actually very well differentiated early adenocarcinomas. The DNA content of oncocytomas is heterogeneous. Rainwater et al (1986) found that 39% of 51 typical specimens of oncocytoma had a marked increase in the DNA tetraploid peak and 11% showed a distinct DNA aneuploid peak. Among 21 grade 2 oncocytomas, 43% showed a marked increase in the tetraploid peak and 24% showed a distinct aneuploid peak. The majority of cases with an abnormal flow pattern had easily identifiable cells, containing large abnormal nuclei on light microscopy. No instances of tumor progression or death were noted in the patients having tumors with normal ploidy or aneuploidy. Three tumors showed evidence of progression from the group with tetraploid flow patterns. These surprising findings, in view of the clinical behavior of these lesions, would appear to preclude the use of flow cytometry on fine needle aspirates for preoperative distinction of oncocytoma from carcinoma.

The identification of oncocytoma by non-invasive means would be useful. Using the central stellate scar seen on ultrasound or CT and the spoke-wheel appearance on angiography, Quinn et al, (1984) reported, in a retrospective analysis,

that 16 of 18 cases of oncocytoma could be correctly diagnosed.
They did note however that the above criteria were of no
value for lesions less than 3 cm in diameter. The average
tumor size in this series was 6.1 cm. A prospective study
of the above criteria in larger lesions is necessary before
definite conclusions can be drawn.

Information about survival can be derived from analysis
of stage at presentation in patients with and without symptoms.
In the current analysis of 3232 histologically confirmed
cases of renal carcinoma, 77.5% of those without symptoms had
disease confined to the kidney and only 9.4% had distant
metastases. By comparison, only 43.9% of those with symptoms
have localized disease and 28% have metastases at presentation
(P < 0.001) (Table 4).

Table 4 Extent of disease compared with symptomatic status
in 3232 malignant renal tumors

	Localized	Direct Extension	Regional Nodes	Distant Mets	Unknown
asymptomatic (n = 489)	77.5*	10.4	1.4	9.4	1.2
symptoms unknown (n=295)	22.8	10.2	1.7	17.6	41.3
symptomatic (n = 2448)	43.9	21.9	4.7	28.0	1.5

* Figures are percentages

There are few available data comparing long term survival
of those with and without symptoms at diagnosis. Skinner et
al (1971 a,b) reported an "overall" survival of 65% in 20
patients with silent tumors compared to an overall 5 year
survival of 44% in 309 patients. Konnack & Grossman (1986)
reported 5 year survival of 85% for 7 patients without
symptoms and 50% overall, for a group of 56 patients.

Survival curves for 62 patients with oncocytomas showed
no difference from an age and sex matched cohort (Lieber
et al, 1981). A distinction has been drawn between grade I
and II oncocytic tumors but the important discovery is that
actuarial survival curves show a significantly poorer prognosis
for patients with grade I clear cell renal tumors compared
to patients with grade I oncocytic lesions (Tomera et al, 1983).

MANAGEMENT OF INCIDENTALLY DIAGNOSED TUMORS

The previous sections have indicated that there are no reliable methods of predicting the behavior of small or incidentally discovered tumors, at least before surgical excision. If there is a solid element to the lesion then whatever size, there exists the potential for destruction of the host. A policy of observation with serial CT scans seems too risky and assuming the patient has a reasonable life expectancy and no significant surgical risk factors, all such lesions should be excised.

The extent of the surgical procedure is currently debated and it is unclear whether the standard radical nephrectomy is indicated in every case. The issue of conservative surgery has been raised by the considerable experience and excellent results with parenchymal preserving surgery in patients with bilateral tumors and those with single kidneys.

Tumor enucleation has been reported to produce a 90% 3 year survival in 33 patients with bilateral disease or tumor in a solitary kidney (Novick et al, 1986). This group of patients was highly selected from 1,286 undergoing treatment for renal tumors over the same time period and contained only low grade lesions. Five of the patients had von Hippel-Lindau's syndrome. After a mean follow-up of 45 months, there were two local recurrences, where one would expect no local recurrence in such well differentiated lesions. In contrast to the latter authors' enthusiastic support for enucleation, is the reported experience of three local recurrences after enucleation (Smith et al, 1984) and the demonstration by Marshall et al, (1986) that there was residual tumor in 6 of 15 kidneys after ex vivo enucleation of the tumor. The size of the tumors in this latter study varied from 5 to 12 cm and all grade 1 tumors had negative tumor beds, whereas all grade 3 tumors were associated with residual disease. In another study, careful microscopic examination revealed that neoplastic cells invaded the pseudo-capsule in 23 of 25 tumors ranging in size between 1.2 and 12 cm. Even in a well differentiated lesion with a diameter of only 1.2 cm, it was possible to demonstrate breakthrough of the pseudo-capsule and spreading into the adjacent normal renal tissue (Rosenthal et al, 1984).

These latter studies indicate that resection of a margin of normal kidney is necessary to avoid leaving malignant cells in the bed and thus partial nephrectomy may be a better procedure. For small well differentiated lesions, enucleation gives results, in terms of non-progression and survival, close to those of radical nephrectomy (Zincke et al, 1985) and it is suggested that partial nephrectomy should improve on this experience and be worthy of further evaluation in patients with suitably placed, small, well differentiated, asymptomatic lesions and a normal contralateral kidney.

Acknowledgements

We thank Dr. Roland Phillips of the Cancer Surveillance Program at the University of Southern California for data and advice.

REFERENCES

Bell ET (1950) Renal Disease. 2nd ed. Philadelphia: Lea & Febiger.

Bennington JL (1973) Cancer of the kidney - etiology, epidemiology and pathology. Cancer 32: 1017-1029.

Bennington JL, Mayall BH (1983) DNA cytometry on four-micrometer sections of paraffin-embedded human renal adenocarcinomas and adenomas. Cytometry 4: 31-39.

Bhatt GH, Bernadino ME, Graham SD (1983) CT diagnosis of renal metastases. J Comput Assist Tomogr 7:1032-1034.

Choyke PL, White EM, Zeman RK, Jaffe MH, Clark LR (1986) Renal metastases: clinicopathologic and radiologic correlation. Radiology 162: 359-363.

Curry NS, Schabel SI, Betsill WL (1986) Small renal neoplasms: diagnostic imaging, pathologic features and clinical course. Radiology 158: 113-117.

Haertig A, Kuss R (1982) Clinical signs in renal neoplasia. A comparison of two series of three hundred cases, in Kuss R, Murphy GP, Khoury S, Karr JP (eds) Renal Tumors: Proceedings of the first International Symposium on Kidney Tumors. Liss AR, Inc, New York, pp 337-340.

Hajdu SI, Thomas AG (1967) Renal cell carcinoma at autopsy. J Urol 97:978-982.

Hellsten S, Berge T, Wehlin L (1981a) Unrecognized renal cell carcinoma. Clinical and diagnostic aspects. Scand J Urol Nephrol 8: 269-272.

Hellsten S, Berge T, Wehlin L (1981b) Unrecognized renal cell carcinoma. Clinical and pathological aspects. Scand J Urol Nephrol 8: 273-278.

Kline MJ, Valensi QJ (1976) Proximal tubular adenomas of kidney with so-called oncocytic features; a clinicopatholo-

gic study of 13 cases of a rarely reported neoplasm.
Cancer 38: 906-914.

Klinger ME (1951) Secondary tumors of the genitourinary
tract. J Urol 65: 144-153.

Konnack JW, Grossman HB (1986) Renal cell carcinoma as an
incidental finding. J Urol 134: 1094-1096.

Lang EK (1986) Current cost-effective diagnosis of asymptomatic renal mass lesions: in deKernion JB, Pavone-
Macaluso M (eds): Tumors of the kidney Vol 13 International
Perspectives in Urology: Williams & Wilkins, Baltimore,
pp 11-33.

Lieber MM, Tomera KM, Farrow GM (1981) Renal oncocytoma.
J Urol 125: 481-485.

Lieber MM, Tsukamoto T (1986) Renal oncocytoma, in deKernion
JB, Pavone-Macaluso M (eds): Tumors of the kidney,
International Perspectives in Urology Vol 13, Williams
& Wilkins, pp 306-319.

Ljungberg B, Stenling R, Roos G (1986) Prognostic value of
deoxyribonucleic acid content in metastatic renal cell
carcinoma. J Urol 136: 801-804.

Marshall FF, Taxy JB, Fishman EK, Chang R (1986) The
feasibility of surgical enucleation for renal cell
carcinoma. J Urol 135: 231-234.

Mostofi FK, Davis C (1986) Tumors and tumor-like lesions
of the kidney. Curr Probl Cancer 10: 53-114.

Novick, AC, Zincke H, Neves RJ, Topley HM (1986) Surgical
enucleation for renal cell carcinoma. J Urol 135: 235-
238.

Pagani JJ (1983) Solid renal mass in the cancer patient:
second primary renal cell carcinoma versus renal metastasis.
J Comput Assist Tomogr 7: 444-448.

Petersen RO (1986) Urologic Pathology, JB Lippincott,
Philadelphia, p 86.

Quinn MJ, Hartmann DS, Friedman AC, Sherman JL, Lautin EM,
Pyatt RS, Ho CK, Csere R, Fromowitz FB (1984) Renal
oncocytoma; new observations. Radiology 153: 49-53.

Rainwater LM, Farrow GM, Lieber MM (1986) Flow cytometry of
renal oncocytoma; common occurrence of deoxyribonucleic
acid polyploidy and aneuploidy. J Urol 135: 1167-1171.

Riches EN, Griffiths IH, Thackray AC (1951) New growth of
kidney and ureter. Brit J Urol 23: 297-356.

Rosenthal CL, Kraft R, Zingg EJ (1984) Organ-preserving
surgery in renal cell carcinoma: tumor enucleation
versus partial kidney resection. Eur Urol 10: 222-228.

Skinner DG, Colvin RB, Vermillion CD (1971) Diagnosis and management of renal cell carcinoma. A clinical and pathologic study of 309 cases. Cancer 28: 1165-1177.

Skinner DG, Vermillion CD, Pfister RC, Leadbetter WF (1971) Renal cell carcinoma. Amer Family Phys. 4: 89-94.

Smith RB, deKernion JB, Ehrlich RM, Skinner DG, Kaufman JJ (1984) Bilateral renal cell carcinoma and renal cell carcinoma in the solitary kidney. J Urol 132: 450-454.

Tomera KM, Farrow GM, Lieber MM (1983) Well differentiated (Grade I) clear cell renal carcinoma. J Urol 129: 933-937.

Zincke H, Engen DE, Henning KM, McDonald MW (1985) Treatment of renal cell carcinoma by in situ partial nephrectomy and extracorporeal operation with autotransplantation. Mayo Clin Proc 60: 651-662.

EORTC Genitourinary Group Monograph 5: Progress
and Controversies in Oncological Urology II, page 357
© 1988 Alan R. Liss, Inc.

Discussion: Incidental Renal Neoplasms: Incidence in Los
Angeles County, Treatment and Prognosis

Jan G.M. Klijn, Rotterdam, The Netherlands

Denis: A small surgical question: what about the ipsilateral
adrenal, can we leave it or have we to take it out?

Ritchie: I am not sure that the data I have shown will help
to answer that question for your. But in my own view it is
probably reasonable to leave the ipsilateral adrenal when
the tumor is in the lower pole. But when it is in the middle
or upper pole then I would suggest that it is taken "en
bloc".

N.N.: Is there any place for frozen section biopsy during
this type of surgery?

Ritchie: Absolutely, yes. I cannot talk from an enormous
personal experience, but in the cases I have been involved
there have been no mistakes from frozen section histology on
the margins.

Huland: Does everybody in this room agree that it is fair to
take a biopsy during operation and to do a frozen section
and rely on that? Any comment about that?

Ritchie: I am talking about frozen sections in the margins.

Huland: I see.

EORTC Genitourinary Group Monograph 5: Progress
and Controversies in Oncological Urology II, pages 359-378
© 1988 Alan R. Liss, Inc.

PROGNOSTIC FACTORS IN RENAL ADENOCARCINOMA

David F. Paulson, M.D.

Division of Urologic Surgery, Duke University
Medical Center, Durham, North Carolina   27710

The accumulated data indicates that the prognosis
of renal cell carcinoma is a function of the anatomic
distribution of disease in the host at risk and strongly
suggests that when the disease is treated by surgical
extirpation, then the anatomic distribution of disease
as it relates to the excised surgical specimen is the
most important risk factor. However, once the disease
becomes disseminated, the survival of the host is
related to the biology of the disease and there appears
to be a direct correlation between either histologic
grade and/or cell type and the biologic aggressiveness
of the tumor. There is also some data which suggests
that the organ site of the metastatic disease may be
important in predicting outcome after treatment. When
looking at the impact of surgical extirpation in the
management of the disease, the data indicates that the
anatomic distribution of disease is the single most
important factor in predicting the impact of surgical
removal of the malignancy (Robson et al., 1969; Skinner
et al., 1972; Rafla, 1970; Boxer et al., 1979; deKernion
and Barry, 1980; Lieber et al., 1981; McNichols et al.,
1981; Murphy and Mostofi, 1965; McDonald, 1982). Prior
to the onset of current sophisticated noninvasive
staging technology which is able to demonstrate disease
at a site distant from the primary site, the histologic
characteristics of the primary malignancy were
of prime importance. This position was partially
correct, current data demonstrating that the histologic
characteristics of the primary malignancy function to
predict the statistical probability of the patient

having distant disease spread. However, within the staging methodology which exists today, the hypothesis that the anatomic distribution of disease is more important than the loss of cellular differentiation or cell type has been adequately demonstrated by several studies.

The data reported by Selli and co-workers, reviewing the survival experience of patients with renal cell carcinoma treated at the Duke Medical Center between January 19, 1970 and December 1981, supports this hypothesis (Selli et al., 1983). In this study, all patients were restaged according to the UICC (TNM) classification (UICC, 1978) and by Robson. The restaging was performed in a retrospective manner, based on an analysis of all the preoperative clinical studies, the operative report, and the pathologic review of the excised surgical specimen. A comparison of the distribution of disease as a function of the TNM system and as a function of the Robson system is very difficult when one notes that, under the Robson system, stage C tumors can be either node positive or node negative and either renal vein and vena cava positive or negative (Table 1). Perinephric fat extension is stage B. As will be demonstrated, this provides a distortion in understanding the impact of the anatomic distribution of disease. Nonetheless, in the Selli review, the surgical specimen of each of the patients was restaged according to the anatomic distribution of disease and the surgical specimen of each of the patients was regraded and reclassified with respect to cell type. Using nuclear features and the cellular pattern of the tumor, the histologic pattern was determined. Four categories were established: Grade 1 (well differentiated) through Grade 4 (anaplastic) (Riches, 1964; Arner, et al., 1965; Bottiger, 1970; Fisher et al., 1976).

Each tumor was also classified with respect to cell type: clear cells, dark cells, oncocytes, sarcomatous cells, and mixed cells. The cell type was considered predominant only when it constituted 80% of the tumor sample or, if mixed with more than one cell type, the predominant cell accounted for 30% of the sample specimen (Riches, 1964; Arner, et al., 1965; Bottiger, 1970). Patients were excluded from data analysis when insufficient information for staging and grading and

COMPARISON OF THE TWO CLASSIFICATION SYSTEMS FOR STAGING OF
RENAL CELL CARCINOMA

	TNM (1978)	Robson
Small tumor, no enlargement of kidney	T_1	A
Large tumor, cortex not broken	T_2	A
Perinephric or hilar extension	T_3	B
Extension to neighbouring organs	T_4	D
Nodal invasion	N_+	C
Renal vein involved	V_1	C
Vena cava involved	V_2	C
Distant metastases	M_+	D

Table 1. (From Selli 1983).

analysis of treatment response was identified. The
prognostic significance of each variable was assessed by
statistical analysis of the survival time. Survival was
measured from the date of surgery and deaths not due to
renal carcinoma were censored observations and these
patients were not considered as treatment failures. The
censored observations, noncancer deaths, and last-alive
followup are indicated in this manuscript by vertical
bars on the survival graphs. All survival curves were
calculated by the Kaplan-Meier method using Cox
regression procedures to determine the simultaneous
significance of the prognostic factors (Kaplan and Meier
1958; Cox, 1972). In the Selli review, 115 patients had
data sufficient for analysis, 96 of these patients were
treated by radical nephrectomy, 8 had simple nephrectomy
and 11 had a partial nephrectomy (4 having bilateral
simultaneous tumors, 3 having a solitary kidney, 2
having contralateral renal atrophy and 2 having small
neoplasms encountered at the time of other surgery)
(Graham and Glenn, 1979). The anatomic extent of
disease, grade and cell type of the renal tumors in the
study population are given in Tables 2, 3 and 4.

Twenty-one patients received adjunctive therapy, 5
patients being treated with radiotherapy preoperatively
and 10 being treated with postoperative radiation to the

NUMERICAL DISTRIBUTION OF CASES IN THE DIFFERENT CATEGORIES
OF THE TWO STAGING SYSTEMS

Robson			UICC				
			N_0M_0	N_+M_0	N_0M_+	N_+M_+	Total
A:72 cases	PT_1		35	–	2	–	37
	PT_2	V_0	37	1	4	1	43
		V_+	5	–	1	–	6
B: 8 "		V_0	8	–	4	–	12
	PT_3	V_+	8	1	2	1	12
C:15 "		V_0	–	–	2	–	2
	PT_4	V_+	2	–	1	–	3
D:20 "							
Total 115	Total		95	2	16	2	115

Table 2. (From Selli 1983).

COMPARISON OF HISTOLOGIC GRADE WITH PRESENCE OF METASTASES

	Grade			
	1	2	3	4
M_0	53	30	8	6
M_1	0	4	12	2
Total	53	34	20	8

Table 3. (Selli 1983).

renal bed or to metastatic site(s). Six additional
patients received postoperative hormonal manipulation
using progesterone and testosterone. All 21 patients
are included in the review, no evidence existing to
suggest that these treatments would impact upon the
treatment course. No patient who received combination
cytotoxic chemotherapy was included in this review.

DISTRIBUTION OF CELL TYPE AND GRADE

Cell Type	Grade				Total
	1	2	3	4	
Oncocytes	4	–	–	–	4
Clear	44	22	3	1	70
Dark	3	7	7	–	17
Mixed	2	5	10	6	23
Sarcomatous	–	–	–	1	1
Total	53	34	20	8	115

Table 4: (From Selli 1983).

Examination of the survival experience as a function of metastatic or no metastatic disease demonstrates the adverse impact of metastatic disease (Figure 1). This agrees with later published data of Bassil (Figure 2). The presence or absence of

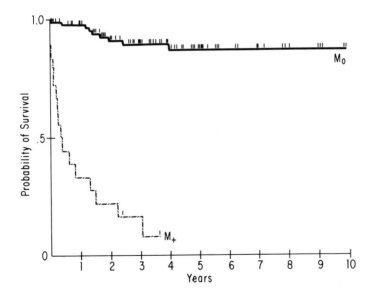

Figure 1: Survival of 115 patients with regard to the presence of metastases. (From Selli 1983)

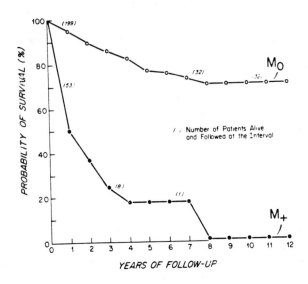

Figure 2: Survival of patients presenting with metastatic disease (Bassil 1985).

metastatic disease at the time of nephrectomy is seen as the most single important factor in determining survival. Of those patients who had metastatic disease at the time of nephrectomy, 80% had died of renal adenocarcinoma within 24 months of surgical intervention. Only 10% of patients who had no demonstrable metastatic disease were dead at 10 months (P 0.001). The survival of patients with no demonstrable metastatic disease seems directly related to the local extent of tumor (Figure 3). In patients who have M_0N_0 disease, the volume of the local tumor seems to be directly related to the survival after surgical extirpation. The published experience of the Cleveland Clinic and the MGH clearly parallels that above (Figures 4 and 5).

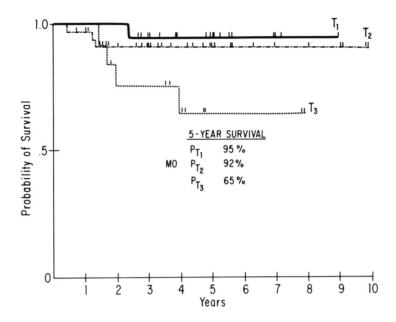

Figure 3: Survival of 115 patients with renal cell carcinoma as a function of local disease (From Selli 1983).

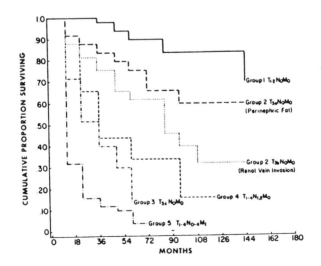

Figure 4: Survival relative to TNM category grouping (From Siminovitch 1983).

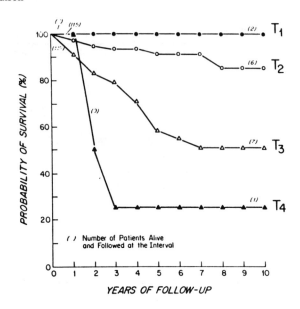

Figure 5: Survival according to pathologic T stage (Bassil 1985).

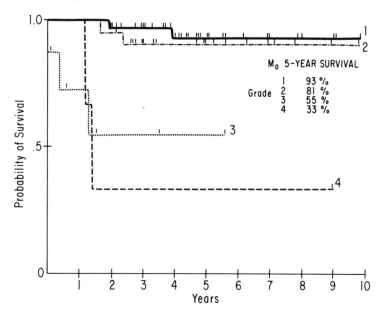

Figure 6: Survival of the patients with regard to grade (From Selli 1983).

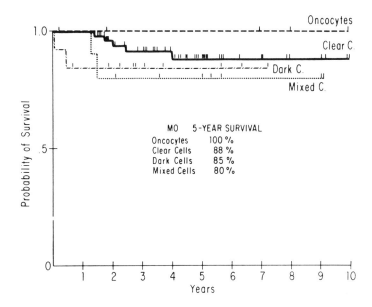

Figure 7: Survival of the nonmetastatic patients with regard to cell type (From Selli 1983).

The pathologic grade of the renal primary does bear some relation to patient survival, even in patients with no demonstrable metastatic disease. However, review of the Selli manuscript suggests that the pathologic grading of the tumor or the cell type itself is a major predictor when the disease is metastatic (Figures 6, 7, 8). Low grade tumors provided an enhanced survival over those whose tumors were of higher grade (P 0.001). While 90% of those patients who were either grade 1 or grade 2 survived 5 years, only 55% of patients whose tumors were pathologic grade 3 and 35% of those patients who were pathologic grade 4, survived an equivalent time. Tumor free survival at 5 years seemed to predict tumor-free survival at 10 years. One concludes that the grade of the tumor functions as a visual predictor of the statistical probability of the patient having metastatic disease which is undetectable by current staging methodology. The relative impact of cell type

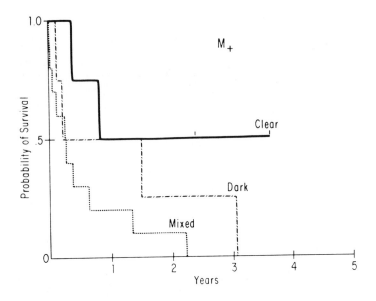

Figure 8: Survival of the metastatic patients with regard to cell type (From Selli 1983).

on survival in M_0 vs. M_+ patients supports the thesis that disease which can be controlled by surgical extirpation provides a survival experience related to the anatomic distribution of disease but, when disease is outside the surgical margins, then the patients survive as a function of tumor biology as reflected in the cell type.

Patients whose disease proceeds by direct extension, either into perinephric fat or renal vein (or vena cava) have a survival experience better than those who have nodal or distant metastatic disease. Extension to perinephric fat may be less ominous than extension to renal vein or vena cava (Figure 9). Venous extension with perinephric involvement is worse than venous extension alone. (Table 5) A similar differential was seen for renal vein involvement (pT_{3b}).

The importance of disease distribution is evident also when one examines the experience of Libertino and coworkers who evaluated the survival experience of 44 patients with renal cell carcinoma extending into the

	$pT_{3c}N_0M_0$	$pT_{3ac}N_0M_0$	$pT_{3b}N_0M_0$	$pT_{3ab}N_0M_0$
Mean Survival	40 mo.	18 mo.	75 mo.	64 mo.

Table 5.

renal vein or inferior vena cava. Actuarial analysis
demonstrates an observed 5 year survival rate of 44 ±
9.1% with an observed 10 year survival rate of 28.9 ±
11%. The observed median survival was 45.8 months
(Libertino et al., 1987). When two perioperative deaths
and two deaths from unrelated disease were censured, the
adjusted 5 and 10 year survival rates were 47.3 ± 9.6%
and 41.4 ± 10% respectively, with an adjusted median
survival time of 57.2 months (Figure 10). The authors

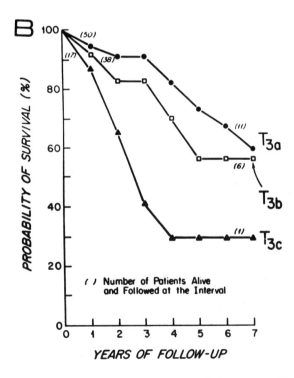

Figure 9: Survival among patients with stage T3 disease
(From Bassil 1985).

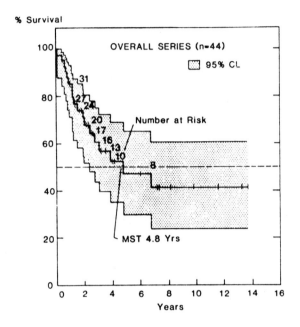

Figure 10: Adjusted survival of 44 patients after resection of renal cell cancer with vena caval extension by Kaplan—Meier curves. Median survival time (MST) is 57.2 months. Stippled area indicates 95% confidence limits. Vertical marks indicate censoring at times of living followup (Libertino 1987).

were unable to detect any difference in survival among patients with regional lymph node involvement and those with distant organ metastasis or continuous organ invasion. They accordingly divided the population into three subgroups: (1) an ideal subgroup of 19 patients whose disease was confined to the kidney and vena cava without extension into perinephric fat, distant metastases, or continuous organ involvement; (2) a favorable subgroup of 13 patients without extrarenal extension other than perinephric fat invasion; and (3) an unfavorable group of 12 patients who had various combinations of regional lymph node involvement, contiguous structure involvement and/or distant metastases. No difference could be identified in the

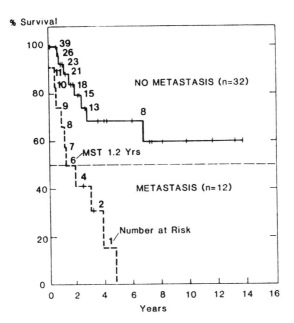

Figure 11: Adjusted survival relative to degree of tumor extension. Tumor extension is limited to subcapsular growth or extension to perinephric fat (solid line indicates ideal and favorable categories). Dashed line (unfavorable category) indicates combination of regional node involvement, distant metastases and contiguous organ invasion (From Libertino 1987).

survival pattern between favorable and ideal groups (P = 0.93). Combining these two groups (32 patients) produced an adjusted 5 and 10 year survival of 68.8 ± 10.1% and 60.2 ± 12%, respectively (Figure 11). In contrast, the 12 patients who had nodal involvement or metastatic disease demonstrated a median survival time of 1.2 years with no survival extending past 4.8 years. The difference in survival was statistically significant (P = 0.002).

The overall 45% survival experience of the entire population is equivalent to that reported previously by other investigators (Table 6). Libertino could not demonstrate any survival difference based on renal extension being either superdiaphragmatic or intradiaphragmatic.

Reference	No Pts	Observed 5-Yr Survival	Observed Mortality
Skinner et al	11	45.0%	Unavailable
Schefft et al	21	28.5%	14.3%
Kearney et al	24	16.6%	4.0%
Libertino et al	44	44.0%	4.5%

Table 6: Study was limited to cancer with renal vein and vena caval extension. The remaining reports included all patterns of cancer growth (Libertino, 1987).

The prognostic significance of lymph node involvement, and the ability to control lymph node involvement by surgical extirpation is debated. The survival rate for patients with lymph node extension varies from 0 to 30% (Hoehn et al., 1983; deKernion, 1980) (Figure 12). Published data also would relate survival among patients with lymph node extension equivalent to the survival of patients who have distant metastatic disease. Thus, the question of the benefit of lymph node dissection remains indeterminant when evaluating the impact of surgical or alternative therapy. The first lymph nodes usually involved are those within the hilum of the kidney (Marshall et al., 1982). Although one might expect that a limited unilateral lymphadenectomy might encompass the only involved nodes, this has not been adequately tested. There remains a theoretical potential for therapeutic gain by performing lymphadenectomy in these patients. However, the presence of lymph node involvement indicates that the patient has a disease process in which the cells have acquired the ability to move from site to site and therefore has a disease which is systemic in nature. Lymphadenectomy does not enhance survival in either T_2 or T_3 tumors (Figures 13A&B). Consequently, it is strongly recommended that patients with lymph node involvement be segregated as to number of lymph nodes involved and level of nodal involvement (be they hilar, or along the great vessels) and they then be substratified with respect to the cell type.

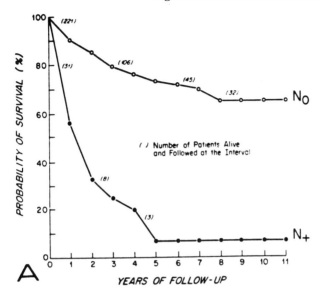

Figure 12: Lymph node status as prognostic indicator (Bassil 1985).

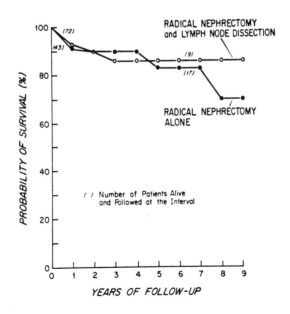

Figure 13A: Choice of surgical procedure had no influence on subsequent course of disease (T_2 tumors) (Bassil 1985).

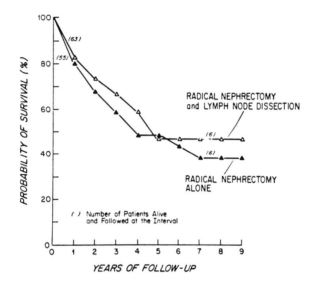

Figure 13B: Choice of surgical procedure had no influence on subsequent course of disease (T$_3$ tumor) (Bassil 1985).

Performance status, site of metastatic disease, and number of organs involved may be reasonable stratification indices in patients who have metastatic disease. DeKernion and co-workers (Maldazys and deKernion, 1986) examined the survival experience of patients with metastatic disease who underwent adjunctive nephrectomy. In more than 100 patients, those who survived longer than 12 months had a good performance status, a limited tumor burden, a completely resected primary lesion, and metastatic disease confined to the lungs (Figures 13A&B). Although the patients within this study received multiple adjunctive treatments after nephrectomy, no specific impact of these adjunctive treatments can be identified in the patient population.

In conclusion, when examining stratification indices in patients with renal cell carcinoma, one must conclude that the anatomic distribution of disease, whether it is confined to the kidney, to the surgical specimen, or whether it has extended to sites which are

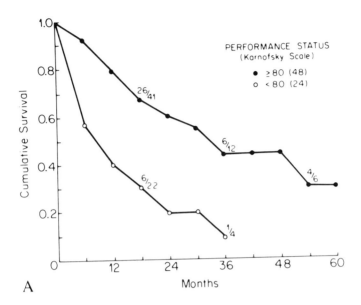

Figure 14A: Survival of patients with metastatic renal cell carcinoma according to performance status. Patients with good performance status survived better than did patients with poor performance status, regardless of therapy (deKernion 1987).

anatomically distinct and do not exist as a function of direct extension from the tumor site are of prognostic importance in determining the impact of surgical therapy. For disease which has extended to sites which are anatomically segregated from the primary organ site (nodal or distant metastatic disease) it would appear that the cell type provides an indication as to prognosis, the cell type indicating the biologic virulence of the tumor within the host. The apparent survival advantage which exists in patients that have lung-only metastatic disease must be recognized and observed with caution. The observation that patients with a single metastatic site experience a survival advantage over those with multiple sites of metastatic disease may reflect only the impact of an increased tumor burden and a probability of other but as yet undetected sites of metastatic extension.

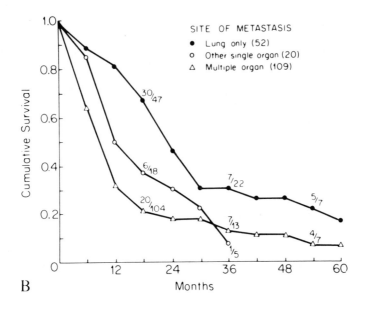

B

Figure 14B: Survival of patients with metastatic renal cell carcinoma according to site of metastases. Patients who had only pulmonary metastases survived better than did those with metastases at other sites (deKernion 1987).

REFERENCES

Arner O, Blanck C, Schreeb T (1965). Renal adenocarcinoma: morphology-grading of malignancy-prognosis. Acta Chir Scand 346:1.

Bassil B, Dosoretz DE, Prout GR (1985). Validation of the tumor, nodes and metastasis classification of renal cell carcinoma. J Urol 134:450.

Bottiger LE (1970). Prognosis in renal carcinoma. Cancer 26:780.

Boxer RJ, Waisman J, Lieber MM, Mampaso FM, Skinner DG (1979). Renal carcinoma: computer analysis of 96 patients treated by nephrectomy. J Urol 122:598.

Cox DR (1972). Regression models and life tables. J R Stat Soc 34:187.

deKernion JB (1980). Lymphadenectomy for renal cell carcinoma: Therapeutic implications. Urol Clin N Am 7:697.

deKernion JB, Barry B (1980). Diagnosis and treatment of renal cell carcinoma. Cancer 45:1947.

deKernion JB (1987). Management of renal adenocarcinoma. In: JB deKernion, DF Paulson (Eds), Genitourinary Cancer Management, Lea & Febiger, Philadelphia, p 187.

Fisher ER, Gregorio RM, Fisher B, et al (1976). The pathology in invasive breast cancer. Cancer 36:81.

Graham DS, Glenn JF (1979). Enucleative surgery for renal malignancy. J Urol 122:646.

Hoehn W, Hermanek P (1983). Invasion of veins in renal cell carcinoma: frequency, correlation and prognosis. Eur Urol 9:276.

Kaplan EL, Meier P (1958). Nonparametric estimation from incomplete observations. J Am Stat Assoc 53:457.

Kearney GP, Waters WB, Klein LA, Richie JP, Gittes RF (1981). Results of inferior vena cava resection for renal cell carcinoma. J Urol 125:769.

Libertino JA, Zinman L, Watkins E (1987). Long-term results of resection of renal cell cancer with extension into inferior vena cava. J urol 137:21.

Lieber MM, Tomera FM, Taylor WF, Farrow GM (1981). Renal adenocarcinoma in young adults: survival and variables affecting prognosis. J Urol 125:164.

Maldazys J, deKernion JB (1986). Prognostic factors in metastatic renal cell carcinoma. J Urol 136:376.

Marshall F, Powell KC (1982). Lymphadenectomy for renal cell carcinoma: anatomical and therapeutic considerations. J Urol 128:677.

McDonald MW (1982). Current therapy for renal cell carcinoma. J Urol 127:211.

McNichols DW, Segura JW, DeWeerd JH (1981). Renal cell carcinoma: long-term survival and late recurrence. J Urol 126:17.

Murphy GP, Mostofi FK (1965). The significance of cytoplasmic granularity in the prognosis of renal cell carcinoma. J Urol 94:84.

Rafla S (1970). Renal carcinoma: natural history and results of treatment. Cancer 25:26.

Riches EW (1964). Monographs on neoplastic disease at various sites. "Tumors of the kidney and ureter", Baltimore, Williams & Wilkins, vol 5.

Robson CJ, Churchill BM, Anderson W (1969). The results of radical nephrectomy for renal cell carcinoma. J Urol 101:297.

Schefft P, Novick AC, Straffon RA, Stewart BH (1978).
  Surgery for renal cell carcinoma extending into the
  inferior vena cava. J Urol 120:28.
Selli C, Hinshaw W, Woodard BH, Paulson DF (1983).
  Stratification of risk factors in renal cell
  carcinoma. Cancer 52:899.
Siminovitch JMP, Montie JE, Straffon RA (1983).
  Prognostic indicators in renal adenocarcinoma. J Urol
  130:20.
Skinner DJ, Vermillion C, Colvin C (1972). The surgical
  management of renal cell carcinoma. J Urol 107:705.
Union Internationale Contre le Cancer (UICC) (1978).
  TNM classification of malignant tumours. In Harmer MH
  (ed): "Union International Contre le Cancer", 3rd ed,
  Geneva.

EORTC Genitourinary Group Monograph 5: Progress
and Controversies in Oncological Urology II, pages 379–380
© 1988 Alan R. Liss, Inc.

Discussion: Prognostic Factors in Renal Adenocarcinoma

Jan G.M. Klijn, Rotterdam, The Netherlands

Paulson: You may notice that I did not address the topic of flowcytometry. I could not find any substantial information which will allow me to make a reasonable statement at this time.

Fair: Dr. Paulson, T1-T2 diseases have minimal risk according to your presentation and N-positive disease is the same as M-positive disease. Could you come down on the question of lymph node dissection with radical nephrectomy? I mean you do not need it in low stage disease and in the high stage it is maybe too late.

Paulson: Well, I tend to probably try to simplify these problems more than I should. I think that the basic statement, that in low grade disease you probably do not need it and in high grade disease it does not do any good, is correct. In fact, if you look into the data of the Massachusetts General Group in which they looked on the subsequent survival for low stage disease, whether or not they had node dissection, and for high stage disease whether or not they had node dissection, the survival curves are almost superimposed one upon the other. However, I think that if we are going to be in there, it is probably appropriate to do a node dissection. Just so if the patient fails we have some idea why the patient fails. Or otherwise, we are in somewhat of a morass with respect to an understanding of the impact of surgical intervention. If there is any possible benefit to removing as much of the tumor burden as possible and, this again is a question that I do not know had an answer, then perhaps removing nodal structures which are tumor-bearing, is of importance. I think that those are questions which we have to address in the future.

N.N.: I would like to ask another surgical question. Is there an advantage of an early transperitoneal vascular division which will minimize metastatic spread, compared to operation via the lumbotomic route which requires renal mass manipulation? In other words, what is the importance of the manipulation of the renal mass with respect to prognosis?

Paulson: The question is, is it important to gain early vascular control to prevent the subsequent dissemination of disease in the host who is undergoing radical nephrectomy. I do not have any data which would show that early vascular control prevents the subsequent appearance of metastatic disease. In fact if you would cannulate the renal vein in any of these tumors and monitored the patient for a period of days prior to nephrectomy, it appears that these tumors are releasing millions of cells over a 24-hour period. Why most of these cells never implant, I do not know. Whether squeezing the tumor, which perhaps increases the circulating tumor burden, or pushing cells out in small clumps would enhance the metastatic potential, I do not know. I personally do not think that early vascular control prevents metastatic disease. What it does it makes the surgeons happier.

Huland: May I have a short comment on your statement about DNA flowcytometry because I somewhat disagree. I think there are accumulating data indicating that DNA measurement is of value, including our own data in 68 patients with T1-T3 renal cell carcinoma with a mean follow-up of 2.5 years. In those who had a diploid tumor the occurrence of metastasis was only in 20% in contrast to those with an aneuploid tumor who had a 81% occurrence of metastases. So I think there is some evidence.

Paulson: I am quite willing to stand correction.

N.N.: Do you favor a simple nephrectomy in patients with T1 and T2 tumors?

Paulson: No, I do not favor a simple nephrectomy in those patients although in retrospect once the specimen is in the pan so to speak and you know it is not a macroscopic T3 lesion, you probably have to go back and do a simple nephrectomy. I think if you go in there and remove the kidney in toto you should make certain that you make every effort to remove the entire kidney and the surrounding fat. Another comment if you are going to do a partial nephrectomy for a polar lesion you should not strip the fat off of that lesion. You should leave that lesion entirely covered by as much peritoneal fatty tissue as possible, so that again the chances of leaving residual disease in your surgical bed is diminished.

EORTC Genitourinary Group Monograph 5: Progress
and Controversies in Oncological Urology II, pages 381–392
© 1988 Alan R. Liss, Inc.

A MULTIVARIATE ANALYSIS OF PROGNOSTIC FACTORS IN DISSEMINATED NON-SEMINOMATOUS TESTICULAR CANCER

G. Stoter[1], R. Sylvester[2], D.Th. Sleijfer[3], W.W. ten Bokkel Huinink[4], S.B. Kaye[5], W.G. Jones[6], A.T. van Oosterom[7], C.P.J. Vendrik[8], P. Spaander[9], M. de Pauw[2], for the EORTC GU Group.

[1]Free University Hospital, Amsterdam, The Netherlands, [2]EORTC Data Center, Brussels, Belgium, [3]University Hospital, Groningen, The Netherlands, [4]Netherlands Cancer Institute, Amsterdam, The Netherlands, [5]Gartnavel Hospital, Glasgow, U.K., [6]Cookridge Hospital, Leeds, U.K., [7]University Hospital, Leiden, The Netherlands, [8]University Hospital, Utrecht, The Netherlands, [9]Red Cross Hospital, The Hague, The Netherlands.

INTRODUCTION

With standard cisplatin combination chemotherapy, the risk of death from disseminated non-seminomatous testicular cancer is approximately 30%, including a 5% toxic death rate from these regimens (Einhorn 1984, Greist et al. 1985, Stoter et al. 1984, Stoter et al. 1986, Williams et al. 1985). This underlines the need to define good risk and poor risk patients prior to treatment in order to decrease the toxicity in the first category and to intensify the treatment in the second group. Several factors have been reported as influencing the prognosis such as: extent of disease (Stoter et al. 1984, Stoter et al. 1986, Williams et al. 1985, Skinner 1982, Ozols et al. 1983, Medical Research Council Working Party on Testicular Tumours 1985), initial serum marker concentrations of HCG, AFP and LDH (Medical Research Council Working Party on Testicular Tumours 1985, Newlands et al. 1983, Bosl et al. 1983, Von Eyben et al. 1982), or their rate of decrease during chemotherapy (Vogelzang et al. 1982, Picozzi et al. 1984), histology (Pugh 1976, Stoter et al. 1979), prior treatment (Stoter et al. 1984, Golbey et al. 1979), treatment protocol, age, time from diagnosis to treatment (Medical Research Council Working Party on Testicular

Tumours 1985), and performance status (Von Eyben et al. 1982).

Since many of these variables may be interrelated, a multivariate analysis of various factors has been performed in order to determine their relative prognostic importance.

MATERIALS AND METHODS

Patients Studied

From July 1979 until March 1983, the EORTC GU-Group entered 214 patients with disseminated non-seminomatous testicular cancer in a randomized prospective study. None of these patients had received prior radiotherapy or chemotherapy. The patients received 4 cycles of induction chemotherapy with cisplatin, vinblastine and bleomycin (PVB), with a randomization between vinblastine 0.4 mg/kg/cycle (100% VBL) or vinblastine 0.3 mg/kg/cycle (75% VBL). One hundred and sixty three patients were evaluable for response. The treatment results of this study have been reported elsewhere (Stoter et al. 1986).

The endpoint for this analysis is the rate of complete response (CR). All patients who did not achieve a CR are categorized as "no CR".

The histological diagnosis was made according to the British classification (Pugh 1976). Staging of the disease was according to the Royal Marsden Hospital classification (Medical Research Council Working Party on Testicular Tumours 1985). However, it was also felt necessary to record the exact number and size of all metastatic lesions.

Serum tumor marker concentrations were measured in each participating institution without a central reference. Radioimmunoassay techniques were used for quantitative determination of βHCG and AFP. Serum concentrations of βHCG $\leq$ 4 ng/ml and AFP $\leq$ 16 ng/ml were considered to be normal. Serum concentrations of LDH were measured by different methods in different institutions where the upper limits of normal varied significantly. For these reasons LDH has been expressed as a numerical factor multiplied by the upper limit of normal for each institution.

Patient Characteristics

Patient characteristics and CR rates with regard to
several of the most important prognostic factors are given
in Table 1.

TABLE 1.   Patient characteristics (N = 163 patients)

Variable			% CR	N (% in each subgroup)	
βHCG	0	– 49	83	99	(61)
	50	– 999	66	35	(21)
	1000	– 9999	39	18	(11)
	10000	– 2000000	18	11	(7)
AFP	0	– 999	76	133	(82)
	1000	– 790000	41	29	(18)
Histology	TD		75	4	(2)
	MTI		73	59	(36)
	MTU		78	76	(47)
	MTT		38	24	(15)
Burden	Low * High		88 58	66 97	(40) (60)
Metastatic sites	0 – 1		80	70	(43)
	2		67	54	(33)
	3 – 5		56	39	(24)
Number of lung metastases	None		75	68	(43)
	1 – 3		94	35	(22)
	4 – 19		60	40	(25)
	> 20		29	14	(9)
Size of lung metastases	None		75	68	(44)
	< 2 cm		89	45	(29)
	< 3 cm		67	15	(10)
	> 3 cm		37	27	(17)

* High tumor burden: lymph node metastases > 5 cm or lung
metastases > 2 cm. TD = teratoma differentiated; MTI =
malignant teratoma intermediate = teratocarcinoma; MTU =
malignant teratoma undifferentiated = embryonal cell
carcinoma; MTT = malignant teratoma trophoblastic.

Sixty-nine patients (42%) had a normal βHCG and 67 patients (41%) had a normal AFP. Only 38 patients (24%) were normal with respect to both markers. Ninety-seven patients (60%) had a high tumor burden (lymph node metastases > 5 cm or lung metastases > 2 cm). Malignant teratoma trophoblastic was found in 15% of the specimens and possible trophoblastic elements were seen in another 7%. Seminomatous components were observed in 16% of the specimens.

Infradiaphragmatic metastases were present in 135 patients (83%), mediastinal metastases in 18 patients (11%), supraclavicular metastases in 35 patients (22%) and lung metastases in 95 patients (58%). Hepatic metastases were observed in 8 patients (5%).

Statistical techniques

Comparisons of the CR rate for the different levels of a given factor were carried out using the classical chi square test for the comparison of proportions. For ordered categorical variables, Kendall's Tau B and C were calculated as a nonparametric measure of correlation or "trend". Kendall and Spearman rank correlation co-efficients were also calculated to determine the degree of correlation between the various prognostic factors (Kendall 1975).

The relative importance of the prognostic factors with regard to the CR rate was studied using a linear logistic regression model (Lee 1980). This model allows many variables to be studied simultaneously (see appendix for a description of the linear logistic model).

RESULTS

A linear logistic regression model was fitted using the variables given in Table 2. Using a step-up procedure to add variables one by one to the model, the single most important factor was LB = $\log_{10}$ (βHCG+1), the logarithm of the βHCG. The final model, using a step-down procedure, is given in the appendix and was composed of the following variables which were all available in 154 patients:

<u>TROPH</u> (trophoblastic elements)
   0 = no or possible
   1 = yes
<u>ALPH</u> (serum concentration of AFP)
   0 = 0-999 ng/ml
   1 = $\geq$ 1000 ng/ml
<u>LUNG</u> (lung metastases)
   0 = no
   1 = yes
<u>SIXNB</u> (size and number of lung metastases)
   0 = none
   1 = 1-3 and $\leq$ 3 cm
   2 = 4-19 and $\leq$ 3 cm or 1-3 and $>$ 3 cm
   3 = $\geq$ 20 or 4-19 and $>$ 3 cm

Once these values are known for any patient, the probability of a CR can be estimated using the formulas in the appendix.

Of special note is the fact that the <u>single</u> most important variable, LB = $\log_{10}$ (βHCG+1), was <u>not</u> retained in the final model. This is because it is highly correlated with all the variables in the model, especially with TROPH and SIXNB. In fact, βHCG appeared to be correlated with most of the other important prognostic factors in contrast to AFP, which is retained in the model. Trophoblastic elements are not correlated with the presence or absence of lung metastases, nor with their size and number. Elevated markers, tumor volume and number of metastatic sites are correlated with AFP and are not retained in the model. Variables other than the 4 included in the final model do not significantly increase one's ability to predict the probability of CR.

As noted in Table 1, patients with 1-3 lung metastases and patients with lung metastases $<$ 2 cm in diameter have a better prognosis than patients with no lung metastases. This may be explained by the fact that 54% of the patients without lung metastases have infradiaphragmatic metastases $\geq$ 5 cm as opposed to only 20% of the patients in each of the 2 most favorable lung subgroups mentioned above. Patients with infradiaphragmatic metastases $\geq$ 5 cm have a response rate of only 56% as compared to a response rate of 84% for the remaining patients.

TABLE 2   Variables analyzed in the logistic regression model

---

1.[*] RT19 (response to treatment): 0=no CR, 1=CR
2.   TROPH (trophoblastic elements in primary tumor); 0=no or possible, 1=yes
3.   TROP (trophoblastic elements in primary tumor): 0=no, 1=possible, 2=yes
4.   TROPP (trophoblastic elements in primary tumor): 0=no, 1=yes or possible
5.   TRT11 (treatment arm): 0=100% VBL, 1=75% VBL
6.   PMAR (elevated markers): 0=normal AFP and HCG, 1=elevated AFP or βHCG)
7.   BURDEN (tumor volume): 0=low volume, 1=high volume
8.   BETA (βHCG): 0=0-49, 1=50-999, 2=10^3-9999, 3=$\geq 10^4$ ng/ml
9.   NBETA (βHCG elevated): 0=no, 1=yes, (>4 ng/ml)
10. LB = $\log_{10}$ (βHCG+1)
11. ALPH (AFP): 0=0-999, 1=$\geq 10^3$ ng/ml
12. NALPHA (AFP elevated): 0=no, 1=yes (>16 ng/ml)
13. LA = $\log_{10}$ (AFP+1)
14. LDH6 (LDH above 2.5 times upper limit of normal): 0=no, 1=yes
15. INFRA (infradiaphragmatic metastases): 0=no, 1=yes
16. SINFRA (size of infradiaphragmatic metastases): 0=none, 1=<5 cm, 2=$\geq$5 cm, 3=$\geq$10 cm
17. MEDIA (mediastinal metastases): 0=no, 1=yes
18. SUPRA (supraclavicular metastases): 0=no, 1=yes
19. LUNG (lung metastases): 0=no, 1=yes
20. SIZE (size of lung metastases): 0=none, 1=$\leq$2 cm, 2=$\leq$3 cm, 3=>3 cm
21. NUMB (number of lung metastases): 0=none, 1=1-3, 2=4-19, 3=>20
22. SIXNB (size by number of lung metastases): 0=none, 1=1-3 and <3 cm, 2=4-19 and $\leq$3 cm or 1-3 and >3 cm, 3=>20 or 4-19 and >3 cm
23. SIZXNB (size by number of lung metastases): 0=none, 1=1-3, 2=4-19 and $\leq$3 cm, 3=>20 or 4-19 and >3 cm
24. SITE (number of metastatic sites): 0=0-1, 1=2, 2=3-5
25. AGER (age >45 years): 0=no, 1=yes
26. HP21 (liver metastases): 0=no, 1=yes

---

[*] Dependent variable

For a given set of patient characteristics TROPH, ALPH, LUNG and SIXNB, a patient can be assigned to one of 4 risk groups based on the predicted probability of CR calculated by the linear logistic regression model. Table 3 presents the composition of the risk groups according to the possible values of these 4 variables and the observed and predicted probabilities of CR by patient characteristics within each group.

TABLE 3   Composition of risk groups based on patient characteristics and the observed and predicted CR rates

Risk Group	Pat. characteristics				Pts N	CR Obs N	CR Pred N	P	
	TROPH	ALPH	LUNG	SIXNB				Obs	Pred
1	no	<1000	yes	1	24	24	24	1.0	0.989
2	yes	<1000	yes	1	3	2	3	0.667	0.914
	no	>1000	yes	1	1	1	1	1.0	0.902
	no	<1000	yes	2	20	20	18	1.0	0.898
	no	<1000	no	0	49	42	43	0.857	0.874
3	yes	>1000	yes	1	0	–	–	–	0.522
	yes	<1000	yes	2	3	1	2	0.333	0.510
	no	>1000	yes	2	10	4	5	0.40	0.475
	no	<1000	yes	3	14	5	6	0.357	0.463
	yes	<1000	no	0	7	3	3	0.429	0.452
	no	>1000	no	0	12	6	5	0.50	0.417
4	yes	>1000	yes	2	0	–	–	–	0.119
	yes	<1000	yes	3	6	2	1	0.333	0.093
	no	>1000	yes	3	4	0	0	0	0.082
	yes	>1000	no	0	0	–	–	–	0.078
	yes	>1000	yes	3	1	0	0	0	0.010

N = number, Pts = patients, Obs = observed,
Pred = predicted, P = probability of CR

Finally the observed CR rate for all patients within each risk group is given in Table 4.

TABLE 4   Response rate by risk group

Risk group	Predicted nr. of CR	Observed nr. of CR	Number of patients	Observed percentage of CR
1 = I	24	24	24	100%
2	65	65	73	89%
3 = II	21	19	46	41%
4 = III	1	2	11	18%
Total	111	110	154	71%

It is seen that the observed CR rate ranges from 100% in risk group 1 to only 18% in risk group 4. From a clinical point of view these 4 groups may be combined into 3 risk groups: group I (=1+2) with a high probability of CR (89-100%), group II (=3) with an intermediate probability of CR (41%) and group III (=4) with a low probability of CR (18%).

DISCUSSION

The main goal of clinical research is to decrease the toxicity of treatment regimens in good risk patients and to intensify the treatment of poor risk patients. For that reason it is of the utmost importance for physicians to be able to prospectively estimate the probability of CR in each one of their patients. The best tool for such an estimation is the linear logistic regression model since it provides an "optimal" subset of variables for use in determining a patient's prognostic category.

Applied to the data in this study the model yielded 4 prognostic variables: TROPH (trophoblastic elements in the primary tumor: yes or no), ALPH (serum level of AFP below or above 1000 ng/ml), LUNG (lung metastases: yes or no) and SIXNB (size and number of lung metastases).

In the initial phase of this analysis, using a step-up procedure, LB = $\log_{10}$ (βHCG+1) appeared to be the <u>single</u> most important variable, not BETA or NBETA (Table 4). When it was decided to omit the Royal Marsden classification of lung metastases and let them take on a continuum of values with regard to size and number, LB fell out of the model using a step-down procedure and LUNG (lung metastases: yes/no) and SIXNB (lung metastases by size and number) remained in the model, with greater predictive power than LB. It became clear that for our patient population the Royal Marsden staging classification of lung metastases should be modified (Table 2, point 22). This did not hold true for retroperitoneal metastases. When a separate category was provided for patients with infradiaphragmatic metastases larger than 10 cm (Table 4, point 16), the variable SINFRA, while significant in a univariate analysis, was not retained by the model.

Investigators in the U.S.A. (Bosl et al. 1983, Birch et al. 1986) and in Europe (Medical Research Council Working Party on Testicular Tumours 1985, Von Eyben et al. 1982, Droz et al. 1986) have performed multivariate analyses with slightly different variables and endpoints. All models yield tumor markers and/or tumor volume as significant variables, although none of the model results are identical. In contrast to the other models, trophoblastic elements in the primary tumor appear to be a prognostic variable in this model.

The multivariate analysis of prognostic factors becomes an increasingly important method for the prospective determination of a patient's risk category. However, due to lack of uniformity in the assessment of laboratory measurements, pathology, and tumor burden, the relative merits of the various models proposed in the literature cannot be determined. For this reason we believe that it is of urgent necessity that such techniques be standardized.

REFERENCES

Birch R, Williams S, Cone A, Einhorn L, Roark P, Turner S, Greco F (1986). Prognostic factors for favorable outcome in disseminated germ cell tumors. J Clin Oncol 4:400-407.

Bosl GJ, Geller NL, Cirrincione C, Vogelzang NJ, Kennedy BJ, Whitmore WF Jr, Vugrin D, Scher H, Nisselbaum J, Golbey RB (1983). Multivariate analysis of prognostic variables in patients with metastatic testicular cancer. Cancer Res 43:3403-3407.

Droz JP, Kramar A, Piot G, Cailland JM, Bellet D, Pico JL, Sanchier-Garnier H (1986). Multivariate logistic regression analysis of prognostic factors in patients with advanced stage non-seminomatous germ cell tumors of the testis. Abstr Proc Amer Soc Clin Oncol 5:98.

Einhorn LH (1981). Testicular cancer as a model for a curable neoplasm: The Richard and Hinda Rosenthal Foundation award lecture. Cancer Res 41:3275-3280.

Golbey RB, Reynolds TF, Vugrin D (1979). Chemotherapy of metastatic germ cell tumors. Semin Oncol 6:82-86.

Greist A, Roth B, Einhorn L, Williams S (1985). Cisplatin combination chemotherapy for disseminated germ cell tumors: long term follow-up. Proc Amer Soc Clin Oncol 4:100.

Kendall M (1975). In: Rank correlation methods. Ed. Kendall M, Charles Griffin and Company, Ltd., London, pp 1-66 and 123-131.

Lee E (1980). Identification of risk factors related to dichotomous data. In: Statistical methods for survival data analysis, Ed. Lee, E., Lifetime Learning Publications, Belmont, California, pp 338-365.

Medical Research Council Working Party on Testicular Tumours (1985) Prognostic factors in advanced non-seminomatous germ-cell testicular tumours: results of a multicentre study. Lancet i:8-11.

Newlands ES, Begent RHJ, Rustin GJS, Parker D, Bagshawe KD (1983). Further advances in the management of malignant teratomas of the testis and other sites. The Lancet i:948-951.

Ozols RF, Deisseroth AB, Javadpour N, Barlock A, Messer-schmidt GL, Young RC (1983). Treatment of poor prognosis non-seminomatous testicular cancer with a "high-dose" platinum combination chemotherapy regimen. Cancer 51:1803-1807.

Picozzi VJ Jr, Freiha FS, Hannigan JF Jr, Torti FM (1984).

Prognostic significance of a decline in serum human chorionic gonadotropin levels after initial chemotherapy for advanced germ cell carcinoma. Ann Int Med 100: 183-186.

Pugh RCB (1976). Testicular tumours - introduction. In: Pathology of the testis. Ed. Pugh, RCB, Blackwell Scientific Publications, Oxford, pp 139-162.

Skinner DG (1982). Advanced metastatic testicular cancer: the need for reporting results according to initial extent of disease. J Urol 128:312-314.

Stoter G, Vendrik CPJ, Struyvenberg A, Brouwers ThM, Sleyfer DTh, Schraffordt-Koops H, van Oosterom AT, Pinedo HM (1979). Combination chemotherapy with cis-diammine-dichloro-platinum, vinblastine and bleomycin in advanced testicular nonseminoma. Lancet i:941-945.

Stoter G, Vendrik CPJ, Struyvenberg A, Sleyfer DTh, Vriesendorp R, Schraffordt-Koops H, van Oosterom AT, ten Bokkel Huinink WW, Pinedo HM (1984). Five-year survival of patients with disseminated non-seminomatous testicular cancer treated with cisplatin, vinblastine and bleomycin. Cancer 54:1521-1524.

Stoter G, Sleyfer DTh, ten Bokkel Huinink WW, Kaye SB, Jones WG, van Oosterom AT, Vendrik CPJ, Spaander P, de Pauw M, Sylvester R (1986). High dose versus low dose vinblastine in cisplatin-vinblastine- bleomycin (PVB) combination chemotherapy of non-seminomatous testicular cancer: a randomized study of the EORTC Genito-Urinary Tract Cancer Cooperative Group. J Clin Oncol 4:1199-1206.

Vogelzang NJ, Lange PH, Goldman A, Vessela RH, Fraley EE, Kennedy BJ (1982). Acute changes of α-fetoprotein and human chorionic gonadotropin during induction chemotherapy of germ cell tumors. Cancer Res 42:4855-4861.

Von Eyben FE, Jacobsen GK, Pedersen H, Jacobsen M, Clausen PP, Zibrandtsen PC, Gullberg B (1982). Multivariate analysis of risk factors in patients with metastatic testicular germ cell tumours treated with vinblastine and bleomycin. Invasion Metastasis 2:125-135.

Williams S, Einhorn L, Greco R, Birch R, Irwin L (1985). Disseminated germ cell tumors: a comparison of cisplatin plus bleomycin plus either vinblastine (PVB) or VP-16 (BEP). Proc Amer Soc Clin Oncol 4:100.

APPENDIX

The Linear Logistic Regression Model

The linear logistic regression model (17) assumes that the relationship between the probability p that a patient achieves a CR and the patient's characteristics X_1, X_2, X_m at entry into the study is given by:

$$p = \frac{e^y}{1 + e^y} \qquad \text{or} \qquad \ln \frac{p}{1 - p} = y \qquad (A)$$

where $y = \sum_{i=o}^{m} B_i X_i$ is a linear function of the patient's characteristics, $X_o = 1$ and the B_i are the unknown regression coefficients that are estimated from the data by the technique of maximum likelihood.

The variables which were analyzed in the model, and their coding, are given in Table 4. Both step-up (variables are added to the model one by one) and step-down (variables are deleted from the model one by one, thus allowing a simultaneous analysis of all the variables and their interactions) methods were used.

The following model was obtained using the step-down method:

$$\hat{p} = \frac{e^{\hat{y}}}{1 + e^{\hat{y}}} \qquad \text{where}$$

$$\hat{y} = 1.9381 - 2.1327 \times \text{TROPH} - 2.2723 \times \text{ALPH} + \qquad (B)$$
$$4.878 \times \text{LUNG} - 2.3212 \times \text{SIXNB} \text{ as an "optimal"}$$
estimate of the CR rate.

Once the values of TROPH, ALPH, LUNG and SIXNB (see Table 3) are known for any given patient, the above formula for $\hat{p}$ gives an estimate of the probability that a patient will have a CR. Risk groups can then be formed based on the value of $\hat{p}$.

EORTC Genitourinary Group Monograph 5: Progress
and Controversies in Oncological Urology II, page 393
© 1988 Alan R. Liss, Inc.

Discussion: A Multivariate Analysis of Prognostic Factors
in Disseminated Non-Seminomatous Testicular Cancer

Ted A.W. Splinter, Rotterdam, The Netherlands

Ten Kate: Can you explain why serum HCG is not a prognostic factor, while histological evidence of trophoblastic elements is?

Stoter: I cannot answer this very interesting question exactly. Initially, we found that serum HCG was the most important prognostic factor regardless of anything else, i.e. patients with an HCG above 10.000 ng/ml consistently had a CR rate of less than 20% and this also remains true in our recent studies. Initially, we had HCG in the model as an independent prognostic factor, but when we omitted the Peckham classification and we introduced the size and number of metastases as a continuum, it appeared that the size and number of lungmetastases overruled the power of HCG because of the close correlation between HCG and the other prognostic factors involved in the model. I realize that this explanation does not answer your question about the relation between serum HCG and histology.

Harland: This study looked at CR rate, while other studies have looked at survival. How did you define CR and how does that relate to survival in the EORTC-studies?

Stoter: We would have liked to use survival as an endpoint, but as you have seen, after 3 years only 20% of the patients had died. Statistically it is not attractive to use that as an endpoint, since the significance of survival curves increases when there are more deaths. That was the reason why we omitted survival as an endpoint. We defined a CR as the presence of normal marker values after chemotherapy, absence of residual lesions on CT-scanning or the histological evidence of necrosis, fibrosis and/or mature teratoma in completely resected residual disease.

EORTC Genitourinary Group Monograph 5: Progress
and Controversies in Oncological Urology II, pages 395–404
© 1988 Alan R. Liss, Inc.

THE ROLE OF RADIOTHERAPY AND CHEMOTHERAPY IN ADVANCED
SEMINOMA

John N. Wettlaufer, M.D.

Division of Urology, Department of Surgery,
    University of Colorado Health Sciences Center,
    Denver, Colorado 80262

Until recently, because of its high radiosensitivity,
seminoma has been primarily treated with post orchiectomy
radiation in all stages. Optimal treatment of seminoma in
clinical early stages has been, for the most part, clear
and uncontroversial with high inguinal orchiectomy
followed by moderate doses of irradiation to the inguinal
and periaortic lymphatics, resulting in high overall cure
rates approximating 100% in clinically confined disease
(Stage I) to close to 90% in patients with small volume
retroperitoneal metastasis (Stage IIA). However, with
rare exceptions, megavoltage irradiation as primary
standard therapy for bulky abdominal (Stage IIB) or
widespread metastatic seminoma (Stages III-IV) has not
been adequate. Accordingly, systemic chemotherapy has
become a logical therapeutic alternative or supplement to
irradiation in patients with advanced metastatic seminoma.
The results of platinum based chemotherapy regimens are
clearly superior in patients with Stages III-IV (5% of all
patients)versus irradiation. However, the ideal treatment
for patients with bulky abdominal seminoma (approximately
10% of all patients with seminoma) remains controversial.
Systemic platinum-based chemotherapy has resulted in
superb over-all, sustained, complete responses in Stage
IIB seminoma which, for the most part, appear to be
superior to that obtained with conventional radiotherapy.
However, there still remains a strong consensus in the
radio-oncology sector to continue to treat patients with
advanced abdominal disease primarily with irradiation.
    This presentation will review treatment of patients

with advanced abdominal and Stage III-IV seminoma.   In
addition, the role of prophylactic mediastinal irradiation
(PMI) in patients with minimal to modest to advanced
abdominal seminoma continues to be controversial and is
reviewed.   The ideal chemotherapy program for advanced
seminoma has yet to be defined, however it appears that
platinum-based programs, either multi-drug or single agent
platinum is indicated.   The preferred treatment for post-
chemotherapy residual masses remains controversial.

RADIOTHERAPY

Patients with retroperitoneal metastasis, designated as
Stage "II" include a group of tumors that are heterogenous
in terms of tumor volume and response to radiotherapy.
Clearly an increase in tumor burden in Stage "II" patients
adversely affects the relapse rate and survival.   The
survival of patients with minimal to modest
retroperitoneal metastasis (Stage "IIA") is 87% compared
to those with "bulky tumor", Stage "IIB" of 65% (Table 1).

Table 1. STAGE II SEMINOMA: RESULTS WITH RADIOTHERAPY

| | | Survival (%) | |
Author	Pts.	IIA	IIB
Doornbos et al (1975)	48	88	75
Van der Werf - Messing (1976) (Orthovoltage)	74	80	55
Van der Werf - Messing (1976) (Supravoltage)	67	90	60
Cionni et al (1978)	59	85	33
Dosoretz et al (1981)	25	100	71
Thomas et al (1982)	86	87	62
Ball et al (1982)	66	79(A+B)	57(C)[*]
Huben et al (1984)	29	100	33
	454	87%	65%

[*]Royal Marsden - Stage IIC (Abdominal Mass >5 cm)

Accordingly, the separation of patients with
retroperitoneal tumor into two groups: "IIA" and "IIB"
defines groups with different prognoses and treatment
plans and seems fully justified.   The Royal Marsden group
(Ball et al, 1982) report no difference in the relapse
rate of 39% between nodal masses > 5 cm and those > 10 cm

in diameter. This observation strongly suggests that Stage "IIB" should include all patients with abdominal masses > 5 cm on CT scan (Royal Marsden classification IIC). Here-to-fore Stage "IIB" has been variously defined as "palpable mass" (Thomas et al, 1982), "bulky tumor metastases" (Dosoretz et al, 1981), "retroperitoneal lymph node > 10 cm" (Doornbos et al, 1975).

The current disease free survival of 87% in data from seven major institutions for Stage "IIA" disease treated with post-orchiectomy irradiation to the subdiaphragmatic ports justifies the continued use of this treatment modality. Relapses should be treated with chemotherapy. The overall survival of patients with bulky "IIB" retroperitoneal metastasis approximates 65%. Patients with bulky retroperitoneal metastasis have routinely received 2000 centiGray (cGy) to the whole abdomen with a boost dose of 2000 to 2500 cGy to the residual bulk disease (Shipley, 1983). There is no evidence that routine use of higher abdominal irradiation doses >3500 cGy will increase the overall disease free control rate (Thomas et al, 1982). Treatment failures in this group do not appear to be dose related, with recurrences or metastasis occurring in a median of four to five months (Thomas et al, 1982). The short time for recurrence of metastasis suggests than many patients with advanced abdominal disease have metastasis at presentation and many of theses failures are from extranodal tumor in addition to local disease outside the radiation ports (Doornbos et al, 1975 and Dosoretz et al, 1981).

Traditionally, patients with clinical retroperitoneal metastasis have received prophylactic mediastinal irradiation (PMI) with doses of 2000 to 3500 cGy. Two recent Canadian studies were reported in which over 1600 cases of seminoma, treated in 18 centers received no PMI (Thomas et al, 1982 and Herman et al, 1983). Uncontrollable mediastinal disease accounted for < 1% of deaths in this group. This study demonstrated that prophylactic mediastinal radiotherapy was not necessary to prevent mediastinal recurrences in low stage retroperitoneal metastasis. They also convincingly demonstrated that although PMI may prevent mediastinal relapse in some instances of advanced bulky abdominal seminoma, it did not significantly improve the survival. PMI has been associated with significant bone marrow hypoplasia (Einhorn, 1982 and Ytredal et al, 1972) which may compromise the use of optimal, curative chemotherapy in patients with high risk for recurrence. Other complications of high dose, multi-field irradiation in advanced seminoma include radiation nephritis, pneumonitis, pulmonary fibrosis and second malignancies. However, two recent reports (Smalley, 1985 and Green, 1983) report 94% and 100% disease free survival in a total of 33 patients with bulky retroperitoneal seminoma treated with abdominal and prophylactic doses of mediastinal and supraclavicular irradiation. Ideally, the question of whether these patients should be initially treated with irradiation or chemotherapy needs to be tested in randomized cooperative group studies. Currently it is our preference to initially treat patients with bulky advanced seminoma with chemotherapy.

The overall survival of patients with Stage III-IV tumor after primary radiotherapy in a literature review (Doornbos et al, 1975) was 136/375 or 36%. The current survival figures obviously are superior to these with the addition of more refined staging techniques and radiotherapy; however, the cure rates (35% - 45%) in patients treated primarily with radiotherapy remains unacceptably low (Ball, 1982, Dosoretz et al, 1981, Thomas et al, 1982).

CHEMOTHERAPY

Systemic chemotherapy has resulted in significant improvement in survival of patients with advanced disease over the past several years. Patients with advanced abdominal and widespread metastatic seminoma treated with platinum based multi-drug chemotherapy can expect an overall sustained disease-free rate of 88% (Table 2). Over the last decade highly successful, multi-drug, platinum based chemotherapy programs for nonseminoma have been used for the most part for advanced Stage II and Stage III/IV seminoma with excellent results and it now appears that seminoma is more sensitive to chemotherapy than nonseminomatous germ cell tumors. Some of these programs have employed post-chemotherapy consolidation radiotherapy or surgical excision of post-chemotherapy residual masses.

Table 2. CISPLATIN CHEMOTHERAPY

Authors	Regimen	No.	CR(%)	Currently NED(%)	Relapses(%)
Van Oosterom et al (1984)	PVB+A	73	51 (70%)	NS	NS
Oliver (1984)	PVB	12	NS	10 (83%)	NS
Stanton et al (1985)	VAB-6	28	24 (86%)	20 (72%)	4 (17%)
Simon et al (1983)	VAB-6	10	10 (100%)	10 (100%)*	3 (30%)
Peckham et al (1985)	BEP	25	24 (96%)	24 (96%)	1 (4%)
Clemm et al (1986)	VIP	16	14 (88%)	14 (88%)	0 (0%)
Wettlaufer (1987)	VcrPC	17	17 (100%)	16 (94%)	1 (6%)
Samuels (1983)	P±C	32	30 (94%)	30 (94%)	0 (0%)
Oliver (1984)	P	16	12 (75%)	13 (81%)*	2 (17%)

* 3 Patients NED with additional other cisplatin based combination chemotherapy

    Van Oosterom and associates in 1984, in a multicenter study, reported a complete response (CR) in 51 out of 73 (70%) patients with advanced seminoma treated with three to four courses of cisplatin, vinblastine and bleomycin (PVB) plus or minus adriamycin. Twenty-four patients also received maintainance therapy with vinblastine and cisplatin. Some patients also recieved consolidation radiotherapy to residual masses or areas of bulk disease. The overall sustained CR (70%) for a minimum of one year was the same for the five participating institutions. Twenty-seven of 33 (81%) with no prior radiotherapy achieved a CR. Myelosuppression and ileus were common, especially in the group with prior irradiation. Other groups have had similar success with PVB in less numbers (Ball et al, 1982, and Oliver et al, 1984). Several other institutions have reported their initial experience with cisplatin-based chemotherapy for advanced seminoma. The Memorial Group recently reported a CR in 24 of 28 (86%) of evaluable patients with advanced seminoma treated with 4 cycles of VAB-6 chemotherapy with surgery in 10 with

residual disease (Stanton, 1985). The overall durable
remission rate in this group was 20 of 24 respondents
(72%). Simon and associates treated 10 patients with VAB-
6 with a CR in all 10. The three relapses are CR with
additional chemotherapy and irradiation. The Royal
Marsden Hospital (Peckham et al, 1985) achieved a
sustained CR in 24 of 25 (96%) patients with advanced
seminoma using platinum, etopside and bleomycin. Clemm et
al in 1986, reported a sustained CR in 14 of 16 (88%)
patients treated with vinblastine, iphosphamide and
cisplatin. Our institution (Wettlaufer, 1984) reported a
CR in 12 of 12 patients (100%) with advanced seminoma
using 2 to 3 courses of vincristine, cisplatin and
cyclophosphamide. This regimen consists of vincristine, 2
mg IV on days 1 and 8, cyclophosphamide 600 mg/m^2, days 1,
3 and 8; and cisplatin 20 mg/m^2, days 1 - 5 with a two to
three week interval between courses of chemotherapy.
Currently we have evaluable data on 17 patients with an
initial CR in all 17 and a sustained complete response in
16 of 17 (94%) with a median and mean follow-up of 50
months. The one recurrence (4 months) and death at 10
months, was in a patient with massive abdominal,
mediastinal, liver and central nervous system metastasis.
Toxicity was minimal, primarily myelosuppression, which
occurred in all 3 patients failing primary radiotherapy.

Cisplatin as a single agent has not been adequately
evaluated, although three recent reports indicate a high
level of activity. The MD Anderson Hospital (Samuels and
Logothetis, 1983) reported their experience with high dose
cisplatin, 100 mg/m^2 weekly in 32 patients for advanced
seminoma. Thirty of 32 (94%) are in CR, 22 for over 2
years. No relapses have recurred in these complete
responses. It is not clear how many of these patients
received cyclophosphamide as well. Many of these patients
experienced severe chronic neurotoxicity. The extent of
prior therapy was not well defined in this abstract. The
London Hospital (Oliver, 1984) reported a CR in 12 of 16
(75%) patients treated with cisplatin 50 mg/m^2 days 1 and
2 every 3 weeks. The two relapses were salvaged with
combination chemotherapy. The Royal Marsden Group
(Peckham et al, 1985) reported 6 of 7 patients free of
disease treated with carboplatin only. A more recent
update (Peckham et al, 1987) reported a CR in over 90% of
33 patients treated with carboplatin. The toxicity of
this regimen is minimal. Clearly cisplatin as a single

agent appears to be effective in the limited studies to date, but further data from other groups is needed to support its use as a single agent.

The optimal chemotherapy for advanced seminoma still remains unclear because of the small number of patients requiring chemotherapy (less than 15% of all seminomas) which has limited the experience in any one treatment center. Currently the evaluation of chemotherapy programs is hindered by the adverse effect of prior irradiation. The chemotoxicity is significantly less and the results are clearly better in patients not pretreated with "curative" radiotherapy (Van Oosterom, 1984; Peckham et al, 1985; Friedman et al, 1985 and Pizzocaro et al, 1986). Although some have questioned the use of alkylating agents in multi-drug regimens for advanced seminoma, they clearly have significant tumor activity as single agents and in combination with cisplatin. Currently, we feel optimal seminoma chemotherapy should include cisplatin and cyclophosphamide.

RESIDUAL BULK TUMOR

The management of residual "bulk tumor" after chemotherapy remains controversial because of the various treatment options (biopsy, surgical excision, radiotherapy, observation), the high frequency of post-treatment residual scar tissue and limited experience. Surgical excision of residual bulk tumor has been detailed by several groups (Table 3).

Table 3. SURGICAL EXCISION OF RESIDUAL "TUMOR" POST CHEMO-SEMINOMA

Chemo	Author	Year	No Tumor	(Scar)
VAB-6	Simon et al	(1983)	7/7	100%
VAB-6	Stanton et al	(1985)	9/10	90%
PVrB	Wolf et al	(1985)	8/8	100%
PVB	Donohue	(1987)	4/4	100%
PVB	Friedman et al	(1985)	3/3[*]	100%
PVB,PEB	Pizzocaro et al	(1986)	13/14	93%
[*]2/3 Post Surgical Death			44/46	96%

Because of the infrequency of positive tumor and the

technical difficulties of surgery, routine excision of residual abdominal and mediastinal masses is not recommended. The role and effectiveness of post-chemotherapy radiotherapy for residual masses or to sites of prior bulk disease are difficult to assess without confirmation of persistant cancer (tissue or positive tumor marker). The Royal Marsden experience (Peckham, 1985) does not support routine radiotherapy for post-chemotherapy residual masses. Currently we follow patients with residual plaque-like masses. Patients with obvious, large volume, bulky disease which does not progressively shrink should probably be treated with radiotherapy. The Memorial Group (Fair, 1987) has demonstrated residual seminoma in 5 patients with bulky cystic masses after VAB-6 chemotherapy.

REFERENCES

Ball D, Barrett A, Peckham J (1982). The management of metastatic seminoma of the testis. Cancer 50:2289-2294.

Cionni L, Diatto S, Pirtoli L, Santoni R, Cappellini M (1978). Radiotherapy of seminoma of the testis. Report of 129 patients. Tumori 64:183-192.

Clemm MD, Hartenstein R, Wollich N, Boening L, Wylmanns W (1986). Vinblastine, ifosfamide-cisplatin treatment of bulky seminoma. Cancer 58:2203-2207.

Donohue JP (1987). Personal communication.

Doornbos JF, Hussey DH, Johnson DE (1975). Radiotherapy for pure seminoma of the testis. Radiology 116:401-404.

Dosoretz DE, Shipley WU, Blitzer PH, Gilbert S, Prat J, Parkhurst E, Wang CC (1981). Megavoltage irradiation for pure testicular seminoma: results and patterns of failure. Cancer 48:2184-2190.

Einhorn LH (1982). Radiotherapy in seminoma: more is not better. Int J of Rad Onc and Biol Phys 8:309-310.

Fair W (1987). Personal Communication.

Friedman EL, Garnick MB, Stomp PC, Mauch PM, Herrington DP, Richie JP (1985). Therapeutic guidelines and results in advanced seminoma. J Clin Oncol 3:1325-1332.

Green N, Broth E, George FW, Kaplan R, Lombardo L, Skaist L, Weinstein E, Petrovich Z (1983). Radiation therapy in bulky seminoma. Urology XX(5):467-469.

Herman JG, Sturgeon J, Thomas GM (1983). Mediastinal prophylactic irradiation in seminoma (abstr). Proc Am Soc Clin Oncol 2:133.

Huben RP, Williams PD, Pontes JD, Panahon AM, Murphy GP (1984). Seminoma at Roswell Park, 1970-1979. Cancer 53:1451-1455.

Oliver RTD (1984). Surveillance for Stage I seminoma and single agent cisplatinum for metastatic seminoma (abstr). Proc Am Soc Clin Oncol 3:162.

Oliver RTD, Hope-Stone HF, Blandy JP (1984). Possible new approaches to the management of seminoma of the testis. Br J Urol 56:729-733.

Peckham MJ, Horwich A (1987). Results of treatment of advanced seminoma with carboplatin. Personal communication at Progress and Controversies in Oncologic Urology II. Amsterdam, The Netherlands, 19-21 March.

Peckham MJ, Horwich A, Hendry WF (1985). Advanced seminoma: treatment with cis-platinum-based combination chemotherapy or carboplatin (JM-8). Br J Cancer 52:7-13.

Pizzocaro G, Salvioni R, Piva L, Zanoni F, Milani A, Faustini M (1986). Cisplatin combination chemotherapy in advanced seminoma. Cancer 58:1625-1629.

Samuels MI, Logothetis CJ (1983). Follow-up study of sequential weekly pulse-dose cis-platinum for far advanced seminoma (abstr). Proc Am Soc Clin Oncol 2:137.

Shipley WU (1983). Radiation therapy for patients with testicular and extragonadal seminoma. Donohue JP (ed): "Testis Tumors", Williams and Wilkins, Baltimore, p 224.

Simon SD, Srougi M, Goes GM (1983). Treatment of advanced seminoma with vinblastine, actinomycin-D, cyclophosphamide, bleomycin, cis-platinum (abstr). Proc Am Soc Clin Oncol 2:132.

Smalley SR, Evans RG, Richardson RL, Farrow GM, Earl JD (1985). Radiotherapy as initial therapy for bulky stage II testicular seminomas. J Clin Oncol 3:1333-1338.

Stanton GF, Bosl GJ, Whitmore Jr WF, Herr H, Sogani P, Morse M, Golbey RB (1985). VAB-6 as initial treatment on patients with advanced seminoma. J Clin Oncol 3:336-339.

Thomas GM, Rider WD, Dempo AJ, Cummings BJ, Gospodarowicz MH, Hawkins NB, Herman JG, Keen CW (1982). Seminoma of the testis: results of treatment and patterns of failure after radiation therapy. Int J Rad Onc Biol Phys 8:165-174.

Van der Werf-Messing B (1976). Radiotherapeutic treatment of testicular tumors. Int J Rad Onc Biol Phys 1:235-248.

Van Oosterom AT, Williams SD, Cortes-Funes H, ten Bokkel Huinink WW, Vendrik CPJ (1984) Treatment of seminomas with chemotherapy. Kurth KH (ed): "Progress and Controversies in Oncological Urology", Alan R. Liss, Inc. p 103.

Wettlaufer JN (1984) The management of advanced seminoma. Semin Urol II(4):257-263.

Wolf RM, Uben RP, Pontis JE (1985). Treatment of advanced seminoma with platinum containing combination chemotherapy (abstr). J Urol 133(4-2):245a.

Ytredal DO, Bradfield JS (1972). Seminoma of the testicle-prophylactic mediastinal radiation versus periaortic and pelvic irradiation alone. Cancer 30:628-633.

EORTC Genitourinary Group Monograph 5: Progress
and Controversies in Oncological Urology II, pages 405–406
© 1988 Alan R. Liss, Inc.

Discussion: The Role of Radiotherapy and Chemotherapy in
Advanced Seminoma

Ted A.W. Splinter, Rotterdam, The Netherlands

Kaye: You say that you would not resect a residual mass. Is
there a cut off in terms of size, which will make you feel
uncomfortable about such a decision?

Wettlaufer: There are two points. Some of my colleagues tell
me that there is a variation of residual disease, so-called
cystic variation, and the MSKCC-group has now reported on
five of these patients, who still have active viable
seminoma. When I see such a variation, I might want to take
biopsies, but I do not think we can remove these tumors. It
is different from non-seminomas; it is a scirrhous mass, it
involves the great vessels and there are no good surgical
planes. I think there may be a role for biopsies in selected
instances.

Fair: I would like to comment on that. The Memorial
experience involves 41 patients with seminomas after
chemotherapy. It looks like that if the residual mass is
just flat and scirrhous, it does not need to be excised. But
in 17 patients with masses larger than 3 cm, 7 had viable
tumor. So our cut off point is a mass of 3 cm or larger on
CT-scan. In that case we try to completely resect the
residual mass, which is difficult but not impossible.

Wettlaufer: Would you not, based on your experience, give
these patients de novo irradiation?

Fair: I think we would prefer surgical excision.

Wettlaufer: Do you have follow-up of those patients, who had
a surgical excision without any additional treatment?

Fair: Of the 7 patients with viable seminoma, 6 are alive
without any further treatment.

Fosså: What is the cut off level of serum HCG, on which you decide to treat the patient as having a non-seminoma?

Wettlaufer: In practice I do not think there is a cut off level. We have seen patients with pure seminoma and an HCG level of 7000 mIU/l, which normalized after orchidectomy. I do not think that the HCG level should determine your therapy. You should ask the pathologist to look very hard for non-seminomatous elements and then make a judgement on how the patient reacts to the therapy. The party-line in several articles is that HCG-levels above 200 mIU indicate that perhaps you have to treat these patients as having non-seminomatous tumors. I want to make a plea for an adjustment i.e. pursue the latter patients as seminomas and treat them with chemotherapy used for non-seminomas.

EORTC Genitourinary Group Monograph 5: Progress
and Controversies in Oncological Urology II, pages 407–416
© 1988 Alan R. Liss, Inc.

IS THERE STILL A PLACE FOR LYMPHADENECTOMY IN CLINICAL
STAGE I NON-SEMINOMA?

L.WEISSBACH, E.A.BOEDEFELD, R.BUSSAR-MAATZ,
K.KLEINSCHMIDT and Testicular Tumor Study Group

Urol.Klinik, Urban Krankenhaus, 1 Berlin 61
(L.W.,R.B.M.,K.K.);Studienzentrale,Med.Univ.Klinik,
53 Bonn (E.A.B.,TTSG), Germany

INTRODUCTION

World wide, some 600 patients with stage I non-seminomatous testis tumor have been managed by surveillance after
orchidectomy. This policy was introduced and promoted by
PECKHAM et al.(1982) and widely adopted by other British
centers. Their results reflect the wealth of experience in
diagnosis and in management of recurrences which has accumulated at the Royal Marsden Hospital and elsewhere in Britain
over the past 8 years. Moreover, the British referral system
and the cooperation between clinics and medical practitioners
seems to be effective enough to permit stringent follow-up.
This may also be true - in varying degrees - for hospitals
or centers in Europe and the USA conducting surveillance
studies. However, outside specialized centers preconditions
may not be adequate to guarantee successful or safe surveillance. Authors from the center in Milano with 59 surveillance
patients have called surveillance "a potentially dangerous
policy" (ZANONI et al.1985).

Based on the results of four prospective multicenter
trials (WEISSBACH et al.1984; WEISSBACH and BUSSAR-MAATZ 1987)
we discuss a modified, ipsilateral lymph node dissection
(RPLND) for purposes of pathological staging and early therapeutic decisions, which we consider to be the standard therapy for patients in stage I disease.

SURVEILLANCE

The analysis of data compiled from recent literature on surveillance suggests an average relapse rate of 28% (range 22-40%) with 17% (15-27%) retroperitoneal recurrences. These figures must be compared to a total recurrence rate of 10-16% and a frequency of retroperitoneal recurrence of less than 2% after ipsilateral RPLND. As the frequency of retroperitoneal relapse indicates the proportion of actually understaged patients, surgical staging is evidently far superior to clinical and radiological staging. The sensitivity of non-invasive techniques depends on the size and site of metastases and on total tumor burden.

Table 1 summarizes sensitivities of various techniques depending on the size of metastases. The results have been verified by subsequent RPLND and histological examination.

Table 1   Sensitivity of Diagnostic Techniques Depending on Size of Metastases (Results of TNM Trial)

Techniques	Mets < 2cm		Mets 2-5cm		Mets > 5cm	
	n	(%)	n	(%)	n	(%)
CT	6/34	(18)	16/32	(50)	12/16	(75)
TM	8/30	(27)	11/28	(39)	7/12	(58)
LAG	19/30	(63)	21/29	(72)	11/13	(85)
CT + TM	11/29	(38)	21/30	(70)	12/14	(86)
LAG + TM	23/31	(74)	26/30	(87)	13/14	(93)
CT+US+TM*	12/28	(43)	23/31	(74)	14/15	(93)
CT+LAG+TM**	23/30	(77)	29/32	(91)	14/15	(93)
CT+LAG+US+TM	24/30	(80)	30/32	(94)	14/15	(93)

CT=computed tomography   TM=tumor markers AFP, HCG
US=ultrasound   LAG=bipedal lymphangiography
* pre-operative staging   ** pre-surveillance staging

In table 2 the overall sensitivity (correct positive diagnosis relative to number of patients with retroperitoneal disease) is compared to the predictive value of negative diagnosis (correct negative diagnosis relative to total number of negative diagnoses) (SEPPELT, 1987).

Table 2 Sensitivity and Predictive Value of Negative
Diagnosis in Retroperitoneal Staging (Results of TNM Trial)

Techniques	Sensitivity n	(%)	Predictive Value n	(%)
CT	34/82	(41)	96/144	(67)
TM	26/70	(37)	82/126	(65)
LAG	51/72	(71)	56/77	(73)
CT + TM	44/73	(60)	78/107	(73)
LAG + TM	62/75	(83)	47/60	(78)
CT + US + TM*	49/74	(66)	73/99	(74)
CT + LAG + TM**	66/77	(86)	46/57	(81)
CT+LAG+US+TM	68/77	(88)	43/52	(83)

*pre-operative staging   **pre-surveillance staging

For metastases less than 2 cm in diameter the detection limit
was, at best, 80% provided 3 imaging techniques (computed
tomography<CT>, ultrasound<US>, and bipedal lymphangiography
<LAG>) were employed in conjunction with tumor marker deter-
mination (TM). In 23% of patients with small metastases, or
14% of all patients with retroperitoneal disease, metastases
were not detected by a combination of CT, LAG, TM. The corresponding overall predictive value of negative diagnosis was
81%, i.e. 19% of clinical stage I patients actually had retroperitoneal disease. Our results confirm previous reports. The
fact that even metastases larger than 5cm were frequently
missed is rather discomforting. With the usual pre-surveillance staging (CT, LAG, TM) the failure rate was 7%; the
combination CT, TM, usually employed in follow-up, had a
failure rate of 14%. In the context of a surveillance protocol this might have serious consequences as the experience
of PIZZOCARO et al.(1985) suggests. Despite monthly controls
and bi-monthly CT, recurrences in 4 of 11 abdominal relapse
patients escaped detection until they had grown to sizes of
more than 5cm in diameter.

    The by no means negligible group of understaged patients
in any surveillance protocol and the patients whose recurrences are detected late carry all the risk and burden of protracted treatment.

While patients with pulmonary metastases are generally cured with 3 to 4 courses of platinum-based chemotherapy, patients with abdominal relapse fare less well requiring more, or more aggressive chemotherapy and often additional surgery of residual tumor. They have been shown by the "Medical Research Council Working Party on Testicular Tumour" to have a 3-year survival of only 65-88% depending on extent of para-aortic node involvement (PECKHAM et al.1985).
Considering the rate and pattern of relapse and the Working Party's detailed 3-year survival figures the estimated survival of total surveillance patients is in the order of 95-96%. This is in agreement with data on patients with early abdominal and chest metastases, by EINHORN and WILLIAMS (1980). The long-term survival of stage I patients after RPLND reported by DONOHUE (1985) is 99-100%. The survival of stage II A (N1, solitary metastasis ≤ 2cm) and stage II B (N2, metastases ≤ 5cm) patients after RPLND, with or without adjuvant chemotherapy, is also 98-100% (EINHORN 1984).

MODIFIED LYMPH NODE DISSECTION

It is for these reasons that we continue to advocate surgical staging. However, a radical lymph node dissection - as it was carried out until the early eighties - is quite unnecessary today. A modified RPLND limited to narrowly defined ipsilateral regions has been shown to be adequate in pathological stage I (WEISSBACH et al.1987). It equals the previously performed radical dissection in diagnostic accuracy, and permits us to preserve the patient's ejaculation in over 80% of cases.
The limited approach is based on the regularity of testicular lymph flow, and thus lymphatic dissemination, and on the knowledge of first sites of nodal involvement. Precise information on the latter,as well as on patterns of metastatic distribution in advanced disease,is obtained through surgical exploration of the retroperitoneum and patho-histological investigation as have, more recently, been carried out by RAY et al.(1974), HERMANEK and SIGEL (1982) and DONOHUE et al.(1982).

We have been particularly interested in the localisation of solitary metastases since they provide the most direct evidence of primary involvement (WEISSBACH and BOEDEFELD 1987) All patients were subjected to radical lymph node dissection and the resected material was histologically examined.

To localize the metastases the dissection was done stepwise
and lymph nodes were labelled according to a grid which par-
titions the retroperitoneum into 15 numbered zones (fig 1).

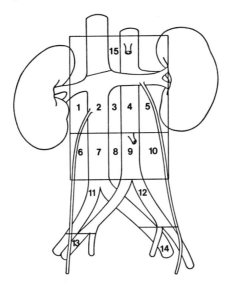

Fig 1   Retroperitoneal subdivisions

Seventy-four of 271 consecutive stage II patients were
found to have solitary metastases of up to 5cm in diameter.
In patients with right testis tumor (table 3) the interaortocaval area is most often the preferred site of metastatic
deposits (45%) whereas the lower pre-aortic field is - in our
series - never primarily involved. This is in agreement with
results of other investigations. The frequency of solitary
metastases in the lower pre- and paracaval areas (11% and 14%
resp.) was unexpected. It contradicts previous assumptions
that they are involved only in rare cases of blockage of up-
ward lymph flow.
In patients with left testis tumor (table 3) the predominant
site of first metastatic deposition is the left upper para-
aortic field (76%). The lower para-aortic (8%) and upper pre-
aortic (11%) areas are less frequently involved. Again, the
lower pre-aortic field is free, also the peri-iliac region.
Two patients with solitary nodes in the lower interaortocaval
and the precaval zone, resp. had previous scrotal lesions.
From our results on primary involvement we define as ipsilateral the areas of regular occurrence of solitary metastases
(fig 2) (WEISSBACH and BOEDEFELD 1987).

Table 3 Localisation of Solitary Retroperitoneal Metastases
< 5cm (Results of Stage II A and Stage II B Trials)

Retroperitoneal Area/Field number		Right Primary (n=36)		Left Primary (n=38)	
		n	(%)	n	(%)
Paracaval	1	2	(6)	–	
	6	5	(14)	–	
Precaval	2	3	(8)	–	
	7	4	(11)	1	(3)
Interaorto-caval	3	10	(28)	–	
	8	6	(17)	1	(3)
Pre-aortic	4	2	(6)	4	(10)
	9	–		–	
Para-aortic	5	–		29	(76)
	10	–		3	(8)
Ri.iliac	11	3	(8)	–	
	13	–		–	
Le.iliac	12	–		–	
	14	–		–	
Supra/hilar	15	1	(3)	–	

In clinical stage I (excluding patients with scrotal violat-
ions) we restrict the surgical staging to these ipsilateral
regions. If they are found to be free of any metastases
—which has to be checked intraoperatively by frozen sections—
and if all other retroperitoneal areas are grossly free,
pathological stage I is established.

Restricting the dissection to ipsilateral areas permits
us to preserve the contralateral sympathetic nerve tracts
which control seminal emission and ejaculation. These are,
in particular, fascicles of the sympathetic chain travelling
lateral to the aorta on either side, nerve fibers originating
from T12 to L4 which travel via paravertebral ganglia into
the hypogastric plexus, and the plexus itself which is situated
below the aortic bifurcation and between the iliac arteries.
The results of the stage I trial on modified vs.radical RPLND
demonstrate that preservation of emission and ejaculation is
indeed achieved, with 72% of patients having antegrade and
11% retrograde ejaculation (table 4).

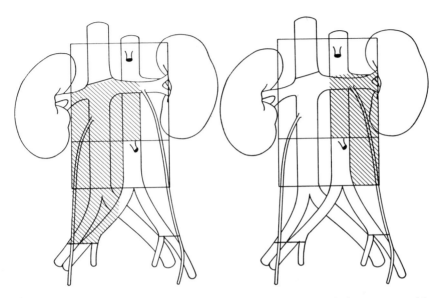

Fig 2   Ipsilateral areas of dissection in modified RPLND if
A primary tumor right   B primary tumor left

Table 4   Ejaculation after Modified RPLND (n=131) and
Radical RPLND (n=53) (Results of Stage I Trial)

Postop. Ejaculation	Modified RPLND		Radical RPLND	
	n	(%)	n	(%)
Antegrade	95	(72)	16	(30)
Retrograde	14	(11)	7	(13)
Lost	22	(17)	30	(57)

The latter group will benefit from treatment with sympatho-
mimetic drugs. Only 17% of patients lost the ability to eja-
culate. (There was no difference in patients with right or
left primary tumor). This compares in our series to a loss of
57% after radical dissection (p < 0.001).
Frequency of relapse after modified and radical lymphadenectomy is shown in table 5. Less than 2% retroperitoneal relapse
after modified RPLND (mean   follow-up is 18 months) support
our claim that it is a highly accurate staging procedure in
clinical stage I. It also provides the basis for immediate

therapeutic measures if retroperitoneal disease is found intraoperatively. In that case, a curative radical dissection is performed. The risk of systemic relapse is minimized with adjuvant chemotherapy (EINHORN 1984).

Table 5 Recurrence after Modified and Radical RPLND in Pathological Stage I (n=225) (Results of Stage I Trial)

RPLND	Total Relapse		Abdom.Relapse		Mean Follow-up
	n	(%)	n	(%)	(months)
Modified (n=160)	26	(16)	3	(< 2)	18
Radical (n=65)	10	(15)	1	(< 2)	21

DISCUSSION

Comparing the latest relevant results of RPLND and surveillance in clinical stage I the argument pro surveillance is today less convincing than it was 5 years ago. The differences between risk/benefit analyses have become rather small. In 1982, PECKHAM et al. stated that with less than 20% relapses under surveillance, RPLND with its unavoidable loss of ejaculation was no longer justifiable. Today, relapse rates under surveillance are up to 40% (with up to 27% retroperitoneal relapse) while the staging RPLND has been successfully modified in such a way as to minimize loss of ejaculation. While true stage I patients run an unneccessary 17% risk to lose ejaculation, 20-30% of clinically understaged patients will receive timely and curative treatment. The cure rate for pathological stage I patients as well as for stage II A/II B patients with RPLND is 99-100%. This has to be weighed against the risk of protracted treatment in case of retroperitoneal disease under surveillance with the possible consequences of more aggressive, more toxic chemotherapy, surgery of residual disease, and less certain outcome. The need for more frequent and more stringent follow-up and the psychological burden of uncertainty on the patient may be added to the debit-side of surveillance.
We conclude that for clinical stage I patients the overall outcome with modified RPLND is as good, or better, as with

surveillance. In a community setting where patients have
limited or no access to specialized centers with the capacities for sophisticated diagnostics, close follow-up, and
salvage therapy in case of progressing disease, the surgical approach is the only safe policy.

REFERENCES

Donohue JP, Zachary JM, Maynard BR (1982). Distribution of
 nodal metastases in non-seminomatous testis cancer.
 J Urol 128:315-320.
Donohue JP (1985). Retroperitoneal lymphadenectomy (RPLND)
 in low stage disease (staging RPLND). (One point of view).
 In: Khoury S, Küss R, Murphy GP, Chatelain C, Karr JP
 (eds.): "Testicular Cancer", New York: Alan R.Liss,
 pp 287-311.
Einhorn LH, Williams SD (1980). The management of dissemi-
 nated testicular cancer. In: Einhorn LH (ed.) "Testicular
 Tumors: Management and Treatment", New York: Masson
 Publishing USA Inc., pp 117-149.
Einhorn LH (1984). Adjuvant therapy of testicular cancer.
 In: Jones SE, Salmon SE (eds.): "Adjuvant Therapy of
 Cancer IV", New York, London: Grune & Stratton pp 549-553.
Hermanek P, Sigel A (1982). Necessary extent of lymph node
 dissection in testicular tumours. Eur Urol 8: 135-144.
Peckham MJ, Barrett A, Husband JE, Hendry WF (1982).
 Orchidectomy alone in testicular stage I non-seminomatous
 germ cell tumours. Lancet II: 678-680.
Peckham MJ and Members of the Medical Research Council Work-
 ing Party on Testicular Tumours (1985). Prognostic factors
 in advanced disease. Lancet I: 8-11.
Pizzocaro G, Zanoni F, Salvioni R, Milani A, Piva L (1985).
 Surveillance of lymph node dissection in clinical stage I
 non-seminomatous germinal testis cancer? Br J Urol 57:
 759-762.
Ray B, Hajdu SI, Whitmore WF jr. (1974). Distribution of
 retroperitoneal lymph node metastases in testicular
 germinal tumors. Cancer 33: 340-348.
Seppelt U (1987). Validierung verschiedener diagnostischer
 Methoden zur Beurteilung des Lymphknoten-Status. In:
 Weissbach L, Bussar-Maatz R (eds.) (ref.below).
Weissbach L, Hartlapp JH, Boedefeld EA (1984). Stage-related
 treatment of non-seminomatous testicular germ cell carcinoma (early stages): Recently activated cooperative clinical trials. In: Denis L, Murphy GP, Prout GR, Schröder F

(eds.): "Controlled Clinical Trials in Urologic Oncology",
New York: Raven Press pp 39-43.
Weissbach L, Boedefeld EA, Hartlapp JH (1987). Prospective
multicenter trials on early-stage non-seminomatous testis
tumor. Progress report after 4 years. Verh.Dtsch.KrebsGes.
Vol 6, Stuttgart, New York: Gustav Fischer Verlag (in press)
Weissbach L, Boedefeld EA (1987). Localisation of solitary
and multiple metastases in stage II non-seminomatous testis
tumor as basis for a modified staging lymph node dissection
in stage I. J Urol 137: ooo (in press).
Weissbach L, Bussar-Maatz R (eds.)(1987): "Die Diagnostik
des Hodentumors und seiner Metastasen", München, Basel:
Karger Verlag (in press).
Zanoni F, Pizzocaro G, Salvioni R, Milani A, Piva L,
Fossati-Bellani F (1985). Orchidectomy alone in clinical
stage I non-seminomatous germ cell tumors (NSGCT) of the
testis: a potentially dangerous policy. Proc. of ASCO
4:110 (Abstract C 430).

ACKNOWLEDGEMENT

The data presented are derived from contributions
of colleagues from 42 German and 6 Austrian clinics
who constitute the "Testicular Tumor Study Group"
(TTSG). The list of names of members of TTSG is
available at Studienzentrale Medizinische Univer-
sitätsklinik Bonn.

The trials were/are supported in part by the
Federal Minister of Research and Technology, Federal Republic of Germany.

EORTC Genitourinary Group Monograph 5: Progress
and Controversies in Oncological Urology II, page 417
© 1988 Alan R. Liss, Inc.

Discussion: Is There Still a Place for Lymphadenectomy in
Clinical Stage I Non-Seminoma?

Ted A.W. Splinter, Rotterdam, The Netherlands

Kaye: Patients with stage II were given adjuvant chemotherapy. What kind of chemotherapy and how many courses?

Kleinschmidt: Patients received PVB. In the stage IIA trial
they were randomized to get 0 vs 2 courses and in the stage
IIB trial 2 vs 4 courses.

Kaye: What about the results?

Kleinschmidt: In the first study with randomization for 0
and 2 courses of treatment patients were followed for 13
months without any difference. In the second study, 223
patients were randomized between 2 and 4 courses with a
median follow-up of 13 months. There is also no difference
between these groups.

Paulson: I would like to know how many of your patients with
a left sided tumor had nodal disease anterior to the vena
cava or in the inter aorta caval area below the take off of
the inferior mesenteric artery?

Kleinschmidt: Two.

Fosså: I would like to emphasize that, in order to find the
right percentage of involved nodes, even with very small
metastases, you need a very attentive pathology department.

EORTC Genitourinary Group Monograph 5: Progress
and Controversies in Oncological Urology II, pages 419–425
© 1988 Alan R. Liss, Inc.

POOR PROGNOSIS GERM CELL TUMORS OF THE TESTES: IMPROVED
RESULTS WITH HIGH DOSE REGIMENS

Robert F. Ozols

Medicine Branch, Clinical Oncology Program,
Division of Cancer Treatment, National Cancer
Institute, Bethesda, Maryland 20892 U.S.A.

INTRODUCTION

Cisplatin based combination chemotherapy has been responsible for the dramatic improvement in survival of patients with testicular cancer observed during the last decade. Complete remission rates of 70-75% can be achieved
for patients even with advanced stage disease. The vast
majority of these patients are cured and the relapse rate is
<10%. However, approximately 1/3 of all patients with ad-
vanced stage testicular cancer present with poor prognostic
features leading to a markedly lower complete response rate.
The overall complete response rate in these patients is approximately 40-60%. The primary clinical feature associated
with a poor prognosis is an increased volume of disease.
The development of more effective treatment for this subset
of patients has been an important goal in the management of
advanced stage testicular cancer.

MATERIAL AND METHODS

We initially treated 10 patients with bulky non-seminomatous testicular cancer with a new regimen termed PVeBV
(Table 1). This regimen consists of cisplatin (at twice the
dose used in previous combination chemotherapy regimens),
vinblastine, bleomycin, and the epidodophyllotoxin VP-16
(Ozols et al., 1983). The rationale for this new drug
regimen was as follows: (a) cisplatin has an important dose
response relationship in testicular cancer, however, dose
escalations beyond 120 mg/ m^2 have not been possible in
the past due to dose limiting nephrotoxicity. The demon-

stration that cisplatin nephrotoxicity, but not the antitumor effect (Litterest, 1981) could be decreased in animals by using hypertonic sodium chloride led to our stu-

TABLE 1. PVeBV Chemotherapy

Cisplatin (P)*	40 mg/m^2 i.v. q.d. x 5	
Vinblastine (Ve)	0.2 mg/kg i.v. day 1	every 21 days
VP-16 (V)	100 mg/m^2 i.v. q.d. x 5	
Bleomycin (B)	30 u i.v. q. wk	

*Administered in 250 ml 3% saline with 6 liters per day
normal saline hydration.

dies of high dose cisplatin administered in 3% sodium chloride following 6 L/day of normal saline hydration (Ozols et
al., 1984). The explanation for the protective effect of
the chloruresis relates to the aquation equilibria of cisplatin and the inhibition of the formation of toxic interme-
diates in the renal tubule by maintenance of a high chloride
ion concentration, (b) VP-16 had been shown to be an active
agent in previously treated testicular cancer patients, (c)
vinblastine and bleomycin were included since previous studies had demonstrated clinical synergy for this combination
in the treatment of advanced stage patients.

All six previously untreated patients receiving treatment with PVeBV in the pilot study achieved a complete remission. Four of these patients achieved a complete remission with three cycles of PVeBV while the other two patients
achieved a complete remission with an additional cycle of
high dose cisplatin plus VP-16 (200 mg/m^2 qd x 5) followed
by autologous bone marrow infusion. There have been no relapses in these patients who achieved a complete remission
and all patients have now been followed-up for more than
5 years.

RANDOMIZED TRIAL OF PVeB vs PVeBV IN THE TREATMENT OF POOR
PROGNOSIS NON-SEMINOMATOUS TESTICULAR CANCER PATIENTS

A prospective randomized trial is currently in progress at the National Cancer Institute for the treatment
of poor prognosis testicular cancer patients. Germ cell

tumor patients with poor prognostic features (Table 2) are randomized to receive either standard therapy with PVeB (cisplatin 20 mg/m^2 iv qd x 5, vinblastine 0.3 mg/kg iv on day 1, bleomycin 30 units q wk) or PVeBV. A randomized trial was necessary since the toxicity of PVeBV in the pilot study was greater than that of PVeB and the relative efficacy must be compared to the increased toxicity of PVeBV. Furthermore, while poor prognostic features in testicular cancer can be defined in general terms, a prospective comparison of PVeBV vs. PVeB is necessary to eliminate any bias due to patient selection. Patients who do not achieve a complete remission with 3-4 cycles of PVeBV receive an additional cycle of intensified chemotherapy with increased doses of VP-16 followed by autologous bone marrow infusion. This study also evaluates the ability of high dose platinum plus VP-16 to salvage patients who do not achieve a complete remission with PVeB or relapse after having achieved a complete remission.

TABLE 2. Eligibility criteria for randomized trial of PVeB versus PVeBV

Advanced abdominal disease
    Palpable mass
    10 cm if not palpable
    Liver metastases

Advanced lung disease
    Mediastinal mass or pulmonary nodule >5.0 cm
    Multiple nodules (>5) with at least one >2.0 cm
    >5 metastases per lung field if each lesion is >1.0 cm
    Pleural effusion
    Hypoxia due to tumor (PO$_2$ < 75 mmHg)

Other
    Pure choriocarcinoma
    Extragonadal primary - including endodermal sinus tumors
    CNS metastases
    Other visceral metastases
    AFP >1000
    HCG >10,000

INTERIM ANALYSIS OF PVEBV VS. PVEB

While this study is still in progress, an interim analysis has been performed (Ozols et al., 1984b). A complete remission, as defined by the normalization of tumor markers and the absence of embryonal elements in any residual masses, was achieved in 26/30 (87%) of patients randomized to receive PVeBV. A complete remission was achieved with 3 cycles of PVeBV in 18/26 (69%) of patients. Seven patients (27%) required an additional cycle of PVeBV and only 1 patient (4%) received high dose VP-16 with autologous bone marrow reinfusion. After the completion of chemotherapy the vast majority of patients (92%) had residual masses and complete surgical removal of the masses was attempted. The relapse rate in those patients who achieved a complete remission has been low and there has been only one relapse (4%) with a median follow-up of 27 months.

Two patients who had achieved a complete remission with PVeBV (8%) developed re-growing masses even though their tumor markers remained normal and at surgery were found to have recurrent teratoma but no evidence of embryonal carcinoma. Two patients died of progressive pulmonary failure and at autopsy had marked pulmonary fibrosis compatible with bleomycin lung toxicity. In both patients there was no evidence of residual embryonal cancer. Consequently, 80% of the complete responders are alive without evidence of recurrent embryonal cancer or re-growth of teratomas with a median follow-up of 27 months.

It should be pointed out that only 4 patients randomized to receive PVeBV did not achieve a complete remission. Two patients presented with massive pulmonary involvement and respiratory failure in addition to other wide-spread metastases and both patients died of irreversible pulmonary failure during their first cycle of chemotherapy.

The complete response rate to PVeB in the interim analysis was 62%. Eighty percent of patients who achieved a complete remission had residual masses. Similar to the observation with PVeBV, however, residual teratoma was found at surgery and there was no evidence of embryonal carcinoma. In the PVeB arm of the study there has been a 20% relapse rate with recurrent embryonal cancer. Patients were subsequently salvaged with high dose cisplatin plus VP-16, although the durability of complete remissions following salvage therapy has been in most cases short. There also has been a 20% recurrence rate with teratoma in this group of patients. In addition, 1 patient died of progressive respiratory failure due to bleomycin induced pulmonary fibrosis.

TOXICITY OF PVEBV VS. PVEB

It is clear that PVeBV is a more toxic reigmen than PVeB. Gastrointestinal toxicity is more severe due to the high dose cisplatin. Peripheral neuropathy was similar with PVeBV and PVeB although clinically significant ototoxicity was observed only with PVeBV.

Myelosuppression was more severe with PVeBV than PVeB. Eighty-seven percent of patients on PVeBV had a white blood cell nadir of <1000 compared to 50% for patients receiving PVeBV. Furthermore, neutropenic fevers requiring antibiotic therapy occurred in 80% of the PVeBV patients compared to 56% of those patients receiving therapy with PVeB. Platelet suppression was also more severe with PVeBV compared to PVeB. It is our policy to monitor patients receiving PVeBV on a daily basis and antibiotics are instituted immediately at the time the patient develops neutropenia with an associated fever.

The major disturbing toxicity in this study has been the 6% incidence of fatal bleomycin induced pulmonary fibrosis seen equally in both arms of this trial. Toxicity occurred even though the patients were carefully monitored using physical examinations, chest X-rays, and pulmonary function tests and bleomycin was discontinued at the earliest sign of any pulmonary toxicity.

DISCUSSION

Several interim conclusions can be made from this study. (1) The selection criteria have identified a group of patients in whom standard therapy is not satisfactory. (2) Patients who do not achieve a complete remission with PVeB are not salvaged by treatment with high dose cisplatin and VP-16. (3) Respiratory failure is a primary characteristic associated with the inability to achieve a complete remission with PVeBV. (4) PVeBV is more myelosuppressive than

PVeB although the short duration of the nadirs and the lack of any cumulative effects together with the necessity for only 3 cycles of therapy in most patients has made this toxicity manageable. (b) The major toxicity from drugs in this study relates to the development of pulmonary fibrosis from bleomycin.

If the preliminary results on the superiority of PVeBV compared to PVeB are confirmed by additional patient entry into this study and with longer follow-up, this will represent important advance in the treatment of patients with poor prognosis testicular cancer. However, as the study is designed, it will not be possible to tell whether the improvement in complete response rate observed with PVeBV is due to the use of high dose cisplatin (twice that used in standard therapy with PVeB) or to the addition of VP-16, or to the combination. Studies are currently in progress in the United States in which poor risk patients are randomized to receive a regimen of high dose platinum plus VP-16 plus bleomycin vs. standard dose cisplatin, VP-16, and bleomycin. In this study the importance of double dose platinum will be ascertained.

Since our initial reports, several other investigators have confirmed the importance of high dose regimens in the treatment of poor prognosis testicular cancer (Schmoll et al., 1984; Daugaard et al., 1985; Trump et al., 1985), Table 3.

TABLE 3. High dose cisplatin regimens in testicular cancer patients

Reference	Regimen	Patients	Results
Schmoll et al., 1984	DPP 40 mg/m^2 iv qd x 5 VP-16 140 mg/m^2 iv qd x 5 Bleo 15 mg/m^2 q wk	15 (previously un-treated)	13/15(87%)CR
Daugaard et al., 1985	DPP 40 mg/m^2 iv qd x 5	23:15 previously untreated and 8 previously treated	15/23(65%)CR
Trump et al., 1985	DDP mg/m^2 iv qd x 5 VP-16 100 mg/m^2 iv qd x 5	12 previously treated	2/16(17%)CR

Future studies in high risk testicular cancer patients will be aimed at developing more effective regimens with less toxicity. The group at Indiana has demonstrated that a combination of VP-16, cisplatin and iphosphamide (VIP) is an active regimen in treatment of refractory germ cell tumor patients (Loehrer et al., 1985). It is possible that this combination with increased doses of cisplatin may prove to be an active regimen in previously untreated patients with poor prognostic features. In particular, the absence of bleomycin in this regimen could be a major advantage.

REFERENCES

Daugaard G, Rorth M (1985) High-dose cisplatin (DDP) and VP-16 in patients with poor prognosis germ cell cancer. Proc Am Soc Clin Oncol 3:163.

Litterst CL (1981) Alterations in the toxicity of cis-di-chlorodiamminestration. Toxicity and Applied Pharmacol 61:99-108.

Ozols RF, Corden BJ, Jacob J, Wesley MN, Ostchega Y, Young RC (1984a) High-dose cisplatin in hypertonic saline. Ann Int Med 100:19-24.

Ozols RF, Deisseroth AB, Javadpour N, Barlock A, Messerschmidt GL, Young RC (1983) Treatment of poor prognosis nonseminomatous testicular cancer with a 'high dose' platinum combination chemotherapy regimen. Cancer 51:1803-1807.

Ozols RF, Ihde D, Jacob J, Steis R, Veach SR, Wesley M, Young RC (1984b) Randomized trial of PVeBV [High dose (HD) cisplatin (P), Vinblastine (Ve), Bleomycin (B), VP-16 (V)] versus PVeB in poor prognosis non-seminomatous testicular cancer (NSTC). Proc Am Soc Clin Oncol 3:155.

Schmoll H-J, Arnold, H, Mayr T (1984) Platinum-ultra high dose/etoposide/bleomycin (DDP-HD/VP16/BLM): An effective regimen for testicular cancer with poor prognosis. Proc Am Soc Clin Oncol 3:163.

Trump DL, Hortvet L: Etoposide and very high dose cisplatin: Salvage therapy for patients with advanced germ cell neoplasms. Cancer Treat Rep 69:259-261.

EORTC Genitourinary Group Monograph 5: Progress
and Controversies in Oncological Urology II, page 427
© 1988 Alan R. Liss, Inc.

Discussion: Poor Prognosis Germ Cell Tumors of the Testes:
Improved Results With High Dose Regimens

Ted A.W. Splinter, Rotterdam, the Netherlands

Akdas: What is your opinion about the high percentage of
ototoxicity? Is it due to higher age?

Ozols: Ototoxicity is due to the high dose Cisplatin and not
to the age of the patients. Maybe in the future high dose
Carboplatin, which does not induce ototoxicity, might replace high dose Cisplatin, if it is shown to have the same
efficacy. In the follow-up of the patients with ototoxicity,
the audiogram remains unchanged, but on clinical grounds
there is an improvement. So the patients acquire some kind
of adaption. No patient uses a hearing aid. In a quality of
life assessment, the patients do not indicate the ototoxicity as a major problem.

Kaye: The improved results could be both due to the Vp16 and
high dose Cisplatin. How are you going to proceed from here?

Ozols: We are going to proceed with a regimen of high-dose
Cisplatin, Vp16 and Ifosfamide. Einhorn's study, comparing
normal and high dose Cisplatin together with Vp16 and Bleomycin, is the only study, which can answer the question
whether high dose Cisplatin is responsible for the results.
It will be increasingly difficult to perform randomized
studies in high risk patients, since the prevalence is
decreasing in the U.S.A.

Horwich: With regard to Vp16, it does appear that the prognostic factors for combinations containing that drug are the
same as for PVB. Therefore, I do not feel that Vp16 is the
sole means of overcoming adverse prognostic factors in your
combination. With regard to Bleomycin, it would appear that
there are relatively low-dose combinations, which are very
effective in advanced disease. Therefore, it may not be
necessary to abandon an active drug entirely in this
subgroup with advanced disease.

EORTC Genitourinary Group Monograph 5: Progress
and Controversies in Oncological Urology II, pages 429–436
© 1988 Alan R. Liss, Inc.

HIGH DOSE CHEMOTHERAPY FOLLOWED BY AUTOLOGOUS BONE MARROW RE-INFUSION IN RELAPSING OR REFRACTORY TESTICULAR CANCER

D.Th.Sleijfer, P.O.M.Mulder, E.G.E. de Vries,
H.Schraffordt Koops, P.H.B. Willemse,C.Th.Smit
Sibinga, N.H.Mulder.

Department of Internal Medicine and Department of
Surgical Oncology, University Hospital Groningen;
Regional Red Cross Blood Bank Groningen-Drenthe,
The Netherlands.

INTRODUCTION

Although a high cure rate in patients with
disseminated germ cell tumors of the testis can be reached
with standard cisplatin-based chemotherapy, a number of
patients fail to achieve a complete remission or relapse
after some time, and approximately 20% of all patients will
die as a result of therapy-resistant disease (Einhorn,
1981). The choice of salvage therapy still remains a
difficult problem. Cyclophosphamide has some clinical
activity as a single agent and has also been used in
remission-induction combination chemotherapy (Jacobs, 1979;
Golbey, 1979). Moreover, it may also be valuable as a part
of salvage chemotherapy (Crispino, 1986). VP 16-213
(etoposide) has also been introduced as an active agent in
first line treatment as well as a part of salvage therapy
in patients with disseminated testicular cancer (Peckham,
1983; Hainsworth, 1985; Bosl, 1985). In a variety of
tumors, a dose-response curve to chemotherapy has been
demonstrated (Frei, 1980). This fact, together with the
present cryopreservation technology make reconstitution
after reinfusion of frozen autologous bone marrow after
marrow ablative therapy possible. It allows to study dose
escalation in relapsing or refractory testicular cancer
using agents with primarily bone marrow toxicity such as
cyclophosphamide, melphalan and etoposide.

In the literature, marrow is usually obtained from the posterior iliac crest under general anesthesia. However, patients with relapsing or refractory germ cell tumors are often in a compromised general condition and general anesthesia can be an additional burden for these patients. Another risk factor can be the pulmonary toxicity of general anesthesia in patients pretreated with bleomycin. It has recently been shown that bone marrow harvesting under mild general analgesia, using meperidine and diazepam, is a safe procedure which can be performed on an out-patient basis (De Vries, 1984). The richness of the collected marrow can be determined by cell count or by the absolute number of myeloid progenitor cells (Postmus, 1984). In most patients a volume of 1000-1500 cc is harvested. After the marrow is centrifuged in an apheresis machine, the buffy coat is separated and cryopreserved in liquid nitrogen with dimethyl sulfoxide as a cryopreservative.

Patients treated with ablative doses of chemotherapy can be nursed in reverse isolation, in a laminar air flow room, but also in a single-patient bedroom without special isolation procedures (Mulder, 1984). Infection prophylaxis can consist of oral non-absorbable antibiotics directed against potential pathogenic flora in the digestive tract (Sleijfer, 1980). Nutritional support consists of enteral tube feeding (De Vries, 1982) or of parenteral nutrition. Platelet transfusions are given prophylactically at a level below 15-20 x 10^9/1. In these patients, autologous cryopreserved platelets can also be used (Van Imhoff, 1983).

A number of drugs have been considered to be suitable for application in high dose regimens in patients with germ cell tumors: melphalan, cyclophosphamide and VP 16-213. One of the major advantages of melphalan is its short half-life. This makes rapid re-infusion of even non frozen autologous marrow possible and shortens the duration of aplasia (McElwain, 1979). Melphalan can be given at a dosage of 180-225 mg/m^2 (Lazarus, 1985). The highest dose of cyclophosphamide that can be given without a high probability of cardiac toxicity is 7 g/m^2 (Gottdiener, 1981). VP 16-213 (etoposide) can be given at a dose level of 3.5 g/m^2, even without autologous bone marrow re-infusion. At this dose, the dose-limiting extramedullary toxicity is oropharyngeal mucositis (Postmus, 1984). In combining high dose cyclophosphamide and high dose VP 16-213, dose limiting extramedullary toxicity was found after 7 g/m^2 cyclophosphamide together with 2.5 g/m^2 etoposide (Postmus, 1984). After completion of the chemotherapy course, the stored marrow is thawed and re-infused. The moment of re-infusion has been established based on clinical experiences (Bruckner, 1972; Lazarus, 1985) or on pharmacokinetic studies (Taha, 1983; Holthuis, 1986) and varies, depending on the cytostatic drugs used, between one and four days after chemotherapy.

RESULTS

There are very few published reports of high dose chemotherapy in patients with refractory or relapsing germ cell tumors of the testis. Frequently, patients with germ cell tumors are described together with other solid tumors in phase I or in broad phase II studies (Spitzer, 1980; Gorin, 1981; Barbasch, 1983).

Blijham et al (1981) treated thirteen patients with testicular cancer with high dose cyclophosphamide (4.5 mg/m^2) and VP 16-213 (600 mg/m^2) with or without BCNU, adriamycin or platinum. Of 10 evaluable patients, four patients achieved a complete and three a partial remission, with a median response duration of 15 weeks. Wolff et al (1984) treated eleven patients with progressive refractory germ cell tumors with VP 16-213 (2.4 g/m^2) with bone marrow reinfusion, every 3-4 weeks followed by 1.2 g/m^2 VP 16-213 without bone marrow support. Of 10 evaluable patients, two complete and four partial responders, all of short duration, were obtained. Biron et al (1985) collected the results of high dose chemotherapy in testicular cancer from several centres in France. Six patients were treated with melphalan 140 mg/m^2, one reached a complete and one a partial response. Nine patients were treated with melphalan (140-200 mg/m^2) together with etoposide (400-1000 mg/m^2). Of these patients, one reached a complete and six a partial remission. The duration of response was short, 10 weeks for evaluable patients. Using etoposide alone, or in combination with cisplatinum, with or without bleomycin and cyclophosphamide , followed by autologous bone marrow transplantation, Pico et al (1986) described eight complete remissions and 8 partial remissions out of twenty-two patients. Mulder et al (1987) reported on three patients treated with cyclophosphamide (7 g/m^2) and etoposide (2.5 g/m^2). Because only one patient achieved a short partial remission, the next eight patients received etoposide 2.5 g/m^2 without marrow support, four weeks later followed by cyclophosphamide (7 g/m^2) and etoposide (2 g/m^2) with marrow re-infusion. Of these eight patients, two reached a complete response for 46 and 66+ weeks and four a partial response (6-22 weeks). Recently, collected data from many centres active in bone marrow transplantation mentioned about 75 patients with testicular cancer treated with different chemotherapy schedules, with a complete response rate of approximately 20% (Bone marrow autotransplantation in man, Report of an International Cooperative Study, 1986).

The toxicity of high dose chemotherapy followed by bone marrow re-infusion is considerable, and includes next to severe and longlasting myelosuppression, nausea, vomiting, alopecia, mucositis, hepatitis, and hemorrhagic cystitis. The myelosuppression, with a number of days with severe leukopenia varying between 2-20 days, can lead to treatment-related infections (Blijham, 1981; Wolff, 1984; Mulder, 1987) and to treatment-related deaths (Blijham, 1981). Thrombopenia, with a duration of 0-18 days depending on the dosages used, is in most cases not complicated by bleeding episodes as a result of prophylaxis with platelet transfusions.

CONCLUSION

The aim of salvage chemotherapy in patients with relapsing or refractory testicular cancer is to achieve a high percentage of complete remissions. The results of ablative chemotherapy for which autologous bone marrow transplantation is indicated, are comparable to other salvage regimens not requiring bone marrow support (Bosl, 1985; Hainsworth, 1985; Einhorn, 1986). From the available data on marrow-ablative chemotherapy in relapsing testicular cancer patients, it is clear that this salvage therapy is not sufficient to cure a substantial number of these patients. Other agents, active in testicular cancer and with primarily bone marrow toxicity such as ifosfamide

(Einhorn, 1986) or carboplatin (Peckham, 1985) can probably be incorporated in order to increase complete response rates of marrow-ablative chemotherapy. Another potential for the application of these regimens is the use as up-front chemotherapy before or as late intensification after standard remission-induction chemotherapy in patients initially presenting with unfavorable prognostic characteristics (Stoter, 1987).

REFERENCES

Barbasch A, Higby DJ, Brass C, Bakri K, Karakousis C, Pontes JE, Wajsman LZ, Beckley S, Freeman A, Killion K, Burnett D (1983). High dose cyto-reductive therapy with autologous bone marrow transplantation in advanced malignancies. Cancer Treat Rep 67: 143-148.

Biron P, Philip T, Maraninchi D, Pico JL, Cahn JY, Fumoleau P, Le Mevel A, Gastaut JA, Carvassonne M, Kamioner D, Herve P, Brunat Mentigny M, Hayat M (1985). Massive chemotherapy and autologous bone marrow transplantation in progressive disease of nonseminomatous testicular cancer: a phase II study in 15 patients. In Dicke KA, Spitzer G, Zander AR (eds). Autologous bone marrow transplantation. The University of Texas, M.D.Anderson Hospital and Tumor Institute at Houston. P.203-210.

Blijham G, Spitzer G, Litam J, Zander AR, Verma DS, Vellekoop L, Samuels ML, McCredie KB, Dicke KA (1981). The treatment of advanced testicular carcinoma with high dose chemotherapy and autologous marrow support. Eur J Cancer 17: 433-441.

Bone-marrow autotransplantation in man. Report of an International Cooperative Study (1986). Lancet II: 960-962.

Bosl GJ, Yagoda A, Golbey RB, Whitmore W, Herr H, Sogani P, Morse M, Vogelzang N, MacDonald G (1985). Role of etoposide-based chemotherapy in the treatment of patients with refractory or relapsing germ cell tumors. Am J Med 78: 423-428.

Buckner CD, Rudolph RH, Fefer A, Clift RA, Epstein RB, Funk DD, Nieman PE, Slichter SJ, Storb R, Thomas ED (1972). High dose cyclophosphamide therapy for malignant disease. Toxicity, tumor response and the effects of stored autologous marrow. Cancer 29: 357-365.

Crispino S, Pizzocaro G, Marchini S, Monfardini S (1986). Chemotherapy with adriamycin and vincristine alternated with cyclophosphamide and actinomycin D in testicular germ cell tumors refractory to cisplatin, vinblastine and bleomycin. Eur J Cancer Clin Oncol 22: 251–256.

De Vries EGE, Mulder NH, Houwen B, De Vries-Hospers HG (1982). Enteral nutrition by nasogastric tube in adult patients treated with intensive chemotherapy for acute leukemia. Am J Clin Nutr 35: 1490–1496.

De Vries EGE, Vriesendorp R, Meinesz AF, Mulder NH, Postmus PE, Sleijfer DT (1984). No narcosis for bone marrow harvest in autologous bone marrow transplantation. Blut 49: 419–421.

Einhorn L (1981). Testicular cancer as a model for curable neoplasm. The Richard and Hinda Rosenthal Foundation Award Lecture. Cancer Res 41: 3275–3280.

Einhorn LH (1986). VP 16 plus ifosfamide plus cisplatin as salvage therapy in refractory testicular cancer. Cancer Chemother Pharmacol 18S: 45–50.

Frei E, Canellos GP (1980). Dose: a critical factor in cancer chemotherapy. Am J Med 69: 585–594.

Golbey RB, Reynolds TF, Vugrin D (1979). Chemotherapy of metastatic germ cell tumors. Sem Oncol 6: 82–86.

Gorin NC, David R, Stachowiak J, Salmon C, Petit JC, Parlier Y, Najman A, Duhamel G (1981). High dose chemotherapy and autologous bone marrow transplantation in acute leukemias, malignant lymphomas and solid tumors. Eur J Cancer 17: 557–568.

Gottdiener JS, Appelbaum FR, Ferrans VJ, Deisseroth A, Ziegler J (1981). Cardiotoxicity associated with high dose cyclophosphamide therapy. Arch Int Med 141: 758–763.

Hainsworth J, Williams SD, Einhorn LH, Birch R, Greco FA (1985). Successful treatment of resistant germinal neoplasms with VP 16 and cisplatin: Results of a Southeastern Cancer Study Group trial. J Clin Oncol 3: 666–671.

Holthuis JJM, Postmus PE, Van Oort WJ, Hulshoff B, Verleun H, Sleijfer DT, Mulder NH (1986). Pharmacokinetics of high dose etoposide. Eur J Cancer Clin Oncol 22: 1149–1155.

Jacobs EM, Muggia FM, Rozencweig M (1979). Chemotherapy of testicular cancer: from palliation to curative adjuvant chemotherapy. Sem Oncol 6: 3–13.

Lazarus HM, Herzig RH, Wolff SN, Phillips GL, Spitzer TR, Fay JW, Herzig GP (1985). Treatment of metastatic malignant melanoma with intensive melphalan and autologous bone marrow transplantation. Cancer Treat Rep 69: 473–477.

McElwain TJ, Hedley DW, Burton G, Clink HM, Gordon MY, Jarman M, Juttner CA, Millar JL, Milsted RA, Prentice G, Smith IE, Spence D, Woods M (1979). Marrow autotransplantation accelerates hematological recovery in patients with malignant melanoma treated with high dose melphalan. Br J Cancer 40: 72–80.

Mulder NH, Meinesz AF, Sleijfer DT, Postmus PE, De Vries EGE, Van der Geest S, Orie JLM, Vriesendorp R (1984). Feasibility of high dose VP 16–213 as single agent or in combination with cyclophosphamide and autologous bone marrow transplantation. Neth J Med 27: 389–392.

Mulder POM, De Vries EGE, Schraffordt Koops H, Splinter TAW, Maas A, Van der Geest S, Mulder NH, Sleijfer DT (1987). Chemotherapy with maximally tolerable doses of VP 16–213 and cylophosphamide followed by autologous bone marrow transplantation for the treatment of relapsed or refractory germ cell tumors. Submitted.

Peckham MJ, Barrett A, Liew KH, Horwich A, Robinson B, Dobbs HJ, McElwain TJ, Hendry WF (1983). The treatment of metastatic germ cell testicular tumors with bleomycin, etoposide and cisplatin. Br J Cancer 47: 613–619.

Peckham MJ, Horwich A, Brada M, Drury A, Hendry WF (1985). Carboplatin in the treatment of testicular germ cell tumors: a preliminary report. Cancer Treat Rev 12S: 101–110.

Pico JL, Droz JP, Gouyette A, Beaujean F, Baume D, Amiel JL, Hayat M (1986). High dose chemotherapy regimens followed by autologous bone marrow transplantation in refractory or relapsed non-seminomatous germ cell tumors. Proc ASCO 5: 111.

Postmus PE, De Vries EGE, De Vries-Hospers HG, Vriesendorp R, Van Imhoff GW, Holthuis JJM, Smit Sibinga CT, Sleijfer DT, Mulder NH (1984). Cyclophosphamide and VP 16–213 with autologous bone marrow transplantation: a dose escalation study. Eur J Cancer Clin Oncol 20: 777–782.

Postmus PE, Mulder NH, De Vries EGE, Van Luyn M, Halie MR (1984). Small cell lung cancer and the influence of chemotherapy on CFU_c's in bone marrow. Cancer 53: 396–400.

Postmus PE, Mulder NH, Sleijfer DT, Meinesz AF, Vriesendorp R, De Vries EGE (1984). High dose etoposide for refractory malignancies, a phase I study. Cancer Treat

Rep 68: 1471–1474.

Sleijfer DT, Mulder NH, De Vries-Hospers HG, Fidler V, Nieweg HO, Van der Waaij D, Van Saene HKF (1980). Infection prevention in granulocytopenic patients by selective decontamination of the digestive tract. Eur J Cancer 16: 859–869.

Spitzer G, Dicke KA, Litam J, Verma DS, Zander A, Lanzotti V, Valdivieso M, McCredie KB, Samuels ML (1980). High dose combination chemotherapy with autologous bone marrow transplantation in adult solid tumors. Cancer 45: 3075–3085.

Stoter G, Sylvester R, Sleijfer DT, Ten Bokkel Huinink WW, Kaye SB, Jones WG, Van Oosterom AT, Vendrik CPJ, Spaander P, De Pauw M (1987). Multivariate analysis of prognostic variables in patients with disseminated nonseminomatous testicular cancer: Results from an EORTC multi-institutional phase III study. Cancer Res, in press.

Taha IAK, Ahmad RA, Rogers DW, Pritchard J, Rogers HJ (1983). Pharmacokinetics of melphalan in children following high dose intravenous injection. Cancer Chemother Pharmacol 10: 212–216.

Van Imhoff GW, Arnaud F, Postmus PE, Mulder NH, Das PC, Smit Sibinga CT (1983). Autologous cryopreserved platelets and prophylaxis of bleeding in autologous bone marrow transplantation. Blut 47: 203–209.

Wolff SN, Johnson DH, Hainsworth JD, Greco FA (1984). High dose VP 16–213 monotherapy for refractory germinal malignancies: a phase II study. J Clin Oncol 2: 271–274.

EORTC Genitourinary Group Monograph 5: Progress
and Controversies in Oncological Urology II, page 437
© 1988 Alan R. Liss, Inc.

Discussion: High Dose Chemotherapy Followed by Autologous
Bone Marrow Re-Infusion in Relapsing or Refractory
Testicular Cancer

Ted A.W. Splinter, Rotterdam, The Netherlands

Fosså: Do you think that your treatment might be used as
primary treatment in bad risk patients?

Sleijfer: I have suggested to use high dose Cyclophosphamide
and Vp16 as a late intensification after introduction
chemotherapy.

EORTC Genitourinary Group Monograph 5: Progress
and Controversies in Oncological Urology II, pages 439–450
© 1988 Alan R. Liss, Inc.

THE ROLE OF IFOSFAMIDE IN THE TREATMENT OF NONSEMINOMATOUS
TESTICULAR CANCER

Max E. Scheulen, Norbert Niederle, Roland Kath,
Ursula B. Wandl, Siegfried Seeber and Carl G. Schmidt

Innere Klinik und Poliklinik (Tumorforschung),
West German Tumour Center, Universitaetsklinikum,
Hufelandstr. 55, D-4300 Essen 1, Fed. Rep. Germany

INTRODUCTION

The treatment results in metastatic nonseminomatous
testicular cancer (NSTC) have dramatically improved during
the last decades by the development of highly effective combination chemotherapy regimens and the optimization of combined modality strategies based on more and more sophisticated diagnostic measures and on the subtle assessment of
prognostic factors. Thus, NSTC today is a curable malignant
disease, even when far advanced.

Nevertheless, cytostatic drugs must be searched for,
which are either
- more effective and/or better tolerable and which
- can be favourably combined with established cytostatics
to further improve the therapeutic index in the course of
induction combination chemotherapy, or which are
- non-cross-resistant with established drug combinations
for the realization of the concept of sequential alternating
chemotherapy (Goldie et al., 1982), or for salvage therapy.

After more than ten years of experience with the oxazaphosphorine ifosfamide (Brock, 1972) at the West German Tumour Center (WGTC), this drug in our opinion is an ideal
candidate to fulfil the forementioned qualifications. Accordingly, we reviewed the role of ifosfamide in the treatment of NSTC with emphasis on its
- single agent activity,
- toxic side effects and their prevention,
- inclusion into sequential combination chemotherapy with

non-cross-resistant substances,
- advantageous addition to or substitution for one of the
  components of cisplatin/vinblastine/bleomycin (PVB), still
  the touchstone in combination chemotherapy of NSTC since
  its introduction by Einhorn and Donohue in 1977.

SINGLE AGENT ACTIVITY OF IFOSFAMIDE IN NSTC

The response rate in NSTC without prior chemotherapy to
ifosfamide alone has been determined in Europe during the
late seventies to be about 80%, including complete remissions of short duration in half of the responders (Table 1).
Thus, ifosfamide compares favourably with the most active
agents in treatment of NSTC (Table 2). In contrast, only 20%
of the patients with NSCT resistant to combination chemotherapy containing cisplatin responded to ifosfamide, with
only one CR in 87 patients (Scheulen et al., 1983). These
results have recently been confirmed at Indiana University
(Wheeler et al., 1986) (Table 1).

TABLE 1. Ifosfamide as a single agent in NSTC

AUTHOR	NO. OF PATIENTS	CR (%)	PR (%)	RESPONDERS (%)
Minimal or no prior chemotherapy:				
Bruehl et al., 1976	39	23(59)	14(36)	37(95)
Schmoll et al., 1978	18	2(11)	13(72)	15(83)
Boutis et al., 1982	16	10(63)	4(25)	14(88)
Weissbach & Kochs, 1982	39	8(21)	14(36)	22(56)
Total	112	43(38)	45(40)	88(79)
Prior cisplatin:				
Scheulen et al., 1983	87	1(1)	16(18)	17(20)
Wheeler et al., 1986	30	1(3)	6(20)	7(23)
Total	117	2(2)	22(19)	24(21)

TABLE 2. Single agent activity in NSTC

DRUG	NO. OF PATIENTS	CR (%)	PR (%)	RESPONDERS (%)
Ifosfamide *	112	43(38)	45(40)	88(79)
Cyclophosphamide	14	4(29)	7(50)	11(79)
Cisplatin **	118	22(19)	43(36)	65(55)
Chlorambucil	8	2(25)	2(25)	4(50)
Etoposide ***	24	3(13)	8(33)	11(46)
Bleomycin	54	6(11)	17(31)	23(43)
Vinblastine	41	5(12)	10(24)	15(37)
Mithramycin	133	12(9)	37(28)	49(37)
Actinomycin D	61	11(18)	9(15)	20(33)
Adriamycin	29	-	5(17)	5(17)

Anderson et al., 1979; * Table 1; ** Rozencweig et al., 1979
*** Fitzharris et al., 1980: pretreated patients

TABLE 3. Comparison of uroprotective measures

AUTHOR	INCIDENCE OF HAEMATURIA (%)	
	MICROHAEMATURIA	MACROHAEMATURIA
RANDOMIZED TRIALS:		
Scheef et al., 1979:		
- Standard prophylaxis *	9/ 9 (100) a	
- Mesna	2/11 (18) a	
Scheulen et al., 1983:		
- Standard prophylaxis *		25/ 92 (27) b
- Mesna		16/398 (4) bc
OTHER TRIALS:		
Wheeler et al., 1986:		
- N-Acetyl-cysteine	21/44 (48)	10/ 44 (23) c

a: p < 0.01; b: p < 0.001; c: p < 0.001
* continuous iv infusion of 3,000-4,000 ml normal saline
  daily and alkalinization of the urine

TOXIC SIDE EFFECTS OF IFOSFAMIDE

In contrast to cyclophosphamide, ifosfamide is less myelotoxic but has more pronounced urotoxic side effects, which are dose-limiting. Other clinical toxic reactions are alopecia, nausea and vomiting and CNS symptoms, such as somnolence, confusion and lethargy (Brade et al., 1985).

Brock and coworkers (1981) have investigated on a number of sulfhydryl compounds to inactivate hydroxy metabolites of ifosfamide and acrolein, which cause haemorrhagic cystitis. Mesna (sodium-2-mercaptoethanesulfonate) proved to be most potent, as it is rapidly eliminated into the urinary tract because of the sulfo group and traps toxic metabolites there because of the mercapto group. On the other hand, as mesna is rapidly oxidized to its inert disulfide during intestinal absorption (po route of administration) or in the plasma (iv route of administration), which is reduced to the pharmacologically active thiol compound in the renal tubular epithelium (Ormstad et al., 1983), it may not interfere with the antineoplastic action of ifosfamide.

The high uroprotective efficacy of mesna could be demonstrated in two randomized clinical studies (Scheef et al., 1979; Scheulen et al., 1983) (Table 3). Furthermore, in conformity with its pharmacology, mesna did not interfere with the antitumour activity of ifosfamide in patients with NSTC (Scheulen et al., 1983). It should be stressed that mesna is significantly more potent than N-acetyl-cysteine (Wheeler et al., 1986) (Table 3). Thus, the concomitant application of mesna with ifosfamide is mandatory in the following setting: mesna in a dose of 20% of ifosfamide iv or 40% po simultaneously with ifosfamide and about four and eight hours thereafter, each time after urination.

IFOSFAMIDE FOR THE AMELIORATION OF COMBINATION CHEMOTHERAPY OF NSTC

Taking into account the single agent activity of ifosfamide in NSTC, it could either be advantageously used
- in a setting of sequential combination chemotherapy with non-cross-resistant drugs,
- in salvage therapy,
- by addition to PVB, or
- by substitution for one of the components of PVB.

TABLE 4. Cross-resistance between vinblastine/bleomycin
(VLB/BLM), adriamycin/cisplatin (ADM/DDP) and ifosfamide
and etoposide alone or in combination (IFO/VP16) in NSTC:
The WGTC experience
(Scheulen et al., 1980; 1983; Bremer et al., 1982; Niederle
et al., 1983; Seeber et al., 1983)

	RESPONDERS/TOTAL (%)	
Sequential combination chemotherapy:		
	VBL/BLM	ADM/DDP
First line therapy	97/116 (84)	60/ 63 (95)
Alternative in case of resistance	14/ 24 (58)	18/ 26 (69)
Salvage therapy:		
Ifosfamide (60mg/kg/dx5)	17/87 (20)	
Etoposide (120mg/sqm/dx5po or x3iv)	4/37 (11)	
IFO/VP16 (40mg/kg/dx5 IFO; 120mg/sqm/dx3iv VP16)	19/63 (30)	

Sequential Combination Chemotherapy

The results of the clinical investigations on ifosfamide and etoposide either alone or in combination in sequential combination chemotherapy of NSTC at the WGTC are
summarized in Table 4. The response rate for ifosfamide is
20% and for ifosfamide/etoposide 30% in patients refractory
to vinblastine/bleomycin and adriamycin/cisplatin, but complete remissions are rare (Table 1). Thus, the contribution
of ifosfamide to a curative concept in this therapeutic setting is rather disappointing. However, better overall results might be obtained by the earlier entry of ifosfamide
during induction therapy of NSTC.

Salvage Therapy

Ifosfamide in combination with either etoposide or cisplatinum has produced complete remissions in about 7% of patients with heavily pretreated NSTC at the WGTC (Niederle et
al., 1983). Other combination chemotherapy regimens including ifosfamide used in salvage therapy of NSTC, such as eto-
poside/ifosfamide/cisplatin, have been shown to be more
effective with a CR rate of 33% and 20% of the patients presently NED (Einhorn, 1986b).

Addition of Ifosfamide to PVB

As PVB must be regarded as a highly effective chemotherapeutic regimen with "maximum tolerable side effects",
further addition of active drugs without dose reduction
might only be feasible at the expense of intolerable toxicity. Thus, as for the addition of adriamycin to PVB (Einhorn,
1981), the administration of ifosfamide supplementary to PVB
has not significantly improved the therapeutic results but
led to more pronounced toxic side effects, with drug-related
deaths of five out of 99 patients (Schmoll et al., 1983)
(Table 5). The significant improvement of the NED rate by
addition of etoposide to PVB might at least partially be due
to the simultaneous doubling of the cisplatin dose in the
PVB+VP16 group (Ozols et al., 1984) (Table 5). Altogether,
instead of the addition of ifosfamide to PVB, the replacement of one of its components by ifosfamide seems to be the
safer way to achieve an improvement in the treatment of
NSTC.

Replacement of One of the Components of PVB by Ifosfamide

Excellent results have been reported for cisplatin/
etoposide/bleomycin (PEB) by Pizzocaro and coworkers (1985),
but no three-drug alternative has been proved to be superior
to PVB in prospective randomized trials up to now (Table 5).
As ifosfamide/vinblastine/bleomycin (IVB) has been shown to
be unfavourable (Schmoll, 1980), the potential benefit of
the replacement of one of the other components of PVB by
ifosfamide is a matter of further studies.

Thus, we have investigated on cisplatin/ifosfamide/
bleomycin (PIB) in patients with advanced abdominal NSTC in

TABLE 5. Ifosfamide in combination chemotherapy of NSTC

STUDY * p < 0.05	NO. OF PATIENTS	CR (%)	NED + SURGERY (%)	NED AT PRESENT (%)	DRUG RELATED DEATH (%)
CISPLATIN/VINBLASTINE/BLEOMYCIN (PVB):					
(Einhorn & Donohue, 1977; Einhorn, 1981; 1986a; Stoter et al., 1984)					
- Original series	47	33(70)	5(11)	27(57)	2(4)
- Later series	225	143(64)	44(20)	174(77)	
- Netherlands	91	49(54)	14(15)	58(64)	5(5)
- Other institutions	226	161(71)	18(8)	162(72)	
Total	589	386(66)	81(14)	421(71)	
FOUR-DRUG-REGIMENS:					
PVB +/- Ifosfamide: (Schmoll et al., 1983)					
- PVB + IFO	99	63(64)	13(13)	69(70)	5(5)
- PVB	97	60(62)	11(11)	62(64)	0(0)
PVB +/- Adriamycin: (Einhorn, 1981)					
- PVB + ADM	84	57(68)	9(11)	62(74)	1(1)
- PVB	87	56(64)	10(11)	59(68)	0(0)
PVB +/- Etoposide: (Ozols et al., 1984; Einhorn, 1986a)					
- PVB + VP16	30	26(87)		21(70)*	1(3)
- PVB	16	10(62)		5(31)*	1(6)
THREE-DRUG-REGIMENS:					
Cisplatin/Etoposide/Bleomycin vs. PVB:					
(Williams et al., 1985; Einhorn, 1986a)					
- PVP16B	121	69(57)	25(21)		
- PVB	116	73(62)	13(12)		
(Pizzocaro et al., 1985)					
- PEB	40	25(63)	12(30)	33(83)	
Cisplatin/Vinblastine/Etoposide vs. PVB:					
(Samson et al., 1986)					
- PVVP16	41	24(59)	8(20)		
- PVB	41	24(59)	6(15)		
Ifosfamide/Vinblastine/Bleomycin: (Schmoll, 1980)					
- IVB	38	18(47)	7(18)	21(55)	

a pilot study: cisplatin 40 mg/sqm d 2-4, ifosfamide 5,000 mg/sqm d 1+5, and bleomycin 15 U/sqm d 1,8,15, q 21d, with adequate supportive measures, such as continuous infusion of normal saline, mesna prophylaxis, corticosteroids and antiemetics.

The preliminary treatment results of PIB are shown in Table 6. Maximum duration of NED is one year, at present. Toxic side effects were pronounced, including distinct leukopenia, alopecia and nausea and vomiting in all patients, as well as two cases of reversible nephropathy and ifosfamide-induced psychoses in two patients. There were two drug-related deaths due to septicaemia and bleomycin--induced pulmonary fibrosis, respectively. Urotoxic side effects of ifosfamide could completely be prevented by concomitant treatment with mesna.

TABLE 6. Treatment results in advanced abdominal disease

STUDY	NO. OF PATIENTS	CR (%)	NED + SURGERY (%)	NED AT PRESENT (%)
PVB				
- Einhorn & Donohue, 1977	16	9(56)		
- Einhorn & Williams, 1980	23	10(43)	8(35)	
- Stoter et al., 1984	35	18(51)		
- Einhorn (SECSG), 1986a	36			12(33)
PVP16B				
- Pizzocaro et al., 1985	33	21(64)	10(30)	27(82)
- Einhorn (SECSG), 1986a	35			17(48)
PVB + VP16				
- Ozols et al., 1984	30	26(87)		21(70)
Sequential VBL/BLM and ADM/DDP				
- Scheulen et al., 1984	52	16(31)	1(2)	6(12)
PIB				
- Pilot study (WGTC)	16	8(50)	2(13)	8(50)

As these results are too preliminary to allow definite conclusions, it remains to be seen whether this marked increase in toxicity of PIB in comparison to standard combination chemotherapies can be justified in poor-prognosis NSTC.

CONCLUSIONS

Ifosfamide is one of the most active cytostatic agents in NSTC (Table 1), which compares favourably with cisplatin, etoposide, bleomycin and vinblastine (Table 2). The dose-limiting urotoxicity of ifosfamide can effectively be prevented by concomitant administration of mesna without interference with its antitumour action (Table 3). According to studies of sequential combination chemotherapy of NSTC at the WGTC, ifosfamide is only partially cross-resistant with the substances mentioned above (Table 4).

Thus, ifosfamide is an ideal candidate to be included in induction regimens to further increase the therapeutic outcome in poor-prognosis NSTC or may be used in salvage therapy. The success of new induction protocols including ifosfamide has to be assessed not only with respect to an improvement of the cure rate but also to a reduction of toxic side effects. However, up to now none of the three- and four-drug combinations including ifosfamide has been proved to be significantly superior to standard regimens (Table 5).

The role of the potent agent ifosfamide in the induction therapy of advanced NSTC still remains to be defined in prospective randomized studies with patient stratification according to prognostic factors and accurate toxicity assessment. Thus, a recipe might be found to combine ifosfamide with other active drugs for the advantageous composition of a safe regimen, which is more effective than PEB in poor-prognosis NSTC.

REFERENCES

Anderson T, Waldmann TA, Javadpour N, Glatstein E (1979). Testicular germ-cell neoplasms: Recent advances in diagnosis and therapy. Ann Intern Med 90:373-385.
Boutis LL, Stergiou-Tavantzis J, Mouratidou D, Papadopoulou-Boutis A, Hatzigogos K, Bouhoris N, Dimi-

triadis K, Koukourikos S (1982). Ifosfamide chemotherapy of disseminated non-seminomatous testicular tumors. Proceedings of the 13th International Cancer Congress, Seattle, Wa, Abstr 1017.

Brade WP, Herdrich K, Varini M (1985). Ifosfamide - pharmacology, safety and therapeutic potential. Cancer Treat Rev 12:1-47.

Bremer K, Niederle N, Krischke W, Higi M, Scheulen ME, Schmidt CG, Seeber S (1982). Etoposide and etoposide-ifosfamide therapy for refractory testicular tumors. Cancer Treat Rev 9 (Suppl A):79-84.

Brock N (1972). Pharmacological studies with ifosfamide - a new oxazaphosphorine compound. In Semonsky M, Heijzler M, Masak S (eds): "Advances in Antimicrobial and Antineoplastic Chemotherapy." Baltimore, Md: University Park Press, Vol 2, pp 749-756.

Brock N, Pohl J, Stekar J (1981). Detoxification of urotoxic oxazaphosphorines by sulfhydryl compounds. J Cancer Res Clin Oncol 100:311-320.

Bruehl P, Guenther U, Hoefer-Janker H, Huels W, Scheef W, Vahlensieck W (1976). Results obtained with fractionated ifosfamide massive-dose treatment in generalized malignant tumors. Int J Clin Pharmacol 14:29-39.

Einhorn LH (1981). Testicular cancer as a model for a curable neoplasm: The Richard and Hinda Rosenthal Foundation Award Lecture. Cancer Res 41:3275-3280.

Einhorn, LH (1986a). Have new aggressive chemotherapy regimens improved results in advanced germ cell tumors? Eur J Cancer Clin Oncol 22:1289-1293.

Einhorn, LH (1986b). VP16 plus ifosfamide plus cisplatin as salvage therapy in refractory testicular cancer. Cancer Chemother Pharmacol 18 (Suppl 2):S45-S50.

Einhorn LH, Donohue J (1977). cis-Diamminedichloroplatinum, vinblastine and bleomycin combination chemotherapy in disseminated testicular cancer. Ann Intern Med 87:293-298.

Einhorn LH, Williams SD (1980). Chemotherapy of disseminated testicular cancer. A random prospective study. Cancer 46:1339-1344.

Fitzharris BM, Kaye SB, Saverymuttu S, Newlands ES, Barrett A, Peckham MJ, McElwain TJ (1980). VP16-213 as a single agent in advanced testicular tumors. Europ J Cancer 16:1193-1197.

Goldie JH, Coldman AJ, Gudauskas GA (1982). Rationale for the use of alternating non-cross-resistant chemotherapy. Cancer Treat Rep 66:439-449.

Niederle N, Scheulen ME, Cremer M, Schuette J, Schmidt CG,

Seeber S (1983). Ifosfamide in combination chemotherapy for sarcomas and testicular carcinomas. Cancer Treat Rev 10 (Suppl A):129-135.

Ormstad K, Orrenius S, Lastbom T, Uehara N, Pohl J, Stekar J, Brock N (1983). Pharmacokinetics and metabolism of sodium 2-mercaptoethanesulfonate in the rat. Cancer Res 43:333-338.

Ozols RF, Ihde D, Jacob J, Steis R, Veach SR, Wesley M, Young RC (1984). Randomized trial of PVeBV (high dose cisplatin, vinblastine, bleomycin, VP-16) versus PVeB in poor prognosis non-seminomatous testicular cancer. Proc Am Soc Clin Oncol 3:155.

Pizzocaro G, Piva L, Salvioni R, Zanoni F, Milani A (1985). Cisplatin, etoposide, bleomycin first-line therapy and early resection of residual tumor in far-advanced germinal testis cancer. Cancer 56:2411-2415

Rozencweig M, Von Hoff DD, Abele R, Muggia FM (1979). Cisplatin. In Pinedo HM (ed): "Cancer Chemotherapy 1979. The EORTC Cancer Chemotherapy Annual 1." Amsterdam: Excerpta Medica, pp 107-125.

Samson MK, Crawford ED, Natale R, Bouroncle B, Altman S (1986). A randomized comparison of cisplatin, vinblastine plus either bleomycin or VP-16 in patients with advanced testicular cancer. Proc Am Soc Clin Oncol 5:96.

Scheef W, Klein HO, Brock N, Burkert H, Guenther U, Hoefer-Janker H, Mitrenga D, Schnitker J, Voigtmann R (1979). Controlled clinical studies with an antidote against the urotoxicity of oxazaphosphorines: Preliminary results. Cancer Treat Rep 63:501-505.

Scheulen ME, Seeber S, Schilcher RB, Meier CR, Schmidt CG (1980a). Sequential combination chemotherapy with vinblastine-bleomycin and doxorubicin-cis-dichlorodiammineplatinum(II) in disseminated non-seminomatous testicular cancer. Cancer Treat Rep 64:599-609.

Scheulen ME, Higi M, Schilcher RB, Meier CR, Seeber S, Schmidt CG (1980b). Sequentiell alternierende Chemotherapie nicht-seminomatoeser Hodentumoren mit Velbe/Bleomycin und Adriamycin/Cisplatin. I. Ergebnisse einer randomisierten Studie bei 71 Patienten mit pulmonaler Metastasierung (Stadium IV). Klin Wschr 58:811-821.

Scheulen ME, Niederle N, Bremer K, Schuette J, Seeber S (1983). Efficacy of ifosfamide in refractory malignant diseases and uroprotection by mesna. Results of a clinical phase II-study with 151 patients. Cancer Treat Rev 10 (Suppl A):93-101.

Scheulen ME, Pfeiffer R, Hoeffken K, Niederle N, Seeber S,

Schmidt CG (1984). Long-term survival and prognostic factors in patients with disseminated nonseminomatous testicular cancer. Proc Am Soc Clin Oncol 3:163.

Schmoll H-J (1980). Heutiger Stand der Chemotherapie des metastasierenden Hodenkarzinoms. Beitr Onkol 3:60-81.

Schmoll H, Rhomberg W, Diehl V (1978). Ifosfamide (NSC 109427): Activity in testicular cancer using mono- and combination therapy. In Siegenthaler W, Luethy R (eds) "Current Chemotherapy." Washington, DC: American Society for Microbiology, Vol 2, pp 1098-1091.

Schmoll H-J, Diehl V, Hartlapp J, Illiger J, Mitrou PS, Bergmann L, Hoffmann L, Bombick BM, Graubner M, Queisser W, Sterry K, Haselberger H, Douwes FW, Schnaidt U, Hecker H (1983). PVB +/- Ifosfamid bei disseminierten Hodentumoren: Ergebnisse einer prospektiv randomisierten Studie. Verh Dtsch KrebsGes 4:703-711.

Seeber S, Schuette J, Niederle N, Schmidt CG (1983). Neue Ergebnisse der Behandlung metastasierter Hodentumoren im Frueh- und Spaetstadium. Tumordiagn Ther 4:45-54.

Stoter G, Vendrik CPJ, Struyvenberg A, Sleyfer DT, Vriesendorp R, Schraffordt Koops H, van Oosterom AT, ten Bokkel Huinink WW, Pinedo, HM (1984). Five-year survival of patients with disseminated nonseminomatous testicular cancer treated with cisplatin, vinblastine, and bleomycin. Cancer 54:1521-1524.

Weissbach L, Kochs R (1982). Monotherapy with ifosfamide in the treatment of testicular tumours (non-seminomas). Proceedings of the 13th International Cancer Congress, Seattle, Wa, Abstr 3596.

Wheeler BM, Loehrer PJ, Williams SD, Einhorn LH (1986). Ifosfamide in refractory male germ cell tumors. J Clin Oncol 4:28-34.

Williams S, Einhorn L, Greco A, Birch R, Irwin L (1985). Disseminated germ cell tumors: A comparison of cisplatin plus bleomycin plus either vinblastine (PVB) or VP-16 (BEP). Proc Am Soc Clin Oncol 4:100.

EORTC Genitourinary Group Monograph 5: Progress
and Controversies in Oncological Urology II, pages 451–457
© 1988 Alan R. Liss, Inc.

INDICATIONS AND RESULTS OF SURGERY AFTER CHEMOTHERAPY OF
TESTICULAR TUMORS (NSGT AND SEMINOMA)

John P. Donohue, M.D.

Department of Urology, Indiana University, 926 W.
Michigan St., University Hospital A112, Indianapolis,
IN 46223, U.S.A.

Advanced testicular cancer is best treated with combination platinum based chemotherapy as primary therapy. Those
with more bulky tumor who obtain a partial remission should
then have residual tumor completely resected by surgery. This
effectively re-stages the patient, provides therapeutic benefit to many and determines the need for additional chemotherapy. If carcinoma is found in the resected specimen,
further "salvage" chemotherapy is required. If the resection
is grossly complete even this group can obtain survival in
the majority of cases.

Clinical experience with over 250 such cases permits
several other observations. Some patients who achieve a partial remission (PR) can still be observed. Those with pure
seminoma in the primary specimen who still have a radiographic abnormality after treatment for bulky metastatic disease usually have necrotic tumor, if resected. Therefore,
several groups have demonstrated a successful conservative
approach in the partial responders. Recently, we have noted
another group who can be observed with a PR. Those who had
pure embryonal cancer in the primary tumor and who had a 90%
or greater reduction in measured tumor volume all had necrosis in the resected specimens. Therefore, these PR's can be
observed, if these two conditions are met (pure embryonal
primary and 90% reduction in volume).

Also, we have noted the relapse potential is related
to three major variables: site of the disease (e.g. mediastinal vs. retroperitoneal), histology (sarcomatous elements
vs. none), and bulk of disease (massive vs. moderate vs.
small).

Indications for Cytoreductive Surgery after Chemotherapy

Two different groups of patients need to be considered. The first group are those who have had a partial remission with primary therapy. The second group are those who once had a complete remission after primary chemotherapy, but who relapsed and then achieved a partial remission after salvage chemotherapy.

The first group who do not have complete resolution of findings on abdominal CAT scan or on abdominal ultrasound after chemotherapy are considered as candidates for radical retroperitoneal lymph node dissection. If the residual mass is high in the abdomen and extends into the retrocrural area or apparently involves the diaphragm and has extension into the chest, a combined abdominal and thoracic approach is indicated. Depending upon the circumstances of the individual case, either a thoracoabdominal incision or a median sternotomy in combination with the midline abdominal incision is used. When patients have residual unilateral chest disease, either in the parenchyma or the mediastinum, a thoracotomy incision alone is sufficient assuming that the abdominal findings have completely normalized or were normal initially. If bilateral chest disease is present particularly in the posterior mediastinum, separate thoracotomy incisions may be indicated. If the bilateral chest disease is in any other location, adequate exposure can frequently be obtained through a median sternotomy. Any of these approaches can be used in combination with a midline abdominal incision if there is residual disease in the abdomen.

If any patient in this group, having undergone primary cytoreductive chemotherapy, has a persistently elevated serum marker, AFP or Beta-HCG, he is treated with salvage chemotherapy rather than surgical resection based upon the knowledge that there is still active disease present.

The second set of patients are those who have undergone salvage chemotherapy. The same indications for surgery are used in this set of patients; that is, they would have evidence of only a partial remission. Again, in general, if the patient had an elevated AFP or Beta-HCG, he would be a candidate for further chemotherapy rather than surgical treatment. There are occasional exceptions to this rule if the patient has exhausted all chemotherapeutic regimens which have any likelihood of success and has a limited focus of disease deemed resectable. Table 1 summarizes the indications for surgery.

TABLE 1. Indications for Surgery After Chemotherapy

Finding	RPLND	Thoracotomy	Median Sternotomy
Residual abd. mass on CAT or Ultrasound	+		
Retrocrural mass on CAT	+	+/0	+/0
Unilateral parenchymal mass on WLT		+	
Unilateral mediastinal mass on WLT		+	
Bilateral parenchymal or mediastinal masses			+
Elevated Serum AFP	0	0	0
Elevated Serum BHCG	0	0	0

Operative Setup and Technical Consideration of Retroperitoneal Lymph Node Dissection after Chemotherapy

The technical portions of the retroperitoneal node dissection have been thoroughly described in the past by Donohue (1977). A full bilateral retroperitoneal lymph node dissection is indicated in most cases. Tissue analysis from full RPLND specimens confirms the diverse nature of histologic change in these patients who have had widespread metastatic disease (Griest et al, 1983). Therefore, a simple "lumpectomy" is a dangerous practice, as it risks missing tumor elsewhere in the retroperitoneum.

Results of Surgery at Indiana University

Earlier, we reported on 123 patients treated at Indiana University who had partial remissions after primary or salvage chemotherapy followed by surgery (Donohue et al, 1980; Donohue et al, 1982; Mandelbaum et al, 1980; Mandelbaum et al, 1983).

Currently, our experience with postchemotherapy dissections
exceeds 250 cases. Table 2 shows the results by location of
the residual mass(es) as evidenced by the surgical approach
(RPLND alone, thoracotomy alone, or combined chest and retroperitoneal procedures).

TABLE 2. Histologic Findings in Surgery After Chemotherapy.

Group	No. Patients	Fibrotic-Cystic- Necrotic Tissue		Teratoma		Carcinoma	
RPLND only 2,5	51*	16	31.5%	16	31.5%	19	37%
Thoracotomy only 12,13	48	14	30%	17	35%	17	35%
RPLND + Thoracotomy 13	24**	4	17%	13	54%	7	29%
	123	34	28%	46	37%	43	35%

* These patients represent partial remissions after primary
  chemotherapy and relapse after complete remission who went
  on to have partial remissions with salvage chemotherapy.
**In 17 patients the pathology in the chest and retroperito-
  neum agreed and in 7 they differed.

Patients with either partial remission after primary chemotherapy or patients who had relapsed after primary therapy
and had a partial response to salvage chemotherapy were present in all groups. There was roughly a 2/5-2/5-1/5 division
in the combined series among the findings of fibrotic-cystic-
necrotic tissue (2/5), teratoma (mature or immature)(2/5), and
carcinoma (1/5)(Donohue et al, 1980).

In general, the patients who have only necrotic or fibro-
cystic tissue at the time of exploration do extremely well
postoperatively. Initially the relapse rate was felt to be 10%
in those patients with teratoma. A recent report by Loehrer
and his associates (1983) reported relapse in 16 of 54 patients with surgically resected teratoma with a minimum follow
up of 18 months.

Nine of these patients relapsed with carcinoma and 7 with
recurrent teratoma. In the group of 9 patients with recurrent

carcinoma, 4 have been rendered disease free with subsequent treatment, 2 are alive with disease and 3 are dead. In the group of 7 with recurrent teratoma, 2 have died of inoperable progressive disease and 5 are disease free although 2 have required multiple surgical procedures. The fact that relapses tend to occur near sites of previous resection, points to the necessity of exhaustive dissection in these patients at the time of their cytoreductive surgery.

Also, it needs to be emphasized that if a patient's diagnosis was originally made by means other than orchiectomy and there has been an abnormal testis either by history, examination, or ultrasound finding, the testicle should be removed at the time of surgery due to the possibility of persistence of primary tumor. The testis should also be removed even if the patient had an apparent complete response from chemotherapy. In 42% of such patients either teratoma or carcinoma were found in the testicle which was removed after chemotherapy (Griest et al, 1983). This data would suggest that there may be a barrier in the testis that inhibits the effectiveness of chemotherapy in this organ.

Despite the increased risks in patients who have undergone primary or salvage chemotherapy prior to resection of residual disease, the complication and death rates are acceptable. Donohue and Rowland (1981) reported 49 patients who underwent surgery for advanced disease, 45 having received previous chemotherapy. The total complication rate in this postchemotherapy group with advanced disease was 26% and the death rate was 2% in this group as compared to an overall complication rate of 12% and a death rate of 0.5% in patients who were operated on for lesser stage disease (Stage I or Stage II). Similar findings were reported by Skinner's group (Skinner et al, 1982). Fifty-two patients in their group were operated on for advanced disease. The complication rate was 23% with a death rate of 4%.

Clinical experience with certain patterns of response to chemotherapy led us to recognize another group of patients who almost invariably will have necrosis alone in the residual tumor. The first group so identified have been the patients with pure seminoma in the primary testis tumor. Many have noted that these patients had only necrosis in resected tumors postchemotherapy; and, if observed without surgery, had stable partial remissions and no progression after treatment of bulky metastatic disease with platinum based chemo-

therapy programs. A second group has now emerged as very likely to have necrosis only in resected tissue. These are patients who had pure embryonal carcinoma in their primary tumor
and who had greater than 90% reduction in the size of their
tumor mass as measured on sequential CT scans following treatment. The much cytoreduced, small lesions resected after chemotherapy were entirely necrotic in this subset of patients
treated. But it was necessary to have these two criteria, e.g.
pure embryonal cancer (MTU) in the primary testis tumor and a
very impressive cytoreductive response to chemotherapy treatment (90% or more), in order to achieve in all patients this
histologic response of necrosis only. In retrospect, we may
conclude that these patients were cured by their chemotherapy.
This somewhat parallels our earlier experience of patients
with seminoma who were found to have necrosis with great regularity when their residual metastases were resected post-
chemotherapy. This led to a general consensus that they could
be followed safely, especially if they had smaller lesions
and some measurable response to earlier treatment. Others
chose to use consolidation radiotherapy, particularly to bulky
residual tumors. Relapses in these seminoma patients with PR's
observed expectantly have been few.

In distiction to the seminoma analogy, however, these patients with pure embryonal cancer and advanced disease must
have a dramatic radiographic response (>90%) in order to be
predictive for necrosis only. Anything less than that runs the
risk for some persistent tumor elements with growth potential.
(See Table 2.)

One of the special challenges in postchemotherapy surgery
is the patient with bulky teratoma. This must be well resected,
in several stages if necessary (e.g. chest, supraclavicular,
abdominal and pelvic) as it will not regress; rather most progress either as "mature and immature teratoma" and some revert
to malignant change as well. We have noted several factors associated with increased relapse and survival risks. Univariate
factors predicting for relapse include tumor burden, immature
teratoma with non-germ cell elements, and site (mediastinum),
whereas only immature teratoma with non-germ cell elements and
site predicted for survival. Immature teratoma and mature teratoma had similar relapse-free intervals and overall survival
intervals.

According to a multivariate analysis, primary tumor site
at the mediastinum is the most significant adverse factor pre-

dictive for both relapse and survival (two of five patients survived). This study appears to support the various preclinical models that demonstrate multipotential capabilities of teratoma. Complete surgical excision of teratoma remains the most effective treatment with continued close follow-up recommended for high-risk patients (immature teratoma with non-germ cell elements, large tumor burden, or primary mediastinal tumors)(Loehrer et al, 1986).

REFERENCES

Donohue JP (1977). Retroperitoneal lymphadenectomy: the anterior approach including bilateral suprahilar dissection. Urol Clin N Amer 4(3):509-521.

Donohue JP, Einhorn LH, Williams SD (1980). Cytoreductive surgery for metastatic testis cancer: considerations of timing and extent. J Urol 123:876-880.

Donohue JP, Rowland RG (1981). Complications of retroperitoneal lymph node dissection. J Urol 125:338-340.

Donohue JP, Roth LM, Zachary JM, Rowland RG, Einhorn LH, Williams SG (1982). Cytoreductive surgery for metastatic testis cancer: tissue analysis of retroperitoneal masses after chemotherapy. J Urol 127:1111-1114.

Griest A, Williams SD, Einhorn LH, Donohue JP, Rowland RG, Estes N (1983). Pathologic findings at orchiectomy following chemotherapy for disseminated testicular cancer. Proc Am Soc Clin Oncol 2:139.

Loehrer PJ, Williams SD, Clark SA, Einhorn LH, Donohue JP, Mandelbaum I, Rohn RJ (1983). Teratoma following chemotherapy for non-seminomatous germ cell tumor (NSGCT): a clinicopathologic correlation. Proc Am Soc Clin Oncol 2: 139.

Loehrer PJ, Hui S, Einhorn LH, Donohue JP (1986). Resection of thoracic and abdominal teratoma in patients after cisplatin-based chemotherapy for germ cell tumor. J Thoracic Cardiovascular Surg 92:676-683.

Mandelbaum I, Williams SD, Einhorn LH (1980). Aggressive surgical management of testicular carcinoma metastatic to lungs and mediastinum. Annals Thor Surg 30:224-229.

Mandelbaum I, Yaw PB, Einhorn LH, Williams SD, Rowland RG, Donohue JP (1983). The importance of one-stage median sternotomy and retroperitoneal node dissection in disseminated testicular cancer. Annals Thor Surg 36:524-528.

Skinner DC, Melamud A, Lieskovsky G (1982). Complications of thoracoabdominal retroperitoneal lymph node dissection. J Urol 127:1107-1110.

EORTC Genitourinary Group Monograph 5: Progress
and Controversies in Oncological Urology II, page 459
© 1988 Alan R. Liss, Inc.

Discussion: Indications and Results of Surgery After
Chemotherapy of Testicular Tumors (NSGT and Seminoma)

Ted A.W. Splinter. Rotterdam, The Netherlands

Kaye: You indicated that the presence of sarcomatous elements in the resected immature teratoma is correlated with a worse prognosis. Does that affect your postsurgical treatment i.e. do you give specific chemotherapy?

Donohue: We feel that we have very little to offer to those who have adenocarcinoma or leiomyosarcoma. Perhaps the embryonal rhabdomyosarcomas may be suitable for additional chemotherapy.

Schröder: You said that no one can be watched except seminomas with a PR and perhaps a small subgroup of embryonal carcinomas. Would you ever just remove a residual mass or do you think that all these patients have to be treated with a complete lymph node dissection?

Donohue: We try always to do the standard template. We have published that viable tumor can be found in perfectly normal looking adjacent nodes. If you are there it is not extraordinarily difficult to widen the template and get good margins, but I doubt that we shall ever be able to make a statistical case for this view.

Debruyne: If a patient has multifocal residual disease e.g. retroperitoneal and pulmonary masses, and you have found no viable tumor in the retroperitoneal nodes, do you still perform a thoracotomy? In our material all residual lesions smaller than 3 cm contained fibrotic tissue. Do you think that in these patients surgery can be omitted?

Donohue: We do not perform a suprahilar dissection in our patients with a modestly sized mass after chemotherapy. Many patients have only a little fibrous tissue above the renal arteries, which we do not pursue. There is, however, no concordance between an abdominal and a pulmonary parenchymal mass!

EORTC Genitourinary Group Monograph 5: Progress
and Controversies in Oncological Urology II, pages 461-468
© 1988 Alan R. Liss, Inc.

POTENTIAL ADVANCES IN COMBINATION CHEMOTHERAPY FOR ADVANCED
TESTICULAR CANCER

S.B. Kaye(1), G. Stoter(2), D. Sleijfer(3), W.
Jones(4), W. Ten Bokkel Huinink(5), T. Splinter(6)
A. Van Oosterom(7), A. Harris(8), E. Boven(9),
M. De Pauw and R. Sylvester(10)

1. Gartnavel General Hospital, Glasgow ; 2.
R.R.T.I., Rotterdam ; 3. Academisch Ziekenhuis
Groningen, Groningen ; 4. Cookridge Hospital,
Leeds ; 5. Netherlands Cancer Institute, Amsterdam
; 6. Erasmus University, Rotterdam ; 7. Academic
Hospital of Antwerp, Antwerp ; 8. Newcastle
General Hospital, Newcastle ; 9. Free University
Hospital, Amsterdam ; 10. EORTC Data Centre,
Brussels : for the EORTC G.U. Group

INTRODUCTION

Over the past 10 years, national statistics indicate
both an increase in incidence and a reduction in mortality
for testicular cancer (Boyle et al, 1986). The reason for
the increased incidence is unknown, but the reduced
mortality is clearly related to the introduction of
cis-platinum-containing combination chemotherapy.

The majority of patients with advanced disease are
now curable. For example, over the past 6 years, 147
patients with testicular cancer have been referred to the
University Department of Medical Oncology in Glasgow, and
those requiring chemotherapy (a total of 99) have been
entered into collaborative EORTC Urology Group Protocols.
Overall 90% of these 99 patients are alive and disease-free
following therapy.

CURRENT EORTC STUDIES

In 1983 two studies were started, and these will be

concluded during 1987. Patients were divided into those with "low volume metastases" and "high volume metastases", as defined in table 1.

Table 1

Low Volume Metastases:
- lymph nodes < 5cm (retroperitoneal
                        mediastinal
                        supraclavicular)
- lung metastases, < 4 in number
                        all less than 2cm
- β HCG < 10,000 i.u./l
- AFP < 1,000 i.u./l

High Volume Metastases:
- lymph nodes ⩾ 5cm (as above transverse diameter)
- lung metastases ⩾ 4 in number
                        or any ⩾ 2cm
- β HCG ⩾ 10,000 i.u./l
  AFP ⩾ 1,000 i.u./l

(a)   Low volume metastases

With the aim of reducing toxicity yet maintaining efficacy in this group of patients with an excellent prognosis, patients were randomized to receive cisplatinum (P) 20mg/m^2 for 5 days, etoposide (E) 120mg/m^2 days 1, 3 and 5, with or without bleomycin (B) 30mg i.v. weekly for 12 weeks. Four cycles of EP or BEP were given at 3 week intervals, at the end of which patients were assessed for response. If radiologically apparent residual masses were present, and tumour markers were normal, surgery was performed for response evaluation; and the finding of mature teratoma, fibrosis and necrosis was classified as a Complete Response (CR). An interim analysis, after 180 patients were randomised, has been performed (Stoter et al, 1987). With regard to CR rate there is no difference between the two treatment arms. For patients treated with EP, 59 out of 62 patients evaluable to date (95%) achieved CR; the corresponding figure for BEP was 64 out of 67 (95%). To date 2 relapses from CR have been noted on the EP arm, and 1 on the BEP arm. Patients treated with BEP experienced significantly more toxicity, in terms of skin toxicity, lung toxicity and myelosuppression. The preliminary conclusion is that bleomycin may not be a necessary component of combination chemotherapy for patients with "low volume" metastastic testicular cancer. However, median follow-up is relatively short (16 months) and the study remains open.

(b)   High volume metastases

For this group of patients, whose prognosis overall is less certain than those in group (a), the aim of the current study has been to increase response rates by the introduction of an alternating combination chemotherapy schedule. A randomised study was thus initiated, comparing 4 cycles of BEP (as above) with 2 cycles of BEP alternating with 2 cycles of PVB (cisplatinum [P] 20mg/m^2 days 1 to 5, vinblastine [V] 0.15mg/kg days 1 and 2 and bleomycin 30mg i.v. weekly for 12 weeks). As before response assessment was performed after 4 cycles with surgical evaluation as necessary. An interim analysis has been performed after the accrual of 205 patients (Stoter et al, 1986). With regard to CR rates there is no difference between the two treatment arms. For patients treated with BEP, 49 out of 63 evaluated to date (78%) achieved CR; for patients treated with PVB/BEP the corresponding figure was 45 out of 62 (73%). To date 2 relapse from CR have occurred on the BEP arm and 4 on the PVB/BEP arm. Patients treated with PVB/BEP experienced more toxicity than those treated with BEP, in terms of myelosuppression and neurotoxicity.

The preliminary conclusion is that the alternating schedule incorporating PVB is not superior to treatment with continuous BEP, and this is in line with a report of the randomised study of the South-Eastern Cancer Study Group of the USA, in which BEP proved superior to PVB at least in terms of reduced toxicity. There was also a trend in favour of BEP towards a higher response rate and longer survival for patients with the most advanced disease (Einhorn, 1986).

FUTURE EORTC STUDIES

(a)   Low volume metastases

It is clear that very high response and cure rates can be achieved in this group. Efforts should therefore

continue towards maintaining these results while attempting
to reduce drug toxicity. The most toxic drug involved is
cisplatinum, in terms of nephrotoxicity, neurotoxicity and
gastro-intestinal toxicity. The platinum analogue
carboplatin is an attractive alternative, since it is less
toxic in all 3 respects; however it is more myelotoxic than
cisplatinum. Preliminary studies from the Royal Marsden
Hospital indicate a high response rate with carboplatin in
advanced seminoma (Peckham et al, 1985), but for advanced
teratoma combination schedules with other myelosuppressive
drugs such as etoposide will require to be developed
carefully before the drug can be routinely substituted for
cisplatinum, without risking sub-optimal therapy. Long term
toxicity from cisplatinum is receiving increasing
attention, and both cardiovascular and renal toxicity have
been documented (Bosh et al, 1986). The development of
this particular toxicity might well relate to the schedule
of cisplatinum used, i.e. high dose over a short duration,
e.g. 100mg/m^2 over 4 hours being possibly more toxic than
low dose over a longer interval, e.g. 20mg/m^2 per day
for 5 days. The next EORTC study will assess the
difference, if any, between these two schedules. Patients
will receive 4 cycles of EP with cisplatinum on two days, or
4 cycles of EP with cisplatinum over (the less convenient)
5 days as in the previous study.

(b)   High volume metastases

The CR rates of 70 - 80% for this group still leave room
for improvement. In particular it is clear that within this
group are a smaller number of patients with the most
advanced disease, for whom the prognosis is rather poor.
These have been defined as those with massive tumour bulk,
(i.e. tumour masses > 10cm in diameter) and grossly raised
levels of β HCG (> 50,000 I.u/l) For this group with
"ultra-high volume" metastatic disease, considerable
intensification of chemotherapy is justifiable and since it
is generally agreed that patients with extragonadal primary
germ cell tumours also carry a poorer prognosis, such
patients are also included in this group. For the remaining
larger group of patients with high volume metastases,
alternative schedules to BEP should be assessed with the
aim of improving the overall cure rate. In the past few
years, very few new drugs have proved to be active in the
face of failure of primary treatment for testicular cancer.
The most promising in this regard is the cyclophosphamide

analogue, ifosfamide, which yielded a 23% response rate as 3rd line treatment in a Phase II study reported by the group at Indiana University (Wheeler et al, 1986). This group went on to demonstrate the feasibility of using a combination of etoposide, ifosfamide and cisplatinum (VIP) as salvage therapy, and clearly this combination is active even after relapse following therapy with BEP (Loehrer et al, 1985). It would therefore appear logical to make a direct randomised comparison between 4 cycles of treatment with BEP or with VIP (which will induce rather more myelo-suppression) as first line therapy for patients with high volume metastatic teratoma (excluding "ultra-high volume"), and this will form the basis of the next EORTC Urology Group Study for this patient population.

For patients with "ultra-high volume" disease several approaches have been suggested. These include the use of high dose chemotherapy, short intervals between cycles, and alternating schedules using multiple drugs (Kaye, 1986). An assessment of the most effective schedule is hampered by the lack of randomised trials and the variation in the criteria chosen for treatment as "ultra-high volume" patients.

In March 1986 we began in Glasgow to develop a protocol named BOP/VIP for this small subgroup of patients. The schedule is depicted in table 2, and the rationale is as follows:
(a) to achieve rapid initial response by shortening the treatment interval between courses of cisplatinum (using a non-myelosuppressive combination).
(b) to introduce 2 further effective drugs once the response was established, i.e. etoposide and ifosfamide.
(c) to complete the treatment in approximately 3 months. Thus patients receive 3 courses of BOP followed by 3 courses of VIP, and go on to surgical evaluation of any residual masses if tumour markers are normal.

Table 2

BOP/VIP

BOP:
bleomycin 30mg (6 hour i.v.) day 1.
vincristine 2mg i.v. day 1
cisplatin 50mg/m^2 days 1 and 2
  - repeat at 9 - 10 day interval for
3 courses.

then approx. 2 weeks interval before:

VIP:
VP16 100mg/m^2 days 1, 3, 5.
          (subsequently reduced to 75mg/m^2)
ifosfamide 1.2gm/m^2 days 1 - 5.
          (subsequently reduced to 1.0gm/m^2)
cisplatin 20mg/m^2 days 1 to 5.
  - repeat at 3 weeks intervals for
    3 courses.

Then surgery for residual masses if
tumour markers normal.

To date 9 patients have been treated. They all
fulfilled the criteria outlined above for "ultra-high
volume" disease, apart from one patient with a primary
seminoma also included because of very extensive retroperitoneal and hepatic metastases.

With regard to toxicity, BOP/VIP proved to be feasible,
the major problem being marked myelosuppression following
the 2nd and 3rd cycles of VIP (median nadir Wbc of 1.1 x
$10^9/l$ with a range of 0.1 to 2.7 x $10^9/l$; median nadir
platelets of 20 x $10^9/l$ with a range of 11 to 115 x
$10^9/l$). These data led to a reduction in doses of
etoposide and ifosfamide as in table 2. One patient went
into renal failure (creatinine rise to 1040 umol/l) after
the first cycle of VIP. This followed a period of
neutropenic septicaemia during which gentamycin was given,
and was thought to be a major contributing factor. No other
significant nephrotoxicity was seen.

Regarding response, 7 patients have achieved CR
confirmed surgically in 6. One patient with an extra-

gonadal primary achieved a PR but died at 6 months (possibly not a germ cell tumour) and one went off protocol because of renal failure (above).

BOP/VIP would appear to be a feasible option for patients with the most advanced disease. To assess the role of this type of intensified therapy in this small subgroup of patients, randomised trials on a collaborative basis are required, and discussions between EORTC and the Medical Research Council in the UK are in progress with this in mind.

SUMMARY

An interim analysis of the current EORTC studies in advanced testicular cancer indicates that (a) for low volume metastatic disease the addition of bleomycin (B) to etoposide (E) and cisplatinum (P) may not be necessary, and (b) for high volume metastatic disease the alternating schedule of PVB/BEP is not superior to treatment with BEP.

Future studies will subdivide patients into 3 groups. Those with low volume metastatic disease will receive EP using 2 dose schedules for cisplatin. Those with high volume metastases will receive either BEP or etoposide, ifosfamide and cisplatinum (VIP). Those with ultra-high volume metastases will receive BOP/VIP, possibly randomised against another intensive chemotherapy schedule.

REFERENCES

Bosh G J, Leitner S P, Atlas S A, Sealey J E, Preibisz J J and Scheiner E (1986). Increased plasma renin and aldosterone in patients treated with cisplatin-based chemotherapy for metastatic germ-cell tumours. J Clin Oncol 4:1684-1689.

Boyle P, Kaye S B and Robertson A G (1986). Improving prognosis of testicular cancer in Scotland. CRCS Med Sci 14:976-977.

Einhorn L H (1986). Have new aggressive chemotherapy regimens improved results in advanced germ cell tumours? Europ J Cancer Clin Onc 22:1289-1293.

Kaye S B (1986). Prospects for improved curability of metastatic germ cell tumours carrying the worst prognosis. In Jones W, Ward A M and Anderson C K (eds): "Germ Cell Tumours II" Pergammon Press, Oxford, pp 363-368.

Loehrer P J, Einhorn L H and Williams S D (1985) Salvage therapy for refractory germ cell tumours with VP16 plus Ifosfamide plus cisplatin. Proc Amer Soc Clin Onc 4:100.

Peckham M J, Horwich A and Hendry W F (1985). Advanced seminoma, treatment with cisplatinum-based combination chemotherapy or carboplatin. Brit J Cancer 52:7-13.

Stoter G, Kaye S B, Sleijfer D, Ten Bokkel-Huinink W, Jones W, Van Oosterom A, Splinter T, Pinedo H, Sylvester R and Keizer J (1986). Preliminary results of BEP versus an alternating regimen of BEP and PVB in HVM testicular non seminoma. Proc Amer Soc Clin Onc 5:106.

Stoter G, Kaye S B, Jones W, Ten Bokkel-Huinink W, Sleijfer D, Splinter T, Van Oosterom A, Harris A, Boven E, De Pauw M and Sylvester R (1987 in press). BEP Vs EP in good risk patients with disseminated non-seminoma. Proc Amer Soc Clin Onc.

Wheeler B, Loehrer P, Williams S and Einhorn L (1986). Ifosfamide in refractory male germ cell tumour. J Clin Onc 4:28-34.

EORTC Genitourinary Group Monograph 5: Progress
and Controversies in Oncological Urology II, page 469
© 1988 Alan R. Liss, Inc.

Discussion: Potential Advances in Combination Chemotherapy
for Advanced Testicular Cancer

Ted A.W. Splinter, Rotterdam, The Netherlands

Debruyne: Why do you include extragonadal germ cell tumors
in the bad risk group?

Kaye: Most patients with extragonadal germ cell tumors show
a bad response to chemotherapy and a bad survival, possibly
because they all present as bulky disease.

Pinedo: At last year's ASCO meeting there was a presentation, which stated that not the bulk of the tumor in extragonadal germ cell tumors was important but the primary
presentation in the mediastinum or retroperitoneum. Did you
include this factor as a stratification?

Kaye: We did not, since we were afraid to end up with very
small groups.

EORTC Genitourinary Group Monograph 5: Progress
and Controversies in Oncological Urology II, pages 471–478
© 1988 Alan R. Liss, Inc.

SURVEILLANCE AFTER ORCHIDECTOMY FOR CLINICAL STAGE I GERM-
CELL TUMOURS OF THE TESTIS

A. Horwich[1] and M.J. Peckham[2]

Institute of Cancer Research and The Royal Marsden
Hospital, Sutton, Surrey, SM2 5PT, U.K.[1] and Bri-
tish Postgraduate Medical Federation, London
WC1N 3EJ, U.K.[2]

INTRODUCTION

A range of clinical approaches are highly successful in
curing patients with Stage I germ-cell tumours of the testis.
In non-seminoma these include radical lymph node dissection
and deferred chemotherapy (Donohue et al, 1978), radical node
dissection and routine chemotherapy (Skinner and Scardino,
1979) and radiotherapy with deferred chemotherapy (Peckham et
al, 1979), and in seminoma the traditional management of Stage
I disease following orchidectomy is infradiaphragmatic lymph
node irradiation. Analysis of historical data would suggest
that subclinical metastatic disease is present in only 20-30%
of patients with non-seminoma (Peckham, 1981) and in an even
smaller proportion of patients with seminoma (Maier et al,
1968). Given the effectiveness of salvage treatments it was
felt appropriate to investigate the policy of surveillance
following orchidectomy with the endpoint of the investigation
being curability with avoidance of unnecessary therapy.

Stage I Testicular Non-Seminoma

Surveillance was introduced in the Royal Marsden Hospital
in 1979. The eligibility criteria included normal CT scan of
thorax and abdomen, normal lymphogram, histological confirmation of non-seminomatous germ-cell tumour of the testis and
either normal serum marker levels or rapid fall of serum marker levels to normal values following orchidectomy. One patient with tumour at the cut end of the spermatic cord was
excluded. The pathological review of the primary tumour included assessment of vascular and lymphatic permeation, assess-

ment of local extension of the tumour and immunological staining for HCG and AFP. Transscrotal biopsy, scrotal orchidectomy
or prior orchidopexy were not considered contraindications to
a surveillance policy.

The surveillance protocol for patients who were confirmed
to have Stage I disease clinically included outpatient visits
with physical examination, chest X-ray and assay of serum tumour markers every month for the first year, every two months
for the second year, every three months for the third year,
every four months for the fourth year. Initially, CT scans of
the thorax and abdomen were performed on alternate visits for
the first two years, but more recently CT scans are performed
less frequently with four scans during the first year and a
further scan at the end of the second year.

The results of surveillance are shown in Table 1 which
illustrates data on 132 patients followed from 12-84 months
(median 43 months) from orchidectomy. Thirty-five patients
(27%) relapsed. All relapsing patients were treated with combination chemotherapy using bleomycin, etoposide and cisplatinum in combination (Peckham et al, 1983). Thirty-four (97%)
are alive and disease-free, however, one patient died in remission from complications of renal failure. Thirty-one (90%)
of relapses occurred within one year of orchidectomy and the
site of initial relapse is shown in Table 2. Relapse was revealed by rising serum marker levels in 26 (74%) of patients.

TABLE 1. Surveillance for Stage I Testicular Non-Seminomatous
Germ-Cell Tumours.

Total Patients	Follow up (months)	Relapses	Time to Relapse (months)	[a]Alive and currently disease free
132	12-84	35	2-44 (median 6)	131

[a] Follow-up of relapsing patients 11-76 months (median 35
months) post chemotherapy.

TABLE 2. Surveillance for Stage I Testicular Non-Seminomatous Germ-Cell Tumours: Relapse Pattern (The Royal Marsden Hospital 1979-1985)

Initial site of relapse	% of relapses
Abdominal nodes only	47
Lung only	17
Abdominal nodes and lung	13
Serum markers only	23

TABLE 3. Surveillance for Stage I Non-Seminomatous Germ-Cell Tumours: Prognostic Factors (The Royal Marsden Hospital, 1979-1985)

	% relapse rate	Log rank p value
Epididymis/rete		
Involved	52	< 0.05
Not involved	26	
Vascular invasion		
Present	46	< 0.01
Absent	23	
Lymphatic invasion		
Present	57	< 0.005
Absent	23	
Pre-orchidectomy serum AFP		
Raised	16	< 0.01[a]
Not raised	48	
Histology		
MTU (Embryonal Ca)	44	< 0.005
MTI (Teratocarcinoma)	20	-
MTT (Trophoblastic)	29	-

Tissue AFP or HCG, distal cord involvement, size of primary, invasion of tunica, age, length of history not significant.

[a] Relapse rate lower if raised serum AFP before orchidectomy

(data from Hoskin et al, 1986)

Presentation characteristics of relapsing and non-relapsing patients have been analysed to define groups with a high risk of relapse who may be candidates for adjuvant chemotherapy and to define groups with a low risk of relapse in whom surveillance may be less intensive (Hoskin et al, 1986). The results of this analysis is illustrated in Table 3 and it can be seen that a significantly higher risk of relapse was associated with the histological subtype malignant teratoma undifferentiated (embryonal carcinoma), with the presence of lymphatic or vascular invasion within the primary tumour, and with local extension involving the epididymis or the rete testis. The presence of raised serum alphafetoprotein level before orchidectomy was associated with a lower risk of relapse. Simplifying this analysis to tumour histology and the presence or absence of lymphatic invasion the risk of relapse is 12% for patients with MTI and no lymphatic invasion, 33% for MTU with no lymphatic invasion, 40% for MTI with lymphatic invasion and 78% for MTU with lymphatic invasion.

Thirty-six patients in the study had scrotal interference before orchidectomy. None of these patients developed scrotal recurrence during surveillance (Kennedy et al, 1986) and the relapse rate in this group (11%) is not high.

Surveillance for Stage I Testicular Seminoma

Historical data based on lymphadenectomy in patients staged mainly by clinical examination suggested that there was a low incidence of occult metastatic disease in patients with Stage I seminoma (Maier et al, 1968). With the recognition of highly effective treatment for more advanced stages of seminoma (Hamilton et al, 1986; Peckham et al, 1985) a surveillance policy in seminoma had been evaluated at the Royal Marsden Hospital since 1983. It was recognised that the relatively slow growth of seminomas and the lack of reliable serum marker would make a surveillance policy difficult to operate, although more recently an isoenzyme of placental alkaline phosphatase has been evaluated in metastatic seminoma and may prove useful as a component of surveillance (Horwich et al, 1985).

Eligibility criteria include histology review confirming pure testicular seminoma, normal serum alphafetoprotein and normal CT scan of thorax and abdomen, negative lymphogram and full informed consent to take part in the study. The surveillance protocol required clinic assessment including serum markers and a chest X-ray, and also abdominal films including obliques while contrast remains in abdominal nodes, every two months for one year, every three months for the second year, every four months for the third year, and then six monthly for two further years. CT scans of the abdomen are performed at the end of the first, second and third year and an abdominal ultrasound is performed at 18 months and 30 months post-orchidectomy.

Preliminary results are reported on 90 patients followed from 4-40 months post-orchidectomy (median 18 months). Ten patients have relapsed from 7-24 months post-orchidectomy (median 11 months) and the relapse frequency was the same in the second as the first year post-orchidectomy. The actuarial relapse-free rate was 90% at one year and 85% at two years. The initial relapse pattern was predominantly within abdominal nodes (9 patients), though one patient relapsed with both abdominal lymphadenopathy and a single small lung metastasis. The nine patients with abdominal relapse were treated with infradiaphragmatic nodal irradiation, however, three of these subsequently relapsed in supradiaphragmatic lymph nodes. The patient with a lung metastasis on relapse and patients relapsing after infradiaphragmatic radiation were treated with chemotherapy using carboplatin as a single agent (Peckham et al, 1985) and all the patients in this study are currently alive and disease-free. These results are summarized in Table 4.

TABLE 4. Surveillance for Stage I Testicular Seminoma (The Royal Marsden Hospital 1983-1987)

Patients entered	Median Follow-up	Initial relapses		Second relapse after radio-therapy	Currently alive & disease free
		Stage II	Stage IV		
90	18 months	9	1	[a]3/9	90

[a] treated with chemotherapy

DISCUSSION

A surveillance policy in Stage I testicular non-seminomatous tumours has been carried out at the Royal Marsden Hospital since 1979 and has been demonstrated to be a safe and nontoxic treatment alternative. Both lymphadenectomy and abdominal radiotherapy are avoided and three-quarters of patients require no further therapy following orchidectomy. The early detection of relapse ensures effective salvage chemotherapy. Between 1980 and 1983 58 patients with small-volume metastatic non-seminomatous germ-cell tumours were treated with combination bleomycin, etoposide and cisplatinum and 56 (97%) are alive and disease-free. Results of chemotherapy are worse for more advanced disease (Medical Research Council Working Party report on Testicular Tumours, 1985) and thus an objective of surveillance is to detect relapsing patients while they are in the best prognostic group of metastatic disease.

Analysis of presentation variables has allowed the prediction of risk of relapse and a subgroup with a high risk of relapse may be a candidate for adjuvant chemotherapy following orchidectomy rather than a surveillance policy. In this context it may be appropriate to use only two courses of chemotherapy, since this situation is analogous to patients managed by lymphadenectomy where the surgical specimen confirms involvement of abdominal lymph nodes and where two courses of PVB chemotherapy prevent relapse in almost all of the 50% of patients who would otherwise do so (Williams et al, 1986). Our study would suggest that this high risk subgroup of Stage I patients would be identified by the presence within the primary of MTU (embryonal carcinoma) with lymphatic invasion. A further method of reducing toxicity may be to reduce or delete bleomycin from the treatment schedule (Bosl et al, 1986) or to substitute carboplatin for cisplatin.

The situation with Stage I seminoma is less clear both because of the difficulty of the surveillance examinations and because of the protracted natural history of the disease. Also, the results of the traditional management of adjuvant abdominal node irradiation are excellent. Of 240 patients with Stage I seminoma treated by adjuvant irradiation at the Royal Marsden Hospital between 1964 and 1983 only 5 (2%) subsequently relapsed and all these five were successfully retreated. The toxicity of adjuvant irradiation is minimal though there is a suggestion of increased risk of peptic ulceration (Hamilton et al, 1986) and non-testicular malignancy (Hay et al, 1984).

Additionally, scattered radiation dose to the contralateral testis may impair spermatogenesis.

The incidence of second relapse in supradiaphragmatic nodes (3 patients) is worrisome since this may have been a consequence of delay in treating subclinical abdominal disease. Surveillance for Stage I seminoma should only be undertaken in the context of a formal prospective study and where a reliable clinical follow-up can be assured. Adjuvant abdominal node irradiation remains standard management.

REFFERENCES

Bosl GJ, Bajorin D, Leitner S and participating investigators Memorial Sloan-Kettering Cancer Center (MSKCC), New York (1986). A randomised trial of etoposide (E) + cisplatin (P) and VAB-6 in the treatment (Rx) of "Good Risk" patients (Pts) with germ cell tumors (GCT). Proc ASCO Vol. 5, Abstract no. 405, p 104.

Donohue JP, Einhorn LJ, Periz JM (1978). Improved management of non-seminomatous testis tumors. Cancer 42:2903-2908.

Hamilton C, Horwich A, Easton D, Peckham MJ (1986). Radiotherapy for Stage I seminoma testis: Results of treatment and complications. Radiother Oncol 6:115-120.

Hay JH, Duncan W, Kerr GR (1984). Subsequent malignancies in patients irradiated for testicular tumours. Br J Radiol 57: 597-602.

Horwich A, Tucker DF, Peckham MJ (1985). Placental alkaline phosphatase as a tumour marker in seminoma using the H17E2 monoclonal antibody assay. Br J Cancer 51:625-629.

Hoskin P, Dilly S, Easton D, Horwich A, Hendry W, Peckham MJ (1986). Prognostic factors in Stage I non-seminomatous germ-cell testicular tumors managed by orchiectomy and surveillance: Implications for adjuvant chemotherapy. J Clin Oncol 4:1031-1036.

Kennedy CL, Hendry WF, Peckham MJ (1986). The significance of scrotal interference in Stage I testicular cancer managed by orchiectomy and surveillance. Br J Urol 58:705-708.

Maier JG, Sulak MH, Mittemeyer BT (1968). Seminoma of the testis: Analysis of treatment success and failure. Am J Roentgenol 102:(3)596-602.

Medical Research Council Working Party report on Testicular Tumours (Chairman: Peckham MJ)(1985). Prognostic factors in advanced non-seminomatous germ-cell testicular tumours: Results of a multicentre study. Lancet I:8-11.

Peckham MJ (1981). Testicular tumours: Investigation and staging: General aspects and staging classification. In Peckham MJ (ed): "The Management of Testicular Tumours," London, Publ Edward Arnold Ltd, pp 89-101.

Peckham MJ, Barrett A, McElwain TJ, Hendry WF (1979). Combined management of malignant teratoma of the testis. Lancet II: 267-270.

Peckham MJ, Barrett A, Liew KH, Horwich A, Robinson B, Dobbs HJ, McElwain TJ, Hendry WF (1983). The treatment of metastatic germ-cell testicular tumours with bleomycin, etoposide and cis-platin (BEP). Br J Cancer 47:613-619.

Peckham MJ, Horwich A, Hendry WF (1985). Advanced seminoma: Treatment with cis-platinum based chemotherapy or carboplatin (JM8). Br J Cancer 52:7-13.

Skinner DG, Scardino PT (1979). Relevance of biochemical tumor markers and lymphadenectomy in the management of non-seminomatous testis tumors: Current perspectives. Trans Am Assoc Genito Surg 87:293-298.

Williams S, Muggia F, Einhorn L, Hahn R, Donohue J, Brunner K, Stablein D, DeWys W, Crawford D, Spaulding J for the Testicular Cancer Intergroup Study (1986). Resected Stage II testicular cancer: Immediate adjuvant chemotherapy versus observation. Proc ASCO Vol. 5, Abstract no. 380, p 98.

EORTC Genitourinary Group Monograph 5: Progress
and Controversies in Oncological Urology II, page 479
© 1988 Alan R. Liss, Inc.

Discussion: Surveillance After Orchidectomy for Clinical
Stage I Germ-Cell Tumours of the Testis

Ted A.W. Splinter, Rotterdam, The Netherlands

Chodak: How frequently are you doing markers, chest X-rays
and CT-scans during your 'wait and see' treatment?

Peckham: Initially we had a very rigorous regime of follow-
up: monthly during the first year, bimonthly during the
second year and every 3 months during the third year. We did
CT-scans on alternate visits during the first two years,
chest X-ray and markers at each visit. We never acted on a
single abnormal result. In the case of marker negative
patients who had an abnormality on an imaging test, we
either watched the patient until we were certain about the
metastatic nature of the abnormality or we tried to obtain
tissue. More recently, we have become much more permissive
regarding CT-scans. Presently, we only get 3 CT-scans during
the first year and further rely on chest X-rays and markers.
However, if the tumor does not produce a marker, you may
well have to continue CT-scans during the second and third
year.

EORTC Genitourinary Group Monograph 5: Progress
and Controversies in Oncological Urology II, pages 481–491
© 1988 Alan R. Liss, Inc.

PATERNITY IN YOUNG PATIENTS WITH TESTICULAR CANCER –
EXPECTATIONS AND EXPERIENCE

Nina Aass and Sophie D. Fosså

Department of Medical Oncology and Radiotherapy,
The Norwegian Radiumhospital, Oslo

In patients with testicular cancer the aspect of future
fathership has become increasingly important. In previous
reports a relationship has been indicated between the
occurrence of germ cell tumors and the incidence of
cryptorchism with testicular atrophy and/or fertility
disturbances (Müller et al, 1984; Ali Kahn et al, 1985;
Skakkebaek, 1978). Furthermore, the sperm cell production is
impaired in two thirds of the patients with testicular
cancer after orchiectomy before further treatment (Fosså et
al, 1984). However, during the last years an increasing
number of patients is reported to have fathered children
after treatment for testicular cancer (Fosså et al, 1985a;
Fosså et al, 1985b; Fosså et al, 1986a; Fosså et al, 1986b;
Senturia et al, 1985). The present report deals with some
aspects of paternity observed in young Norwegian patients
with testicular cancer.

PATIENTS AND METHODS

Study Group 1

From November 1, 1985, to October 31, 1986, 77
consecutive patients (15-45 years old) with a newly
diagnosed testicular cancer underwent a semi-structured
interview dealing with general "quality of life" questions
and aspects of paternity. In addition, the patients
themselves filled in a questionnaire dealing with similar
questions concerning fathership. All patients had been
orchiectomized and were referred to the Norwegian Radium
Hospital (NRH) for further treatment. There were 37 seminoma

and 40 non-seminoma patients with a median age of 32 and 27 years, respectively (Table 1).

Study Group 2

One hundred and twenty-two patients, treated at the NRH after 1977, and without activity of testicular cancer for at least 3 years, answered a mailed questionnaire containing questions about post-treatment paternity. Twenty-nine patients with pathological stage I had undergone unilateral retroperitoneal lymph node dissection (RLND) only (Table 2). Twenty-four seminoma patients had received abdominal irradiation (36-40 Gy). Forty-three patients, mainly those with non-seminoma, had been treated by 3-4 cycles chemotherapy (CVB: Cisplatin 20 mg/m2, Day 1 to 5; Vinblastine 0.15 mg/kg, Day 1 and 2; Bleomycin 30 mg Day 1, 5 and 15), often in combination with retroperitoneal lymph node dissection (RLND). Thirteen patients had also received other cytostatic drugs as Cyclophosphamide, Adriamycin, CCNU and/or Vinblastine (Klepp et al, 1984). In the remaining 26 patients treatment had consisted of CVB chemotherapy and abdominal irradiation, sometimes also combined with other cytostatic drugs.

Study Group 3

In 1985 the post-irradiation paternity was also evaluated by a questionnaire which was mailed to 118 relapse-free testicular cancer patients who had undergone abdominal radiotherapy from 1970 to 1978 (median target dose 40 Gy). About two thirds of the patients had had a seminoma, and one third a non-seminoma. The median age of these patients was 32 years (range 18-44). One hunderd and thirteen patients answered the questions about paternity.

RESULTS

Before Treatment

Pre-treatment fathershipp was recorded by 62% of the seminoma patients and in half of the non-seminoma patients from Study Group 1 (Table 1).

TABLE 1. Paternity in Young Patients With Newly Diagnosed Testicular Cancer (Study Group 1).

	Seminoma	Non-seminoma
No. of patients	37	40
Median age (range)	32 (17–44)	27 (16–44)
No. of patients with at least one child (1)	22/36	19/38
Mean no. of children per patient (2)(range)	2.0 (1–3)	1.9 (1–4)
No. of patients wishing children after treatment (3)	21/34	26/36

(1) No. of patients with fathership/evaluable patients.
(2) Only for patients with fathership.
(3) No. of patients wishing children/evaluable patients.

Fifty-seven per cent of the seminoma and 72% of the young non-seminoma patients stated that they would like to have children after their treatment for testicular cancer. Post-treatment paternity was wished even by men above the age of 40 and by men who had more than 2 children (Table 2).

After Treatment

Sixty-three of 122 patients from Study Group 2 had fathered children before treatment for testicular cancer (Table 3).

Twenty-six men had become fathers to 29 children after treatment. Nineteen of these patients had undergone retro-peritoneal lymph node dissection, mostly unilateral RLND. None of the patients in subgroup 4 (i.e. the patients treated with both chemotherapy and radiotherapy) had fathered children after treatment. The patients who had not become fathers were asked about possible reasons. Thirty-five patients stated that they did not want to have

Table 2

Expectations concerning post-treatment paternity in young testicular cancer patients (Study Group 1).

a) Relation to pre-treatment fathership.

No of children	Post-treatmemt fathership planned ?		
before treatment	NO	YES	TOTAL
0	3	27	30
1	0	12	12
2	15	4	19
> 2	5	4	9
Total	23	47	70

b) Relation to age at diagnosis.

	Post-treatment fathership planned ?		
Age (years)	NO	YES	TOTAL
< 20.0	0	9	9
20.1 - 25.0	1	7	8
25.1 - 30.0	6	12	18
30.1 - 35.0	2	10	12
35.1 - 40.0	7	6	13
40.1 - 45.0	7	3	10
Total	23	47	70

Table 3

Patients details and paternity in young patients treated for testicular cancer and with NED $\geq$ 3 years (Study Group 2).

The total number of alternatives can be less than the total number of patients within each sub-group due to lack of answers.

	Sub-group 1 (29)	Sub-group 2 (24)	Sub-group 3 (43)	Sub-group 4 (26)	Total (122)
Mean age[1] (range)	30 (18–40)	33 (17–44)	27 (17–44)	31 (20–44)	30 (17–44)
Seminoma	–	18	1	9	28
Non-seminoma	29	6	42	17	94
CVB[1] x $\leq$ 4	–	–	30	8	38
CVB x $\leq$ 4 + other chemoth.	–	–	13	18	31
Radiotherapy					
$\leq$ 40 Gy	–	17	–	16	33
$>$ 40 Gy	–	7	–	10	17

( ) Total number of patients in each sub-group.
1 At treatment start.

Table 3 cont.

	Sub-group 1 (29)	Sub-group 2 (24)	Sub-group 3 (43)	Sub-group 4 (26)	Total (122)
Paternity before treatment	17	15	17	14	63
Paternity after treatment	14	5	7	–	26
No of children born after treatment	15	6	8	–	29
Reasons for not fathering children after treatment:					
Children not wanted	6	14	9	6	35
"Infertile"	5	1	20	16	42
Partner "infertile"	–	–	1	–	1
Ambiguous	2	1	3	4	10

( ) Total number of patients in each sub-group.

children. Significantly more patients from subgroup 2 did not want to father children after treatment as compared with patients from the other subgroups. A total of 53 patients did, however, not exclude that they in future perhaps would like to father children. Forty-two patients thought that they were infertile, most of them within the subgroups 3 and 4. Thirty-two of the 113 evaluable patients from Study Group 3 fathered at least one child after abdominal radiotherapy (Table 4).

Thirteen males stated that they had tried to have children but no pregnancy had resulted. Ten abortions were recorded after radiotherapy, one of them among the former 13 patients. Fifty-four of the 79 patients who were fathers before radiotherapy did not want to have more children after their treatment for testicular cancer. Twenty of the remaining 25 patients (80%) had additional children after radiotherapy. Ten of the 31 patients who did not have children before radiotherapy had children afterwards, but none of the 4 patients with known fertility problems before the diagnosis of testicular cancer fathered a living child (1 abortion among these 4 patients).

Three of the 68 patients who did not want to have children after treatment stated that they were afraid of possible malformations of the offspring (due to radiotherapy), or that they did not dare to take the responsibility of having a child after their diagnosis of a malignant disease. As many as 13 of 67 evaluable patients who did not want to have children after treatment were not fathers before treatment.

At least 52 patients were born after radiotherapy in the patients from Study Group 3. Nineteen patients had one child, 11 patients 2, and 2 patients 3 children after abdominal radiotherapy. Five additional men stated that they had become fathers after treatment, but did not record the number of children born. The median interval between the start of radiotherapy and the birth of the first child was 42 months (range: 17-150 months). Only one malformation was recorded: There was one case of coxa valga (with a predisposition for this malformation in the mother's family).

Table 4.

Paternity and frequency of abortions before and after abdominal radiotherapy for testicular cancer. (Study Group 3)

Paternity before treatment	Paternity after treatment			
	NO		YES	TOTAL
	Children wanted	Children not wanted		
Yes	5	54	20	79
NO Not tried	6	11	10	27
NO Tried, but unsuccessful	2	2		4
No information		1	2	3
Total	13	68	32	113
Number of abortions	1	5	4	10

DISCUSSION

Our results are in good agreement with previous studies which show maintenance or recovery of fertility after modern treatment for testicular cancer (Berthelsen, 1984; Thachil et al, 1981; Drasga et al, 1983). However, only limited information exists about the patient's expectations and wishes concerning post-treatment fathership. The present observations indicate, that at the time of the diagnosis, 67% of the patients want to have children after their treatment, especially the younger non-seminoma patients.

After single modality cytotoxic treatment (radiotherapy only or cisplatin based chemotherapy only) 25–30% of the patients can become faters. Even more pregnancies can be expected as time elapses after such cytotoxic treatment. Sufficient recovery of the spermatogenesis is observed in most patients 3 years after radiotherapy or 3–4 cycles cisplatin based chemotherapy (Fosså et al, 1985b; Fosså et al, 1986a), but can be delayed in individual patients, especially if the gonadal dose is above 100 cGy.

After unilateral RLND without any cytotoxic treatment paternity is achieved in 60% of the patients. By unilateral RLND, especially in patients with right-sided tumors, most of the presacral sympathic fibres are spared thus avoiding severe ejaculatory disturbances (Fosså et al, 1985a). Dry ejaculation occurs in about 80% of the patients with bilateral RLND (Fosså et al, 1985a). In order to increase the chances of post-treatment fathership in patients with advanced non-seminoma one should develop techniques for bilateral RLND, which spare the sympathic fibres responsible for emission/ejaculation. The combination of cisplatin based chemotherapy with radiotherapy significantly reduces the chances of post-treatment recovery of the spermatogenesis and of future fathership. In addition, the chance of post-treatment paternity is low in patients who already before treatment have fertility problems.

In conclusion, post-treatment paternity should be taken into account and discussed with the patient when planning the initial treatment. Unnecessary overtreatment should be avoided. Optimal radiation techniques are mandatory during radiotherapy, optimally keeping the gonadal dose below 50 cGy. New techniques for RLND should be developed which spare the sympathic fibres responsible for the ejaculatory function.

REFERENCES

Ali Kahn S, Srinivas V, Gonder MJ (1985). Seminoma in an atrophic testis. Urol Int 40:282-283.

Berthelsen JG (1984). Sperm counts and serum follicle-stimulating hormone levels before and after radiotherapy and chemotherapy in men with testicular germ cell cancer. Fertil Steril 41:281-286.

Drasga RE, Einhorn LH, Williams SD, Patel DN, Stevens EE (1983). Fertility after chemotherapy for testicular cancer. J Clin Oncol 1:179-183.

Fosså SD, Abyholm T, Aakvaag (1984). Spermatogenesis and hormonal status after orchiectomy for cancer and before supplementary treatment. Eur Urol 10:173-177.

Fosså SD, Ous S, Abyholm T, Loeb M (1985a). Post-treatment fertility in patients with testicular cancer: I. Influence of retroperitoneal lymph node dissection on ejaculatory potency. Br J Urol 57:204-209.

Fosså SD, Ous S, Abyholm T, Norman N, Loeb M (1985b). Post-treatment fertility in patients with testicular cancer: II. Influence of Cis-platin-based combination chemotherapy and of retroperitoneal surgery on hormone and sperm cell production. Br J Urol 57:210-214.

Fosså SD, Abyholm T, Normann N, Jetne V (1986a). Post-treatment fertility in patients with testicular cancer: III. Influence of radiotherapy in seminoma patients. Br J Urol 58:315-319.

Fosså SD, Almaas B, Jetne V, Bjerkedal T (1986b). Paternity after irradiation for testicular cancer. Acta Radiol Oncol 25:33-36.

Klepp O, Fosså SD, Ous S, Lien H, Stenwig JT, Abeler V, Eliassen G, Høst H (1984). Multi-modality treatment of advanced malignant germ cell tumours in males: I. Experience with cis-platinum-based combination chemotherapy. Scan J Urol Nephrol 18:13-19.

Müller J, Skakkebaek NE, Nielsen OH, Graem N (1984). Cryptorchidism and testis cancer. Atypical infantile germ cells followed by carcinoma in situ and invasive carcinoma in adulthood. Cancer 54:629-634.

Senturia YD, Peckham CS, Peckham MJ (1985). Children fathered by men treated for testicular cancer. The Lancet Oct.5, 766-769.

Skakkebaek NE (1978). Carcinoma in situ of the testis: frequency and relationship to invasive germ cell tumours in infertile men. Histopathology 2:157-170.

Thachil JV, Jewett MAS, Rider WD (1981). The effects of cancer and cancer therapy on male fertility. J Urol 126:141-145.

EORTC Genitourinary Group Monograph 5: Progress
and Controversies in Oncological Urology II, pages 493–496
© 1988 Alan R. Liss, Inc.

ROUND TABLE DISCUSSION: TESTICULAR CANCER (Chairmen: H.M.
Pinedo and S. Fosså)

T.A.W. Splinter

Department of Oncology, Erasmus University
Hospital, Rotterdam, The Netherlands

SEMINOMAS STAGE I AND LOW VOLUME STAGE II

Standard therapy for stage I and low volume stage II
seminoma is still radiotherapy. Although the results of the
wait and see study of Peckham et al are very interesting,
the efficacy and relative lack of toxicity of radiotherapy
in stage I disease raises the question whether it should
ever be more than an intellectual exercise. This attitude
might change in the future when the compelling data of
single agent Carboplatin (vide infra) are confirmed, so that
even bulky stage II seminoma can be effectively treated with
a relatively non-toxic chemotherapy. According to Peckman,
CT-scan and ultrasound are sufficient and lymphangiography
can be omitted as a staging procedure and only
infradiaphragmatic radiotherapy is indicated in stage I and
II seminomas.

SEMINOMAS STAGE II BULKY DISEASE. ROLE OF CHEMOTHERAPY

Seminomas are very chemosensitive tumors. Impressive
results have been obtained with combinations of
Cyclophosphamide - Cisplatin - Vincristin (COC) and Vp16 -
Bleomycin - Cisplatin (BEP). Very interesting are the
results obtained with Carboplatin as a single agent.
According to Horwich, 33 patients with advanced stage
seminoma e.i. bulky abdominal disease, stage III and stage
IV, have been treated so far with Carboplatin 400 mg/m2
every 4 weeks for 4-6 courses. Twenty-two patients have been
followed for a median time of 21 months. The treatment is

exceedingly well tolerated and is given on an outpatient
basis. Eighty-six per cent of these 22 patients have
continuously been free of disease. Some of them had residual
masses, which were monitored by CT-scanning only and
remained stable for the whole period of follow-up. These
data raise the interesting question whether much more toxic
chemotherapy combinations such as BEP, PVB and COC should be
reserved for patients failing on single agent Carboplatin.
Furthermore, more studies with single agents in advanced
seminoma are certainly warranted. The monotonous histology
of most seminomas might be a reflection of the homogeneity
of the tumor and the surprisingly high sensitivity for
single agents such as Cyclophosphamide, Cisplatin and
Carboplatin.

ROLE OF RADIOTHERAPY

No consensus exists about the role of radiotherapy in
bulky stage II disease. In the U.S.A., an intergroup study
is randomizing patients with bulky stage II disease between
radiotherapy and radiotherapy plus BEP. It is expected that,
in view of the data from Peckham on the efficacy of BEP
alone, this study will not recruit enough patients to answer
the question. Fossá from Oslo commented that, out of 55
advanced seminoma patients treated with BEP, 11 have
relapsed. All these patients had some kind of radiotherapy
and all relapses occurred outside the radiation field.
Donohue reported that the SWOG-group is doing a longterm
study of radiotherapy in patients who still have a
significant residual mass after chemotherapy. All 16
patients with a minimal follow-up of more than 3 years are
still relapse-free.

SURGICAL EXPLORATION OR NO EXPLORATION OF RESIDUAL DISEASE

The opinions about the need for surgical exploration of
residual disease after chemotherapy for bulky seminoma
differ widely. The Royal Marsden group monitors residual
disease by CT-scan. In contrast, the Memorial Sloan
Kettering group advocates surgical excision if the residual
mass is larger than 3 cm and claims that 6 out of 7 patients
with viable tumor have been cured. Wettlaufer proposes to do
biopsies in case of residual disease larger than 3 cm,

followed by irradiation if viable tumor is still present. The SWOG-group gives radiotherapy to patients with 'bulky' residual disease. This question of how to handle residual disease is a very important one and may be solved by two randomized trials: one comparing surgical exploration (both excision and multiple biopsies) and radiotherapy, the other comparing clinical monitoring by CT-scan and radiotherapy.

NON-SEMINOMAS: STAGE I

At this moment there are several ways to treat a patient with non-seminoma stage I, e.g. retroperitoneal lymph node dissection (unilateral or complete), radiotherapy, adjuvant chemotherapy, 'active surveillance' or combinations of these. There is no standard method which has to be followed, and the choice of treatment is quite often determined by local historical practice and experience. The key question is what is the . least toxic method to achieve a 100% cure rate in this group of patients, of whom approximately only 25% need more treatment than orchidectomy alone. Therefore, according to Peckham, the main issue for the future is to distinguish those patients, who have micrometastases and treat them with chemotherapy, from those patients, who have a very small probability of having micrometastases and treat them with an active surveillance program, which may be a bit more permissive. Furthermore, it would be very interesting to identify those patients who have only retroperitoneal metastases. Independent of which treatment policy is chosen, it is extremely important that patients with a non-seminoma stage I are treated in a center in order to obtain all documentation necessary to distinguish patients without from patients with metastases. Especially when active surveillance is used as a treatment, it has to be done in an experienced center.

NON-SEMINOMAS: METASTATIC DISEASE

The results of the EORTC study comparing BEP and EP in patients with low-volume metastases of non-seminoma (see Kaye et al, this issue), show that the toxicity of treatment can be reduced without loss of efficacy by omitting Bleomycin. So the standard chemotherapy for this group of patients at this moment is EP. More investigations are needed to find even less toxic therapies e.g. by using Carboplatin instead of Cisplatin. The major problem is the high risk group of patients with bulky metastatic disease. It has been shown by Ozols et al that Vp16 is an important drug together with a normal or double dose of Cisplatin. Sleijfer et al showed that at this moment high-dose Vp16 and Cyclophosphamide combined with autologous bone marrow transplantation is probably not an effective approach in this group of patients. So the question was raised whether debulking surgery, performed after one course of chemotherapy in patients who show a clear shrinking of the tumor but an abnormal decline of the markers i.e. not according to their half-life, might be a useful approach, when followed by a salvage chemotherapy regime. According to Donohue, the large experience in Indianapolis has taught them that you should resist the temptation to perform debulking surgery at the time when markers are still positive. It is preferable, by using salvage chemotherapy early and/or by increasing the number of courses, to reach a marker negative status and then to perform surgery.

A very interesting point was raised by Peckham, who emphasized that rapid scheduling, as was first published by Wettlaufer et al and which is taken up by the EORTC group, may be more important than the introduction of higher doses or new drugs. The experience of the Denver group with the BOP (Bleomycin, Oncovin, Cisplatin) regime followed by salvage chemotherapy in bulky disease patients is based on 63 patients up to now. They still have a 85% CR-rate. Important is the relative lack of toxicity in this group of patients, who often present themselves in a general bad condition.

EORTC Genitourinary Group Monograph 5: Progress
and Controversies in Oncological Urology II, pages 497–507
© 1988 Alan R. Liss, Inc.

BCG IN CARCINOMA IN SITU AND SUPERFICIAL BLADDER TUMORS

Donald L. Lamm, M.D.

WVU Medical Center, Urology Dept.
Morgantown, WV   26506

BCG immunotherapy for recurrent superficial bladder cancer has been highly successful and is perhaps the most successful form of immunotherapy for human malignancy. Current data in fact suggest that BCG immunotherapy is the most effective intravesical treatment of carcinoma in situ and the most effective prophylactic agent for the prevention of recurrence of transitional cell carcinoma. It is presumably the combination of an immunocompetent host with an accessible, antigenic, microscopic or submicroscopic malignancy which has accounted for the surprising success of BCG immunotherapy in bladder cancer in the face of it's failure in most other cancers.

Based on animal studies that had demonstrated BCG to be effective in eradicating small, antigenic tumors when administered in close proximity to the tumor, Morales et al in 1976 were the first to report the clinical use of BCG to prevent bladder tumor recurrence. Nine patients with Stage T-0(O) or T-1(A) transitional cell carcinomas were treated with six weekly vaccinations of 120 mg Armand-Frappier BCG in 50cc saline intravesically plus 5 mg of BCG percutaneously using the multiple puncture technique. (Morales, et al 1976). BCG treatment resulted in a 12 fold reduction in the number of tumors per patient month. Based on these encouraging preliminary results two prospective randomized clinical trials of intravesical BCG using Morales' technique were begun in 1978. My initial results,which were presented in 1979,(Lamm et al 1980) have become more impressive with time. A total of 94 patients enrolled in early randomized studies. Only 10 of 54 (18.5%) patients treated with BCG had recurrent tumor compared with 19 of 40 (47.5%) control patients (P=0.003, Chi square). The disease free interval was prolonged from a mean of 31 months in controls to 58 months with BCG treatment (P=0.0017).

The second prospective randomized trial was performed at Memorial Sloan-Kettering Cancer Center (Camacho et al 1982). The same treatment schedule was used but patients were quite different and were at very high risk for tumor recurrence as evidenced by the 100% recurrence rate by 8 months in the untreated control group. Tumor recurrence was reduced from 2.37 tumors per patient month in control to 0.7 tumors per patient month in the BCG group and continued follow up has demonstrated not only continued protection from recurrence but also significant reduction in tumor progression (Herr et al 1983).

Multiple investigators have now confirmed the efficacy of BCG in the prevention of bladder tumor recurrence. In 1980 Martinez-Pineiro noted 21% tumor recurrence in 29 patients followed for 5 to 42 (mean 15.1) months.(Martinez-Pineiro, 1980) In 1982 Brosman noted no tumor recurrence in 49 patients treated with maintenance intravesical BCG and followed for over 2 years (Brosman, 1982). In 1983 Adolphs and Bastien observed only 9% tumor recurrence in 90 patients treated with a single injection of cyclophosphamide and a 6 week course of intravesical and percutaneous BCG (Adolphs & Bastien, 1983) and Netto and Lemos reported 6% tumor recurrence in 16 patients treated with high-dose oral BCG (Netto & Lemos, 1983). Similar protection from tumor recurrence has been reported by Babayan,(Babayan & Krane, 1985) deKernion,(deKernion et al, 1985) Haaff,(Haaff et al, 1986) Schellhammer,(Schellhammer et al, 1986) and others.

Treatment of Existing Tumor

Despite the observation from animal studies that BCG is rarely effective when tumor burden exceeds 100,000 cells, BCG has been used to treat patients with residual bladder cancer. Surprisingly, such treatment has been remarkably effective and compares very favorably with response rates reported for intravesical chemotherapy. A variety of treatment techniques and BCG substrains have been used. Complete response rates range from 36 to 83 per cent, with a mean complete response rate of 58% in 118 reported cases (Lamm, 1987). While the complete response rate to BCG is excellent, animal data and clinical experience suggest that best results will be seen if every effort is made to remove existing visible tumor prior to initiating therapy.

Table One

BCG Response Rates in Residual Tumor

Primary Author	Number Cases	Complete Response	Per cent
Douville	6	4	67%
Morales	17	10	59%
Lamm	10	6	60%
Brosman	12	10	83%
deKernion	22	8	36%
Kojima	29	16	55%
Schellhammer	22	14	64%
Total	118	68	58%

Responses in 118 patients with solid or papillary tumors treated with intravesical BCG.

BCG Therapy for Carcinoma in situ

Carcinoma in situ, is a poorly differentiated, presumably antigenic, small volume, widely dispersed tumor. When confined to the bladder, CIS is most accessible to direct contact with BCG. The complete response rate of 83 per cent in a combined experience with 180 patients with CIS of the bladder treated with Armand-Frappier, Connaught, and Tice substrains of BCG is higher than that reported with any other intravesical agent. Reported responses range from 68 percent to 100 percent. Evidence suggests that continued treatment, often to up to 6 months, will improve response rates. Brosman(Brosman, 1985), for example, increased his complete response rate from 67% at 12 weeks to 89% at 18 weeks and 100% at 24 weeks in 27 patients who were able to tolerate weekly intravesical BCG treatment.

Responses are frequently long term, and in Brosman's report 87% of patients achieving complete response remained disease free during the 5.25 year average follow up period. Excellent responses have been observed with Tice, Armand-Frappier, and Connaught substrains of BCG (Lamm, 1987).

The excellent long term complete response rate to BCG treatment of carcinoma in situ is making us rethink our treatment strategies. While invasive or metastatic disease can progress despite a complete response to CIS in the bladder, and caution must be exercised with meticulous follow up and bladder biopsy to rule out occult invasive disease, long-term complete responses now clearly make BCG rather than cystectomy the initial treatment of choice in patients with CIS. If and when treatment failure occurs it does so locally in the bladder unless patients have preexisting occult metastatic disease. Therefore, in most patients cystectomy can be reserved for those who fail BCG treatment.

Ongoing studies suggest that the superior response rate of BCG in patients with CIS from historical series will prove to be true in randomized prospective comparisons of BCG and intravesical chemotherapy. Adriamycin has a reported complete response rate in CIS of 59 per cent in five series totalling 76 patients. In our ongoing multicenter Southwest Oncology Group trial, BCG has been compared with Adriamycin. Patients randomized to BCG have had an 80% complete response rate compared with a 47% complete response rate in patients treated with Adriamycin ($p < 0.0001$).

Table Two
BCG Therapy for Carcinoma In Situ

Primary Author	Number	Complete Response	Percent
Morales	7	5	71
Lamm	23	22	96
Herr	47	34	72
Brosman	33	31	94
deKernion	19	13	68
Schellhammer	6	6	100
S.W.O.G. (*)	64	51	80
Total	180	149	83

*Current data from ongoing studies.

BCG Immunotherapy vs. Chemotherapy

While the mechanism of action of BCG is not completely defined, it is clearly different from that of chemotherapy. Most intravesical chemotherapies are alkylating agents, and resistance to one agent increases the likelihood of resistance to the second. Such cross resistance has not been identified with BCG. In our experience with 22 patients who had failed intravesical chemotherapy, 82 per cent responded favorably to BCG (Lamm, 1987). Fortunately, patients who fail BCG treatment will also commonly respond to intravesical chemotherapy.

Two studies have found BCG to be superior to Thiotepa chemotherapy. In Brosman's randomized comparison of intravesical maintenance BCG with Thiotepa, no recurrences were observed in 27 randomized or 12 nonrandomized patients treated with BCG. In patients treated with Thiotepa 9 of 19 patients (40 per cent) had tumor recurrence (Brosman, 1982). Very similar results were reported by Netto and Lemos with a markedly different BCG treatment protocol (Netto & Lemos, 1983). Using Moreau BCG in oral doses of 200 to 800 mg. three times a week, only 1 of 16 patients (6%) had tumor recurrence compared with a 43 per cent incidence of tumor recurrence in patients treated with Thiotepa.

The Southwest Oncology Group has an ongoing multicenter trial comparing intravesical and percutaneous Connaught BCG with Adriamycin. Early results in this study suggested a marked advantage for the BCG group.(Lamm & Crawford, 1985) Forty-six institutions have cooperated in this study and currently 250 patients are evaluable. Overall, 96 of 125 patients (77%) randomized to receive BCG are disease free compared with 53 of 125 patients (42%) randomized to receive Adriamycin. In patients with CIS 80% of patients treated with BCG had complete response compared with 47% of patients treated with Adriamycin. In patients without CIS only 26% in the BCG group developed recurrent tumor compared with 45% in the Adriamycin group. The observed difference could not be explained on the basis of decreased response to Adriamycin due to previous chemotherapy treatment, since the advantage of BCG treatment was similar in patients who had and had not received prior chemotherapy.

BCG Inhibition of Tumor Progression

BCG and intravesical chemotherapy with Thiotepa,
Epodyl, Adriamycin, and Mitomycin C have been found to
reduce tumor recurrence. Some evidence suggests that
Thiotepa and Mitomycin C decrease tumor progression when
compared to untreated controls (Green et al, 1984 ; Huland
et al, 1984). Our experience with 90 patients with stage Ta
or T1 transitional cell carcinoma enrolled in BCG protocols
suggests that BCG treatment reduces tumor progression
(Reynolds et al, 1985). Twenty - six patients served as
controls and initially did not receive chemotherapy or
BCG. Sixty - four patients were enrolled in randomized BCG
protocols. Both groups have been followed for a median of
27 months. The BCG group actually comprised a higher risk
population, since only 23% of the control group had lamina
propria invasion compared with 69% of the BCG group. In
the control group 65% had tumor recurrence, 23% progressed
to stage A or greater, and 8% progressed to stage B or
greater. In the BCG group 16% had tumor recurrence
(p<0.001), 6% progressed to stage A or greater (p<0.05),
and 3% progressed to stage B or greater (not statistically
significant). Progression from stage A to stage B occurred
in 17% of our controls, 30% of controls in the Group A
study (Heney et al, 1983) and only 4% of our patients
treated with BCG. Inhibition of recurrence was significant
at the p=0.0035 level by log-rank testing. Importantly,
the incidence of tumor progression in patients with CIS was
not significantly different from that of patients with
papillary tumors, suggesting that BCG abrogated the poor
prognosis of CIS. Supporting this observation, Herr
observed no complete responses in 26 patients with CIS
treated with fulguration alone, compared with a 65%
complete response rate at 3 or more years duration in
patients treated with intravesical and percutaneous BCG.
Cystectomy for progressive or intractable disease was
required in 65% of patients who did not receive BCG and
only 17% of those who did (Herr et al, 1986). These
preliminary data, if confirmed by other investigators, may
herald marked improvement in survival of superficial
bladder cancer. For example, if only 30 per cent of the
10,600 deaths that occur annually in the United States
result from progression of superficial disease, and
prophylactic intravesical treatment can reduce progression,
as suggested by our data, to only one fourth the current
rate, deaths in this group of patients would be reduced
from 3,180 to 795 per year.

BCG Immunotherapy Technique

Patients with solitary grade I, stage Ta tumors will rarely have tumor progression and therefore generally require no further therapy. However, for most patients the benefit of BCG treatment would appear to far outweigh the risk. Ideal candidates are those with documented tumor recurrence, carcinoma in situ, high grade tumor, or tumor invading the lamina propria. Non-invasive carcinoma of the prostatic urethra has not been a contraindication to BCG immunotherapy,since complete and long term resolution of CIS of the prostatic urethra has been documented.

Clinically effective BCG intravesical vaccines include Armand-Frappier, Connaught, and Pasteur preparations in doses of 120 mg, Tice (50 mg), Japanese (40 mg), and RIVM ($1x10^9$ viable units). Patients have been treated weekly empirically for six weeks. The necessity of maintenance BCG immunotherapy remains debatable, but increasing evidence suggested that a single 6 week course of intravesical BCG is suboptimal treatment. In theory since it is known that the immune stimulation induced by BCG wanes with time and the proclivity of the urothelium to tumor formation persists, periodic retreatment with BCG should improve long term results. In my experience the initiation of maintenance BCG immunotherapy in patients followed for at least one year or until tumor recurrence reduced the rate of tumor recurrence four-fold, from 1.9 to 0.49 tumors per 100 patient months (Lamm 1985). Preliminary results of Catalona's prospective randomized comparison of maintenance and no maintenance BCG immunotherapy have to date not revealed an advantage for maintenance therapy (Lamm 1985). One would, of course, not expect to see any advantage of maintenance therapy until the protective effect of primary treatment has waned. Preliminary observations in such an investigation may therefore be misleading. Moreover, it is clear that protocols using just intravesical BCG for 6 weeks have inferior responses. Haaff et al found that while 56% of patients responded to a single 6 week course, an additional 56% of those who fail will again respond to a second course (Haaff et al, 1986). The highest response rate for the treatment of carcinoma in situ and the lowest long-term recurrence rate for patients given prophylactic BCG occur with the maintenance protocol described by Brosman (Brosman, 1985). In CIS complete responses were increased from 67% after 12 weekly treatments to 88-100% with an additional 6 to 12 weeks of treatment. With monthly maintenance BCG immunotherapy only 11% of patients had tumor recurrence. This recurrence rate can be compared with historical series without maintenance that range from 19 to 54%.

Equally undecided is the advantage of concurrent percutaneous BCG administration. Clearly excellent results can be obtained with high-dose intravesical BCG alone, as documented by Brosman and others. Flamm and Grof, on the other hand, observed no significant reduction in tumor recurrence with 6 to 12 weekly Connaught BCG treatments given by the intravesical route alone (Flamm et al 1981). My experience with Armand-Frappier BCG given only intravesically was equally disappointing, with 40 per cent of patients developing tumor recurrence (Lamm 1985). However, Herr has observed excellent reduction in tumor recurrence with Armand-Frappier BCG given intravesically alone (Lamm 1985). Antitumor responses to BCG appear to be related at least in part to systemic immunity as measured by PPD skin test conversion. Our experience and that of Kelly and co-workers (Kelly et al, 1985) suggests the PPD skin test conversion correlates with response to BCG treatment. We observed tumor recurrence in only 1 of 22 patients (4.5 percent) who converted to PPD skin test positive compared with a 32% incidence of tumor recurrence in 38 patients who were skin test positive before BCG or remained negative after treatment (p=0.017) (Lamm 1985). One should not conclude that patients who are PPD skin test positive are not candidates for BCG immunotherapy since these patients, as well as those who fail to convert to skin test positive with BCG, have recurrence rates which are still significantly lower than those who are not treated with BCG. Many patients who remain skin test negative after intravesical BCG, or have tumor recurrence, will respond to continued treatments with both skin test conversion and freedom from tumor recurrence. However, only prospective randomized studies will be able to answer these questions, since Herr has observed prolonged protection from tumor recurrence with a single course of intravesical BCG despite the absence of PPD skin test conversion.

Conclusions

BCG immunotherapy significantly reduces the incidence of tumor recurrence when compared to no treatment or chemotherapy with Thiotepa or Adriamycin. Responses in the treatment of carcinoma in situ of the bladder average 83%, and a multicenter study has found BCG to be superior to intravesical chemotherapy with Adriamycin. Fifty-eight per cent of patients with unresectable or residual tumors within the bladder respond with complete resolution of disease. Early experience suggests that disease progression to muscle invasion or metastasis is reduced five fold with BCG treatment. If confirmed, such reduction in progression would result in major improvement in the survival of patients presenting with superficial bladder cancer.

BIBLIOGRAPHY

Adolphs HD, Bastian HP (1983). Chemoimmune Prophylaxis of Superficial Bladder Tumors. J Urol 129:29.

Babayan RK, Krane RS (May 1985). Intravesical BCG for Superficial Bladder Cancer. Abstract 393, Am. Urol. Assoc., 80th Ann Mtng., Atlanta, Ga.

Brosman SA (1982). Experience with Bacillus Calmette-Guerin in Patients with Superficial Bladder Cancer. J Urol 128:27.

Brosman S (1985). The Use of Bacillus Calmette-Guerin in the Therapy of Bladder Carcinoma in situ. J Urol 134:36.

Camacho F, Pinsky CM, Kerr D, Braun DW Jr., Whitmore, WF Jr., and Oettgen HP (1982). Treatment of Superficial Bladder Cancer with Intravesical BCG in Immunotherapy of Human Cancer. Terry WT, and Rosenberg SA, editors. Elsevier, North Holland, New York, p. 309.

deKernion JB, Huang MY, Lindner A, Smith RB, Kaufman JJ (1985). The Management of Superficial Bladder Tumors and Carcinoma in situ with Intravesical Bacillus Calmette-Guerin. J Urol 133:598.

Green DF, Robinson MRG, Glashan R, Newling D, Dalesio O, and Smith PH (1984). Does intravesical chemotherapy prevent invasive bladder cancer? J Urol 131:33.

Haaff EO, Dresner SM, Ratliff TL, and Catalona WJ (1986). Two courses of intravesical Bacillus Calmette-Guerin for transitional cell carcinoma of the bladder. J Urol 136:820.

Henry NM, Ahmed S, Flanagan MJ, Frable W, Corder MP, Hafermann MD, Hawkins IL (1983). Superficial bladder cancer: progression and recurrence. J Urol 130.

Herr HW, Pinsky CM, Whitmore WF Jr., Oettgen JF, Melamed MR (1983). Intravesical Bacillus Calmette-Guerin (BCG) Therapy of Superficial Bladder Tumors. Abstract 307, Am Urol Assoc 78.

Herr HW, Pinsky CM, Whitmore WF Jr., Sogahi PC, Oettgen JF, and Melamed MF (1986). Long-term effect of Intravesical Bacillus Calmette-Guerin in flat carcinoma in situ of the bladder. J Urol 135:265.

Huland H, Otto U, Droese M, & Kloppel G (1984). Long term Mitomycin C instillation after transurethral resection of superficial bladder carcinoma: influence of recurrence, progression and survival. J Urol 132:27.

Lamm DL, Thor DE, Harris SC, Reyna JA, Stogdill VD, Radwin HM (1980). Bacillus Calmette-Guerin Immunotherapy of Superficial Bladder Cancer. J Urol 124:38.

Lamm DL (1985). BCG Immunotherapy in Bladder Cancer. J Urol 134:40.

Lamm DL, Crawford ED (March 1985). BCG Versus Adriamycin in Bladder Cancer. A Southwest Oncology Group Study. Proc. A.S.C.O. 4:109-(c424).

Lamm DL (1987). BCG Immunotherapy in Bladder Cancer. Urology Annual, Vol 1, p 69-86.

Martinez-Peneiro JA (1980). BCG Vaccine in the Treatment of Non-infiltrating Papillary Tumors of the Bladder. In: Bladder Tumors and Other Topics in Urologic Oncology. Pavone-Macaluso, Smith M, Edsmyr F (editors) New York. Plenum Press, p 173.

Morales A, Eidinger D, Bruce AW (1976). Intracavitary Bacillus Calmette-Guerin in the Treatment of Superficial Bladder Tumors. J Urol 116:180.

Netto NR Jr., Lemos CG (1983). A Comparison of Treatment Methods for Prophylaxis of Recurrent Superficial Bladder Tumors. J Urol 129:33.

Reynolds RH, Stogdill VD, Lamm DL (April 1985). Disease Progression in BCG-Treated Patients with Transitional Cell Carcinoma of the Bladder. A U A Proc 133:390(392).

Schellhammer PF, Ladaga LE (1986). Bacillus Calmette-Guerin for Therapy of Superficial Transitional Cell Carcinoma of the Bladder. J Urol 135:261.

EORTC Genitourinary Group Monograph 5: Progress
and Controversies in Oncological Urology II, pages 509–510
© 1988 Alan R. Liss, Inc.

Discussion: BCG in Carcinoma In Situ and Superficial
Bladder Tumors

Jan H.M. Blom, Rotterdam, The Netherlands

Fair: We looked at a randomized trial of maintenance and
non-maintenance. There were 46 patients on maintenance and
47 on non-maintenance therapy, which means one 6 week
course. The mean follow-up time was 22 months. There were no
differences in disease-free results. As a result of that we
just gave a single 6 week course. The same is true in
looking at time to progression. There is no difference in
the curves as far as progression to invasive disease is
concerned.

One other aspect that may be a little bit different from Dr.
Lamm's study is that in our patients we did not find that
the PPD conversion actually was correlated with a better
response. In truth, the patients that had a positive PPD to
start with had a better response than any other group. This
was true whether one looked at the maintenance aspect of PPD
conversion which others have commented on.

There is also another current controversy in the States
about giving multiple courses of treatment. The only thing
that I want to say here is: If one is going to compare the
results of one course or two courses, or BCG first, followed
by Thiotepa, or something like that, it is very important to
use controls and these are the reasons why: We just concluded a multivariate analysis on 212 patients. At 3 months,
that is, the first evaluation after 6 weeks of BCG, or 3
months after the BCG was started, 114 of these patients had
a positive finding of either a visible tumor, a positive
biopsy or a positive cytology. We did not include flow
cytometry in this. With no other treatment except just
cauterizing or biopsing the visible tumor (the standard
urologic treatment), but giving no more BCG or no other
intravesicle therapy, at 6 months only 78 were positive.
That means that 31% converted from a positive to a negative
finding with nothing more than just cystoscopy and resection
of tumor. Therefore, if you are going to say that a second

course is valuable or Thiotepa is valuable or something like that, you must have a control group because the natural history is, that at least a third of these patients will convert between 3 and 6 months.

Lamm: I think this is an excellent study and one may try to correlate the results with our experience in both the clinic and laboratory. You cannot go from the mouse to the man, but I think our evidence does clearly suggest that maintenance, as you would expect, is of value only after the initial treatment has had a time to wane. We know that these patients do in fact maintain at proclivity for tumor recurrence for many years. We do not know whether perhaps some of these patients have in fact a specific immunity developed to bladder tumor and have maintained that immunity. That non-specific aspect of the immunotherapy, however, we know, does decrease with time.

EORTC Genitourinary Group Monograph 5: Progress
and Controversies in Oncological Urology II, pages 511–524
© 1988 Alan R. Liss, Inc.

BCG-RIVM INTRAVESICAL IMMUNOPROPHYLAXIS FOR SUPERFICIAL BLADDER CANCER

F.M.J. Debruyne[1], A.P.M. van der Meijden[1], L.M.H. Schreinemachers[2], A.D.H. Geboers[1], M.P.H. Franssen[1], M.J.W. van Leeuwen[3], P.A. Steerenberg[4], W.H. de Jong[4], E.J. Ruitenberg[4]. Dep. of Urology, University Hospital Nijmegen[1], Dep. of Urology, Groot Ziekengasthuis, Den Bosch[2], IKO Cancer Center, Nijmegen[3], Dutch National Institute of Public Health and Environmental Hygiene, Bilthoven[4], The Netherlands

INTRODUCTION

It is now widely acknowledged that prophylactic intravesical therapy after transurethral resection (TUR) of superficial bladder cancer (pTa, pT1 and CIS) significantly reduces the tumor recurrence rate and is beneficial in preventing tumor progression.

Intravesical chemotherapy has been used for these purposes for almost two decades and different agents have proven to be effective (Soloway, 1980). Since the first report in 1976 by Morales et al. on the use of BCG intravesical immunotherapy, it has become evident that this form of prophylaxis is also effective and more recent reports claimed that BCG is even superior to intravesical chemotherapy and hence could be the most effective agent presently available for the (prophylactic) treatment of superficial bladder cancer (Brosman, 1982; Lamm et al., 1982). This suggestion, however, is not fully evidenced by results of prospective randomized clinical trials in which intravesical immuno- and chemoprophylaxis are compared.

On the other hand several types of BCG-vaccines prepared from different BCG-strains have been used in different studies and it is not clear yet if all strains have a similar effectivity.

The present paper deals with the use of the new strain BCG-RIVM in the prophylactic management of superficial bladder cancer.

BCG-RIVM

In the Netherlands a BCG-vaccine has been produced at the "Rijksinstituut voor Volksgezondheid en Milieuhygiene, RIVM" (National Institute of Public Health and Environmental Hygiene). The BCG-strain used for the RIVM-vaccine was originally derived from a seedlot of the institute Pasteur in Paris. This vaccine is produced as a homogeneously dispersed culture under continuous stirring. This method ensures a relatively high ratio of viable organisms and a small quantity of subcellular debris and dead microorganisms. For intravesical immunoprophylaxis BCG-RIVM is provided in 30 ml vials containing 1×10^9 lyophilized viable units. As a stabilizer for lyophilization 833 mg Haemacel, 500 mg D-glucose and 0.5 mg Tween 80 are added. The vials are closed under vacuum. For intravesical use the dry cake is resuspended by adding 10 ml sterile physiological saline and a homogeneous suspension is obtained by swirling of the vial.

Immunostimulation and antitumor activity by the BCG-RIVM was observed both in experimental and spontaneous animal tumors (De Jong et al., 1983; 1984; Klein et al., 1982; Kreeftenberg et al., 1981; Lagrange and Gheorghiv, 1982; Ruitenberg et al., 1981). In man, this BCG preparation was studied as adjuvant immunotherapy in melanoma patients (EORTC protocol 18781) and in bronchus carcinoma (Jansen et al., 1980). From these studies it became clear that also an immunostimulating effect could be achieved in man.

BCG-RIVM toxicity studies

Before attempting the use of BCG-RIVM for intravesical immunoprophylaxis in superficial bladder cancer in man, local and systemic toxicity studies were performed both in animals (dogs) and in man.

For the animal study female Beagle dogs were used. After coagulation of the bladder wall the dogs were treated with 6 weekly intravesical instillations of BCG-RIVM, once a week for 6 consecutive weeks. In one group of dogs a simultaneous intradermal BCG scarification using a multi-puncture apparatus was performed. The conclusion of this study was that BCG-RIVM intravesical instillation with or without intradermal scarification causes no significant systemic toxicity. The immunostimulatory effect was observed in post-therapy bladder biopsies which showed follicular accumulation of lymphocytes and small granuloma's. The latter were only found in the dogs treated both intravesically and intradermally (v.d. Meijden et al., 1986).

A phase I study in man also proved that intravesical instillation of BCG-RIVM can be used safely with regard to local and systemic toxicity. In 30 patients the toxic side effects of BCG-RIVM were evaluated after intradermal and intravesical administration. All patients had a history of recurrent multiple non-invasive superficial bladder cancer and were previously unsuccessfully treated with intravesical chemotherapy. BCG-RIVM (1×10^9 culturable particles) was instilled in the bladder in combination with intradermal BCG-RIVM (8×10^7 culturable particles) administration once a week for six consecutive weeks. BCG was applied intradermally by a multi-puncture technique. The conclusions of this study were that no systemic toxicity was observed whereas the local vesical toxicity was minimal. Only the skin reactions after intradermal multipuncture application were distinct but well tolerated. The urine was almost completely cleared from BCG particles within 24 hours after instillation. The immunostimulating activity of BCG was clear from the conversion of the PPD (Purified Protein Derivate) reaction to positive in 95% of the patients who had negative skin tests before BCG treatment (Schreinemachers et al., 1987).

Comparative study with BCG-RIVM

In January 1985 a clinical trial comparing BCG-RIVM with Mitomycine C (MMC) (protocol 30845) was started as a joint study of the EORTC GU-group and the Dutch South-Eastern Urological Cooperative Group. In this trial comparison with MMC was chosen since at that time this drug was assumed to be the most potent and less toxic for intravesical chemotherapy (Huland and Otto, 1983; Soloway, 1984).

The objective of this two armed prospectively controlled and randomized trial was to compare the prophylactic effect of intravesically administered BCG-RIVM to Mitomycine-C in patients with primary or recurrent superficial bladder tumors including CIS on:

- recurrence rate, including evaluation of the number and size of recurrent tumors
- duration of disease free interval
- the rate of progression to a higher stage (T category) of the disease
- the incidence and severity of side effects.

Intradermal scarification with BCG, initially thought to act synergistically with the intravesical administration and thus to be necessary to obtain optimal prophylactic immunostimulation was omitted in agreement with the obser-vations by Brosman (1982) and Herr et al. (1986), suggesting that percutaneous sensitisation with BCG before the intravesical administration of the agent, may not be necessary to achieve its effect.

All patients with a primary or recurrent resectable pTa and pT1 papillary transitional cell carcinoma of the bladder proven by histopathological investigation could be admitted to the study. All visible lesions had to be com-pletely removed by differentiated transurethral resection which had to be associated by at random biopsies of the mucosa with normal appearance. Also eligible were patients with carcinoma in situ (CIS). Previous intravesical or systemic therapy with cytotoxic drugs excluded patients to entry as well as untreated urinary tract infections or a recurrent severe bacterial cystitis.

Patients were randomly allocated to BCG-RIVM or MMC intravesical instillation which started between 7 and 15 days after the complete transurethral resection (TUR) of all papillary superficial tumors. The therapeutic regimen is shown in fig. 1. BCG was given once a week for 6 conse-cutive weeks. MMC was instilled once a week for one month (week 1-4) and thereafter once a month for a total of 6 months. Control cystoscopy was performed three and six months after TUR. If recurrence was observed at 3 months in the BCG group, the tumor was again completely resected and additional intravesical BCG therapy was restarted for six weekly instillations. If recurrence was observed in the MMC group, the tumor was totally resected and the MMC treatment was continued monthly. If, however, at 3 months an increase in T category to T2 or higher was observed the patient went off-study. After 6 months control cystoscopy was performed every 3 months for three years. Patients went off-study at their first recurrence after completion of intravesical

Figure 1

THERAPEUTIC REGIMEN

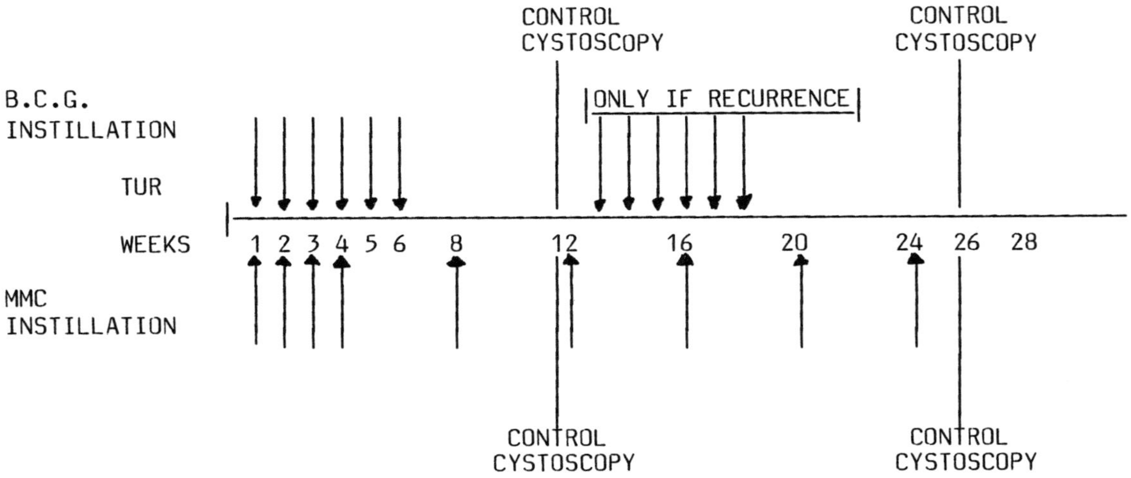

treatment, i.e. at 6 months or thereafter.

A total number of 269 patients have been entered into this study, which was closed on October 1st 1986. The data of 183 patients entered by the Dutch South-Eastern cooperative group (enrolled by 10 Institutions) have been analysed in Januari 1987 with regard to toxicity and (preliminary) efficacy.

Stratification for CIS, pTa and pT1 as well as for primary and recurrent tumors was similar in both treatment arms. Local and systemic toxicity are shown in Table 1-3. Tables 1 and 2 compare the occurrence of bacterial and substance induced cystitis by patients and number of instillations. No difference between the two treatment groups was observed. Systemic toxicity was absent in both treatment arms.

TABLE 1. Protocol 30845:   no. of occurrences of chemical cystitis

	BCG	MMC
NO. OF PATIENTS	78	87
NO. OF OCCURRENCES	13 (16.7%)	12 (13.8%)
NO. OF INSTILLATIONS	510	727
NO. OF OCCURRENCES	32 (6.3%)	28 (3.9%)

(data cooperative group) Jan. 1987

The number of occurrences of allergic reactions is shown in Table 3. This analysis shows a more frequent allergic reaction in the MMC arm.

The first and (very) preliminary result with regard to recurrence is shown in Table 4. This table demonstrates no statistically significant difference between the two therapeutic regimens, although the figures suggest a slightly higher recurrence rate in the BCG-RIVM group. An analysis of the total number of patients followed for a longer period of time must confirm these preliminary data. Therefore, these data have to be handled with caution and do not allow any conclusion at this moment at all.

TABLE 2. Protocol 30845: no. of occurrences of bacterial cystitis

	BCG	MMC
NO. OF PATIENTS	78	87
NO. OF OCCURRENCES	17 (21.8%)	16 (18.4%)
NO. OF INSTILLATIONS	510	727
NO. OF OCCURRENCES	29 (5.7%)	23 (3.2%)

(data cooperative group) Jan. 1987

TABLE 3. Protocol 30845: no. of occurrences of allergic reactions

	BCG	MMC
NO. OF PATIENTS	78	87
NO. OF OCCURRENCES	1 (1.3%)	6 (6.9%)
NO. OF INSTILLATIONS	510	727
NO. OF OCCURRENCES	2 (0.4%)	14 (1.9%)

(data cooperative group) Jan. 1987

TABLE 4. Protocol 30845: available follow-up as of January 1987

	BCG	MMC
PTS WITH FOLLOW-UP	75	84
MEAN FOLLOW-UP (MONTHS)	6.00	6.00
TOTAL NO. OF CYSTOSCOPIES	141	151
TOTAL NO. OF RECURRENCES	19	11
RECURRENCE RATE	0.54	0.29

(data cooperative group) Jan. 1987

DISCUSSION

BCG immunoprophylaxis has become a more and more useful and used therapy in intravesical bladder tumors. Prerequisites for effective intravesical BCG prophylaxes are (amongst other factors such as the ability of the host to react to mycobacterial antigens): small tumor load and adequate numbers of living bacilli, especially the close contact between the bacilli and the bladder wall (Zbar and Rapp, 1974).

The clinically relevant mechanisms of action of immunotherapeutic agents are still unknown and although they can be characterized by their capacity to modulate the immune system and host defense mechanisms their use remains largely empirical. The immunostimulating effect of intravesical BCG therapy is, however, clearly demonstrated by the local reaction of the bladder as well as by the conversion of the PPD skin reactions, from negative to positive, which can be regarded as an expression of the systemic immunostimulating effect of BCG.

Different vaccines prepared from BCG have been used for intravesical immunoprophylaxis. Apart from the BCG-RIVM vaccine used in our study several reports on other vaccines such as BCG-Tice, BCG-Frappeur, BCG-Connaught, BCG-Glaxo,

BCG-Pasteur have been published. All vaccines seem to have some effectiveness with the exception of the BCG-Glaxo preparation, probably due to a low number of viable organisms (Lamm, 1987).

Kelley et al. (1986) investigated the efficacy of different strains. They showed that there was a correlation between the development of a delayed hypersensitivity response to PPD antigen and treatment results. Patients whose skin test converted from negative to positive remained significantly more free of tumor recurrence.

It was also demonstrated that there was a relationship between treatment results and different lots of BCG. Striking differences in the number of colony-forming units between lots of BCG of the same preparation and among different preparations were revealed ranging from 10^6 colonies till 10^{12} colonies per ampule (Kelley et al., 1985). Furthermore not only the number of bacilli present in the vaccine is important but also the activity to multiply in vivo, i.e. the viability.

It is not known whether the culture method of BCG might influence the efficacy in the prophylactic treatment of superficial bladder cancer. In general two different culture methods are used. The first (classic) way of preparing BCG is to grow it as a surface culture. This surface pellicle is subsequently homogenized in a ball mill. This means that together with viable bacilli subcellular debris and dead bacilli are harvested. In the second method BCG is grown in a homogeneously stirred liquid culture medium. Bacteria are collected by centrifugation and resuspended. This culture method ensures a relatively high ratio of viable organisms and a small quantity of subcellular debris and dead microorganisms. BCG-RIVM is prepared according to the second method. Other preparations (Tice, Connaught, Armand Frappier) are cultured as a surface pellicle. It is possible that the difference in culture method is responsible for the significant difference in local side effects between BCG-RIVM and other vaccines. In the present study agent induced cystitis was only seen in 16.7% of the patients (comparable with the local toxicity of intravesical chemotherapy) whereas about 90% of the patients complain of (transient) cystitis when the other strains are used (Lamm et al., 1986). On the other hand the question arises whether the efficacy of the preparation is not related to its local toxicity. The adherence of the bacilli to the bladder wall is probably an important factor by which BCG exerts its effect. It is possible that subcellular debris or cell products are necessary to achieve attachment of BCG to the bladder wall (Nickel et al., 1985). Ratliff et al. (1987) demonstrated that the protein fibronectin could play a role in the attachment of BCG.

The results with regard to recurrence rate obtained so far in our study, although still very preliminary, do not indicate superiority of BCG-RIVM over MMC. This is in contrast with other randomized trials in which it has been demonstrated that BCG strains are superior to intravesical chemotherapy. (Brosman, 1982; Lamm et al., 1985; Netto and Lemos, 1983; Shapiro et al., 1984). However, additional prospective studies are indispensable to prove the superiority of one agent over another and of one regimen over another. It is not yet clear whether 6-weekly instillations are suboptimal as suggested by Haaff et al. (1986) and whether maintenance therapy is necessary or not. In general, treatment results have been more favourable with intensive regimens (Brosman, 1982; 1985). However, the toxicity also has been substantially greater with intensive regimens. Recently Badalement et al. (1987) showed that in their group of patients BCG maintenance therapy is not improving the results, and Catalona et al. (1987) showed that more than two courses of BCG therapy was not beneficial in patients failing to respond.

These data just indicate how many questions with regard to intravesical BCG therapy still remain open. These questions can only be solved by conducting further prospective randomized clinical trials with regard to the prophylactic use of BCG in superficial bladder cancer. As far as the BCG-RIVM vaccine is concerned, the most urgent question to be solved is whether this preparation with minimal toxicity is as effective as the other vaccines. Therefore a comparative protocol is now studied by the Dutch South-Eastern Cooperative Group in which two different BCG preparations are compared with a standard intravesical chemotherapy. One BCG vaccine (Tice) has proven its efficacy but side-effects cannot be ignored. The RIVM preparation with less frequent side-effects has also proved antitumor activity. As in the first protocol MMC is chosen as standard intravesical chemotherapy. This and

and other studies will certainly contribute to further elucidation of the exact value of active intravesical immunotherapy with BCG in superficial bladder cancer.

REFERENCES

Badalement RA, Herr HW, Wong GY, Gnecco C, Pinsky CM, Whithmore WF, Fair WR, Oettgen HF (1987). A prospective randomized trial of maintenance versus nonmaintenance intravesical Bacillus Calmette-Guérin therapy of superficial bladder cancer. J Clinic Oncol 5: 441-449.

Brosman SA (1982). Experience with Bacillus Calmette-Guérin in patients with superficial bladder carcinoma. J Urol 128: 27-30.

Brosman SA (1985). The use of Bacillus Calmette-Guérin in the therapy of bladder carcinoma in situ. J Urol 134: 36-39.

Catalona WJ, Hudson MA, Gillen DP, Andiole GL, Ratliff TL (1987). Risks and benefits of repeated courses of intravesical bacillus Calmette-Guérin therapy for superficial bladder cancer. J Urol 137: 220-224.

Haaff EO, Dresner SM, Ratliff TL, Catalona WJ (1986). Two courses of intravesical Bacillus Calmette-Guérin for transitional cell carcinoma of the bladder. J Urol 136: 820-824.

Herr HW, Pinsky CM, Whitmore WF jr, Sogani PC, Oettgen HF, Melamed MR (1986). Long-term effect of intravesical Bacillus Calmette-Guérin on flat carcinoma in situ of the bladder. J Urol 135: 265-267.

Huland H, Otto U (1983). Mitomycin instillation to prevent recurrence of superficial bladder carcinoma. Results of a controlled prospective study in 58 patients. Eur Urol 9: 84-86.

Jansen HM, The TH, Orie NGM (1980). Adjuvant immunotherapy with B.C.G. in squamous cell bronchial carcinoma. Thorax 35: 781-787.

de Jong WH, Ursem PS, Kruizinga W, Osterhaus ADME, Ruitenberg EJ (1983). Effects of Bacillus Calmette-Guérin on natural killer cell activity in random bred rats. In: Cancer etiology and prevention. RG Crispen ed. Elsevier Science publishing Co. Inc. Amsterdam p. 123.

de Jong WH, Steerenberg PA, Kreeftenberg JG, Tasjema RH, Kruizinga W, van Noorle-Jansen LM, Ruitenberg EJ (1984). Experimental screening of BCG preparation produced for cancer immunotherapy: safety and immunostimulating and antitumor activity of four consecutively produced batches. Cancer Immunol Immunoth 17: 18-27.

Kelley DR, Haaff EO, Berich M, Lage J, Bauer WC, Dresner SM, Catalona WJ, Ratliff TL (1986). Prognostic value of purified protein derivate skin test and granuloma formation in patients treated with intravesical Bacillus Calmette-Guérin. J Urol 135: 268-271.

Kelley DR, Ratliff TL, Catalona WJ, Shapiro A, Lage JM, Bauer WC, Haaff EO, Dresner SM (1985). Intravesical Bacillus Calmette-Guérin therapy for superficial bladder cancer: effect of Bacillus Calmette-Guérin viability on treatment results. J. Urol. 134: 48-53.

Klein WR, Ruitenberg EJ, Steerenberg PA, de Jong WH, Kruizinga W, Misdorp W, Bier J, Tiessema RH, Kreeftenberg JG, Teppema JS, Rapp HJ (1982). Immunotherapy by intralesional injection of BCG cell walls or live BCG in bovine ocular squamous cell carcinoma: a preliminary report. J Nat Cancer Inst 69: 1095-1103.

Kreeftenberg JG, de Jong WH, Ettekoven H, Steerenerg PA, Kruizinga W, van Noorle-Jansen LM, Sekhuis J, Ruitenberg EJ (1981). Experimental screening of two BCG preparations produced according to different principles. Immuno-stimulating properties, safety and antitumor activity. Cancer Immunol Immunoth 12: 21-29.

Lagrange PH, Gheorghiu M (1982). Antitumor activity of two BCG vaccine preparations against the levis lung carcinoma in mice. Cancer Immunol Immunoth 12: 217-224.

Lamm DL, Thor DE, Stogdill VD, Radwin HM (1982). Bladder cancer immunotherapy. J Urol 128: 931-935.

Lamm DL, Crawford ED, Montie JE, Scardino PT, Stanisie TH, Grossman HB, Sullivan JW (1985). BCG versus adriamycin in the treatment of transitional cell carcinoma in situ: a South-west Oncology Group Study. J Urol 133: 184A.

Lamm DL, Stogdill VD, Stogdill BJ, Crispen RG (1986). Complications of Bacillus Calmette-Guérin immunotherapy in 1278 patients with bladder cancer. J Urol 135: 272-274.

Lamm DL (1987). Personal communication.

Meijden van der APM, Steerenberg PA, Jong de WH, Bogman MJJT, Feitz WFJ, Hendriks BT, Debruyne FMJ, Ruitenberg EJ (1986) The effects of intravesical and intradermal application of a new B.C.G. on the dog bladder. Urol. Res. 14: 207-210.

Morales A, Eidinger D, Bruce AW (1976). Intracavitary Bacillus Calmette-Guérin in the treatment of superficial bladder cancer. J Urol 116: 180-183.

Netto MR, Lemos GC (1983) A comparison of treatment methods for the prophylaxis of recurrent superficial bladder tumors. J Urol 129: 33-34.

Nickel JC, Morales A, Heaton JPW, Costerton JW (1985). Ultrastructural study of the interaction of B.C.G. with bladder mucosa after intravesical treatment of bladder cancer. J Urol 133: 268A

Ratliff TL, Palmer JO, McGarr JA, Brown EJ (1987). Intravesical Bacillus Calmette-Guérin therapy for murine bladder tumors: Initiation of the response by fibronectin-mediated attachment of B.C.G. J Urol in press.

Ruitenberg EJ, de Jong WH, Kreeftenberg PA, Kruizinga W, van Noorle Jansen LM (1981). BCG preparations, cultured homogeneously dispersed or as surface pellicle, elicit different immunopotentiating effects but have similar antitumor activity in a murine fibrosarcoma. Cancer Immunol Immunoth 11: 45-51.

Schreinemachers LMH, Meijden van der APM, Wagenaar J, Steerenberg PA, Feitz WFJ, Groothuis DG, Tiesjema RH, Jong de WH, Debruyne FMJ, Ruitenberg EJ (1987). BCG intravesical and intradermal application. A phase I study to the toxicity of a Dutch B.C.G. preparation in patients with superficial bladder cancer. Eur Urol in press.

Shapiro A, Ratliff TL, Oakley DM, Catalona WJ (1984). Comparison of the efficacy of intravesical Calmette-Guerin with thiothepa, mitomycin-C, poly I: C/Poly L-Lysin and cisplatinum in murine bladder cancer. J Urol 131: 139-143.

Soloway M (1980). Rationale for intensive intravesical chemotherapy for superficial bladder cancer. J Urol 123: 461-466.

Soloway M (1984). Rationale for intensive intravesical chemotherapy for superficial bladder cancer. In: Progress and controversies in oncological Urology. KH Kurth, FMJ Debruyne, FH Schröder, TAW Splinter and TDJ Wagener (Eds.) Alan R Liss, New York p. 608.

Zbar B, Rapp HJ (1974). Immunotherapy of guinea pig cancer with BCG. Cancer 34: 1532-1536.

ACKNOWLEDGEMENTS

The authors wish to thank all collaborating urologists and their nursing staffs for their excellent contributions to this study, B.Th. Hendriks for his assistance in performing the dog bladder instillation, Dr. M.J.J.T. Bogman for examining the pathology of the dog bladders and Mrs. D.M. Litjens-de Heus for assisting in preparing and typing the manuscript.

Participating Institutions:

Ziekenhuis De Stadsmaten, Enschede
Ziekenhuis Ziekenzorg, Enschede
Juliana Ziekenhuis, Apeldoorn
Lukas Ziekenhuis, Apeldoorn
Malberg Ziekenhuis, Arnhem
Ziekenhuis Rivierenland, Tiel
St. Ignatius Ziekenhuis, Breda
St. Maartens Gasthuis, Venlo
De Wever Ziekenhuis, Heerlen
St. Radboudziekenhuis, Nijmegen

EORTC Genitourinary Group Monograph 5: Progress
and Controversies in Oncological Urology II, pages 525-532
© 1988 Alan R. Liss, Inc.

IS THERE AN OPTIMAL TREATMENT SCHEME FOR ADJUVANT INTRA-
VESICAL THERAPY?
PRELIMINARY ANALYSIS OF AN EORTC PROTOCOL COMPARING EARLY
AND DELAYED INSTILLATION WITH AND WITHOUT MAINTENANCE OF
EITHER ADRIAMYCIN OR MITOMYCIN-C IN PATIENTS WITH SUPERFI-
CIAL TRANSITIONAL CARCINOMA OF THE BLADDER.

K.H. Kurth (1), C. Bouffioux (2), R. Sylvester
(3), M. de Pauw (3), and members of the EORTC GU
Group (3)

1. Dept. of Urology, Erasmus University Rotterdam,
   The Netherlands,
2. Dept. of Urology, University of Liege, Belgium,
3. EORTC Data Center, Brussels, Belgium.

Superficial transitional cell bladder carcinoma includes a broad spectrum of heterogeneous tumors. Subcatego-
ries are critical for the natural history of the tumor. The
likelihood to recur is clearly related to such prognostic
factors as the number of tumors present, the recurrence rate
prior to entry into a study and tumor stage and grade
(Kurth, 1984).

The concept of intravesical adjuvant chemotherapy has
undergone rapid changes. Ideally an agent locally instilled
would have an acceptable toxicity and prevent all recurrences, thus progression into a higher stage would never be
observed. Of course, no agent fulfills these requirements.

Next to the agent used, dose and treatment schemes may
be of some importance for the outcome of adjuvant or prophylactic intravesical chemotherapy. In this chapter we will
concentrate on treatment schemes. Many treatment schedules
are reported as for example preoperative instillation
(Mishina, 1982), instillation immediately or hours after TUR
(Zincke, 1983; Kurth, 1983), intensive instillation repeated
daily (Flüchter, 1983) or several times weekly (England,
1981; Schulman, 1983; Gavrell, 1978), delayed instillation 1
to 4 weeks post-TUR (Schulman, 1982; Huland, 1985) or continued instillation after 12 months (Huland, 1985).

Results as achieved with early intensive chemotherapy strongly suggest that the percentage of patients with recurrences will be markedly reduced (Schulman, 1983). On the other hand, Devonec and co-workers (1983) instilled 40 mg Mitomycin-C for 10 days and noted that a recurrence was seen in 88% (22/26 patients) after a mean follow-up of 12.2 months, suggesting that such short and intensive therapy is likely to be inadequate.

Longterm instillation gained much attention, especially through the results reported by Huland and coworkers (1985), who instilled Mitomycin-C 20 mg every 2 weeks for 1 year and then every 4 weeks for 2 years. After a mean follow-up of 30.5 months they observed a recurrent tumor in 10.4% only (5/48). However, in this study, as in other studies, the time and duration of instillation of the cytostatic drug was not a matter of randomization. Therefore it cannot be stated with certainty, that the duration of treatment was of crucial importance for the results achieved.

Hence the EORTC GU Group started two parallel randomized protocols in September 1983 to compare the effect of immediate or delayed instillation with and without maintenance of either Mitomycin-C 30 mg or Adriamycin 50 mg on the percentage with recurrence, the recurrence rate per year and the tumor rate per year. The drug was instilled within 6 hours or 7 days after TUR, instillation was continued 3 times weekly and 5 times monthly. Thereafter patients were randomized for continued 6 times monthly instillations or no further instillations.

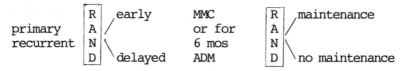

Prot. 30831, 1983-1985
Prot. 30832, 1983-1985

Figure 1

The local toxicity in patients who were treated early was acceptable. Mitomycin-C led to chemical cystitis in 5% after 1923 instillations, whereas in the group of patients with the start of treatment 1 week after TUR the occurrence of chemical cystitis was 4% after 2043 instillations (one patient may report several occurrences of chemical cystitis).

In the Adriamycin study likewise the occurrence of chemical cystitis was not higher in patients treated with early instillation (2% after 1344 instillations) than in patients with delayed instillations (3% after 1270 instillations). Thus, early instillation hours after TUR did not lead to an unacceptable increase of local side effects.

A first and preliminary analysis of the parallel protocols was performed in March 1987. 446 patients in protocol 30831 with a mean follow-up of 10.4 and 11.2 months respectively were analysed for per cent with recurrence, recurrence rate per year and tumor rate per year. There was no significant difference for patients treated by early or delayed instillation (table 1).
Three hunderd and fifty patients were analysed for the effect of continued instillation after 6 months. Again there were no significant differences in the recurrence rate and the tumor rate per year (table 2).

TABLE 1. Protocol 30831 Comparison Early vs Delayed Instillation (p = n.s.)

| | Mitomycin-C | |
	Early	Delayed
Patients with follow-up	221	225
Mean follow-up (months)	10.4	11.2
Per cent with recurrence	31	32
Recurrence rate per year	0.4	0.4
Tumor rate per year	1.2	1.3

EORTC 30831, 3.87

If early instillation with or without maintenance was compared with delayed instillation with and without maintenance, the figures for the recurrence rate per year and the tumor rate per year were very similar. The statistical comparison did not deliver any significant differences (table 3).

TABLE 2. Protocol 30831 Comparison Installation for 6 Months
       (nm) vs Instillation for 12 Months (m), p = n.s.

| | Mitomycin-C | |
	No maintenance	Maintenance
Patients with follow-up	180	170
Mean follow-up (months)	13	13
Per cent with recurrence	31	29
Recurrence rate per year	0.41	0.35
Tumor rate per year	1.1	0.8

EORTC 30831, 3.87

TABLE 3. Protocol 30831 Comparison of All Treatment Groups,
       p = n.s.

| | Mitomycin-C | | | |
| | Early | | Delayed | |
	No main-tenance	Main-tenance	No main-tenance	Main-tenance
Patients with follow-up	85	86	95	84
Mean follow-up (months)	12.2	13	13.4	13
Per cent with recurrence	31	31	31	27
Recurrence rate per year	0.4	0.37	0.39	0.33
Tumor rate per year	1.1	0.8	1.1	0.8

EORTC 30381, 3.87

The same analysis was performed for the protocol 30832
(Adriamycin). Three hunderd and sixty-six patients with a
mean follow-up of 12 months were included in the analysis to
study the effect of early or delayed instillation. Although
the percentage with recurrence and the recurrence rate per
year is smaller in the group of patients treated by early

instillation, statistical analysis did not show a significant difference in favour of one or the other treatment schemes (table 4).

TABLE 4. Protocol 30832 Comparison Early vs Delayed Instillation, p = n.s.

| | Adriamycin | |
	Early	Delayed
Patients with follow-up	188	178
Mean follow-up (months)	12	12.3
Per cent with recurrence	17	26
Recurrence rate per year	0.25	0.35
Tumor rate per year	0.68	0.67

EORTC 30832, 3.87

The same is true for patients treated for 6 or 12 months (table 5).

TABLE 5. Protocol 30832 Comparison Instillation for 6 Months (nm) vs Instillation for 12 Months (m), p = n.s.

| | Adriamycin | |
	No maintenance	Maintenance
Patients with follow-up	147	146
Mean follow-up (months)	14.5	14.5
Per cent with recurrence	24	19
Recurrence rate per year	0.28	0.22
Tumor rate per year	0.59	0.41

EORTC 30832, 3.87

If early instillation with or without maintenance is compared to delayed instillation with and without maintenance, best results were achieved in patients treated early and patients treated for 12 months. Only 14% had a recurrence after a mean follow-up of 14 months, the recurrence rate per year was 0.18 compared to 0.34 in patients treated delayed and only for 6 months, the tumor rate was lowest and only half of the tumor rate observed in patients treated delayed for 6 months (table 6).

TABLE 6. Protocol 30832 Comparison of All Treatment Groups, p = n.s.

| | Adriamycin | | | |
| | Early | | Delayed | |
	No main-tenance	Main-tenance	No main-tenance	Main-tenance
Patients with follow-up	80	70	67	76
Mean follow-up (months)	14.5	14.2	14.4	14.9
Per cent with recurrence	19	14	30	24
Recurrence rate per year	0.22	0.18	0.34	0.26
Tumor rate per year	0.58	0.32	0.61	0.48

EORTC 30832, 3.87

However, if the subgroups are statistically compared there is no statistical difference in favour of one of the subgroups. Comparison of the group with the best and the worst results, namely early with maintenance versus delayed instillation without maintenance, delivered a p-value of 0.08.

CONCLUSION

Although early post-TUR instillation with maintenance seems to be superior to delayed instillation without maintenance the differences between the treatment arms are not significant.
Later analysis after a longer follow-up may or may not show statistically significant differences. When observed, however, such differences are expected to be small. The pa-

tients in the parallel protocols were stratified for primary or recurrent tumor. Other prognostic factors like the number of tumors present, size of the tumors, T- and G-category will be stratified retrospectively. These variables, which certainly influence the outcome of treatment, were not yet analysed. However, as already stated, one may not expect a completely changed picture.

The optimum frequency and duration of adjuvant chemotherapy is as yet incompletely defined.

Recommendation for intravesical adjuvant chemotherapy for superficial bladder cancer should be based on the outcome of randomized studies. From the results reported here we cannot conclude that the natural history of superficial bladder tumor is favourably influenced by early instillation or continued instillation for longer than 6 months. Because a treatment course of 6 months seems to be as safe for the patient as treatment over 12 months one would be in favour of a scheme which lowers the inconvenience for the patient and costs.

REFERENCES

Devonec M, Bouvier R, Sarkissian J, Bendimerad O, Gelet A, Dubernard JM (1983). Intravesical instillation of Mitomycin-C in the prophylactic treatment of recurring superficial transitional cell carcinoma of the bladder. Brit J Urol 55: 382.

England HR, Flynn JT, Paris AMI, Blandy JP (1981). Early multiple-dose adjuvant thiotepa in the control of multiple and rapid Tl tumor neogenesis. Brit J Urol 53: 588-592.

Flüchter StH, Harzmann R, Hlobil H, Erdmann W, Bichler KH (1982). Lokale Chemotherapie des Harnblasenkarzinoms und Mitomycin. Urologe A 21: 24-28.

Gavrell GJ, Lewis RW, Meehan WL, Leblanc GA (1978). Intravesical thiotepa in the immediate postoperative period in patients with recurrent transitional cell carcinoma of the bladder. J Urol 120: 410-411.

Huland H, Otto U, Droese M, Klöppel G (1984). Long-term mitomycin-C instillation after transurethral resection of superficial bladder carcinoma: influence on recurrence, progression and survival. J Urol 132: 27-29.

Kurth KH, Maksimovic PA, Hop WCJ, Schröder FH, Bakker NJ (1983). Single-dose intravesical epodyl after TUR of Ta TCC bladder carcinoma. World J Urol 1: 89-93.

Kurth KH, Schröder FH, Tunn U, Ay R, Pavone Macaluso M,

Debruyne FMJ, de Pauw M, Dalesio O, ten Kate F, and members of the EORTC GU Group (1984). Adjuvant chemotherapy of superficial transitional cell bladder carcinoma: preliminary results of a European Organization for Research on Treatment of Cancer randomized trial comparing doxorubicin hydrochloride, ethoglucid and transurethral resection alone. J Urol 132: 258-262.

Mishina T, Watanabe H, Fujiwara T, Kobayashi T, Maegawa M, Nakao M, Nakagawa S (1982). Prophylactic use of mitomycin-C bladder instillation for preventing the recurrence of bladder tumors. In Ogawa M, Rozencweig M, Staquet MJ (eds): "Mitomycin-C, Current Impact on Cancer Chemotherapy", Amsterdam-Princeton-Geneva-Tokyo: Excerpta Medica, pp 153-161.

Schulman CC, Robinson M, Denis L, Smith P, Viggiano G, de Pauw M, Dalesio O, Sylvester R, and members of the EORTC GU Group (1982). Prophylactic chemotherapy of superficial-transitional cell bladder carcinoma: an EORTC randomized trial comparing thiotepa, an epipodophyllotoxin (VM26) and TUR alone. Eur Urol 8: 207-212.

Schulman CC, Denis L, Oosterlinck W, De Sy W, Chantrie M, Bouffioux C, Van Cangh PJ, Van Erps P (1983). Early adjuvant adriamycin in superficial bladder carcinoma. World J Urol 1: 86-88.

Zincke H, Benson RC, Hilton JF, Taylor WF (1985). Intravesical thiotepa and mitomycin-C treatment immediate after transurethral resection and later for superficial (stages Ta and Tis) bladder cancer: a prospective, randomized, stratified study with crossover design. J Urol 134: 1110-1114.

EORTC Genitourinary Group Monograph 5: Progress
and Controversies in Oncological Urology II, pages 533–537
© 1988 Alan R. Liss, Inc.

Discussion: Is There an Optimal Treatment Scheme for
Adjuvant Intravesical Therapy? Preliminary Analysis of an
EORTC Protocol Comparing Early and Delayed Instillation
With and Without Maintenance of Either Adriamycin or
Mitomycin-C in Patients With Superficial Transitional
Carcinoma of the Bladder

Jan H. M. Blom, Rotterdam, The Netherlands

Pavone-Macaluso: I think that the EORTC urological group has
made a very interesting contribution to the study of how to
treat recurrent tumors. I would like to stress the fact that
it is not yet possible to compare the Adriamycin study with
the Mitomycin-C study, because the majority of the patients
treated with Adriamycin had primary tumors versus the vast
majority of the patients included in the Mitomycin-C trial,
who had recurrent tumors, and so this explains why the
overall recurrence rate in the Adriamycin treated patients
is much lower than that found with Mitomycin-C. So, these
are not studies to be compared one with the other, but they
were devised to have two possibilities using two different
drugs to see whether early was better than delayed or vice
versa and whether short-term was better than long-term or
vice versa. In spite of the fact that it has been mentioned
that early versus delayed treatment had more or less the
same number of patients suffering from chemical cystitis, I
think it is also fair to mention that there were a few
patients who were obliged to stop treatment in the early
scheme and no patient stopped treatment in the delayed
scheme. Perhaps this is not of great importance for
Mitomycin-C or Adriamycin, but perhaps when BCG is employed,
I think that it is much better to wait some time after the
TUR before the treatment can be started. What is your experience about that, Dr. Lamm?

Lamm: Certainly in a patient who has an extensive tumor
resection I think it would be safer to wait before initiating BCG. However, in patients who have just but a biopsy or
a resection of a small tumor we find it quite safe to give
treatment within 24-28 hours in patients who travel considerable distances to the hospital. But in a patient who
has continued hematuria, a traumatic catheterization or a
bladder perforation, it is very risky to give BCG early.

Mensink: It is nice to hear that we have the expectation of a favorable response towards tumor recurrence by pumping in many baccilli into a patient. But, occasionally the patient might have a toxic or an allergic reaction. I would like to ask Dr. Lamm and Dr. Debruyne: is there any chance that, when a patient has this severe reaction one might have better expectations of the therapy? In other words: is there a correlation between this toxic effect and the tumor response?

Lamm: I have no data to suggest that that is true or false. However, I would be concerned about the patient who has a toxic reaction, and the objective should be to be able to prevent toxicity. We have not seen any reduction in efficacy by treating the toxic reaction. Again, there is a possibility to overwhelm the immune system and reduce the antitumor effect. The patient with a systemic infection may be a better candidate for having a reduced effect than an increased effect.

Debruyne: There are some severe side effects, although they are recorded in a very limited number of patients so far. There are two types of side effects. First of all the systemic side effects to which you alluded to. These side effects are very minimal and have in fact hardly been seen. When they are present they can easily be treated by conventional tuberculostatic therapy and no patient so far, as far as I know, has had life threatening situations. A precaution that we have included in our trials, and certainly in the combination trials with intradermal scarification, although we are not sure if it is necessary, is that patients with a history of previous tuberculosis were excluded for such a trial. But as far as we feel, it should not be an obligation for further studies to exclude these patients. A severe toxicity, and Dr. Lamm already mentioned it, was seen in our study in one patient and concerned a local reaction, but that is not directly due to the infectious reaction of BCG itself, but rather to the inflammatory reaction of the bladder mucosa. We have seen in one patient a severely scarred bladder. At the last annual meeting of the AUA there were more reports on these severe local side effects.

Kurth: Dr. Lamm, your results look so impressive that anybody who is involved with the treatment of superficial bladder tumor might ask: "Why should I go on with other drugs?" I have the following question: you told us that you stratified your patients according to different prognostic factors. Could you tell us whether all patients with any prognostic good or poor risk factor are likely to respond or are there differences? Can you identify a group of patients who have a higher chance to respond? My question is in fact a remark. You suggested a little bit that because Adriamycin is as good as Epodyl and Thiotepa is as good as Mitomycin-C it will make no difference if you work with Adriamycin or any other drug. This is not true.

Jakse: Since we have now at least five BCG strains and some of the companies or some of the investigators claim that their strain is the best one, do we have to go through the same procedure as we did with chemotherapeutic agents or is there any relevant animal system which is useful to look for the best strain and for the best dosage and schedule?

Harland: I wanted to ask about the local reaction - this is a question for Dr. Lamm - following BCG. I have the impression that, on occasion, it can give a very nasty cystitis. I do not think it is of any long-term consequence, but it is unpleasant for the patient at the times. I was wondering if you could tell us how the local side effects compared in the Adriamycin versus intravesical BCG randomized study.

Schröder: I would like to extend Dr. Kurth's question and ask Dr. Lamm if he has analysed whether the prognostic factors that are of any importance in this disease were equally distributed in the two arms of his Adriamycin/BCG study.

Hall: I just wanted to ask a follow-up to Dr. Jakse's question. I think Dr. Lamm stated that the Glaxo strain was inactive against tumor in the U.S.A. and I want a clarification of that. Is this also applicable to the Glaxo strain available elsewhere in the world and if so, on what basis do you make that statement?

Lamm: We actually have two inquiries about the prognostic factors in the Adriamycin and the BCG study. Patients were required to have two recurrences per 12 months for entry into the study. They were all documented histologically to have pTa or pTl tumors. All tumor grades were included and they were not stratified on the basis of tumor grade. Patients were stratified according to the presence or absence of previous chemotherapy: those numbers were equal. They were also stratified by the presence or absence of carcinoma in situ.

In terms of prognostic criteria I would ask the questioners if there is any prognostic criterion which will distinguish recurrence at a level of 0,00008.

In terms of: is there a best strain? I think, most of the strains are comparable. There are in fact animal studies which compare the different strains. The Glaxo preparation that is available in the U.S. through the local pharmacy contains 2-26 x 10^6 organisms which is 2% of the commonly used intravesical dose. We in our animal model, comparing Tice, Armand Frappier and Glaxo BCG, were unable to give the mouse enough Glaxo BCG to produce an antitumor effect. There are, however, clinical studies using Glaxo BCG that are reporting to observe an antitumor response. We also in the laboratory observed that Glaxo appeared to be inferior in inducing NK-response in vitro using human lymphocytes.

Debruyne: With regard to Dr. Jakse's question: of course there are not so many differences between the strains itself. It is not only the number of colony-forming units of bacteriae, but also their viability. There has been a publication in the Journal of Urology last year in which it was clearly demonstrated that the different lots can contain different amounts of baccillae, not only between the strains, but also within one strain. That could cause some differences with regard to results.

With regard to Dr. Kurth's question: there are, of course retrospectively, some indications that the patient will respond to BCG therapy. First of all, and I must agree here with Dr. Lamm, Dr. Fair's data are rather conflicting. But anyway, the patients in whom the PPD converted seem to react better, and there is an indication that patients in whom the urine after intravesical immunotherapy produced Interleukin-respond favourably to the BCG treatment. But this second method is rather sophisticated to use at the moment as a response criteria.

Kurth: One short comment to Dr. Lamm. When you look at the "time to first recurrence" curves shown by Dr. Fair, they looked rather different from yours. Maybe this was a very bad prognostic group. But your group too had no favourable prognostic signs, still your results are very impressive. We need repetition of these results. We need several nicely performed studies to show without any doubt that BCG is the best and the first drug for intravesical prophylaxis.

Lamm: Certainly I agree that more studies are needed. And I think the comment about the Memorial series being a highly select high risk group is very true. In their original control study all patients in the control group developed tumor recurrence by eight months and even with BCG the majority of patients developed tumor recurrence.

EORTC Genitourinary Group Monograph 5: Progress
and Controversies in Oncological Urology II, pages 539-548
© 1988 Alan R. Liss, Inc.

PROGRESS AND CONTROVERSIES IN CHEMOTHERAPY OF ADVANCED
UNRESECTABLE AND/OR METASTATIC CARCINOMA OF THE BLADDER

Hideyuki Akaza

Department of Urology, Faculty of Medicine,
The University of Tokyo
7-3-1 Hongo, Bunkyo-ku, Tokyo 113, Japan

INTRODUCTION

Striking advances have been made in chemotherapy of
cancers in recent years, and our conception of cancer
chemotherapy has undergone great change. In the field of
urology, for instance, in the last 10 years it has become
possible to cure testicular cancer even in cases with
distant metastases (Chabner, 1984).

Prior to 1980, chemotherapy of advanced unresectable
and/or metastatic bladder cancer was able to achieve a
temporary beneficial effect, but it was not considered to
be capable of achieving a clear life-prolonging effect
(Devita, 1982). However, in recent years, the results of
clinical trials employing combination chemotherapy have -
at least in terms of the response rate - documented a
degree of efficacy which apparently requires us to
reconsider our prevailing conception regarding chemotherapy (Yagoda, 1983).

In the near future, will chemotherapy of bladder
cancer be able to achieve success comparable to that
attained in relation to testicular cancer?

From this viewpoint, I would like to analyze the main
clinical trial results that have been reported to date.

COMPARISON OF RESULTS OF STUDIES ON CHEMOTHERAPY OF
ADVANCED UNRESECTABLE AND/OR METASTATIC BLADDER CANCER

There have already been a number of excellent reviews (de Kernion, 1977; Yagoda, 1983; Stoter, 1985) published with regard to the efficacy rates of single-drug chemotherapy and combination chemotherapy in the treatment of advanced unresectable and/or metastatic bladder cancer. Thus, there is no reason to perform yet another similar review here since space is limited. Instead , it is intended to properly select from the many recent reports studies which comprised a comparatively large number of cases and employed an established evaluation method, and to carry out a comparison of those studies so as to achieve a clearer understanding of the actual current status of chemotherapy of advanced unresectable and/or metastatic bladder cancer.

Table 1 compiles, for those selected studies, the data on the administered drugs, number of evaluable cases, response rates (complete response (CR) + partial response (PR)), 95% confidence limits (in the case that these data were not provided in the published report, they were calculated on the basis of the number of cases and the response rate and presented in Table 1), median duration of response, median survival length and references.

Comparison of the response rates shows large variations among the studies. For single-drug chemotherapy, from 14% to 43%, and for combination chemotherapy, from 17% to 71%. In addition, the range of 95% confidence limits was broad. There were no statistically significant differences among the trials (by the chi-square test) if one excludes from the comparison those studies which showed extremely low response rates, i.e., on Adriamycin (ADM) (by Yagoda, 1977), cisplatinum (CDDP) + ADM + cyclophosphamide (CTX) (by Maru, 1987), and methotrexate (MTX) (a trial on patients with recurrent tumors; by Oliver, 1984), and a study which showed a very high response rate, i.e., MTX + vinblastine (VBL) + ADM + CDDP (M-VAC therapy; by Sternberg, 1985).

If the median duration of response is compared, the longest duration was 17 months and the shortest duration was 2.5 months; all the other studies showed durations within the range of 4 months to 9 months. This tendency to uniformity in the median duration of response in the studies is even clearer in the case of comparison of the median survival length. That is, in the ADM single-drug

Table 1. Results of Chemotherapy on Advanced Bladder Cancer

Agent(s)	No. of patients	Response rates* (CR+PR)	95% confidence limits	Median duration of response (CR+PR)	Median survival length	Investigators
1) ADM	35 measurable	14%	4.7%~30%	2.5 mos	CR+PR+MR+Stab: 21 mos	Yagoda 1977
2) CDDP	21 measurable	43%	22%~66%	average CR:17 mos PR:5.7 mos		Herr 1980
MTX 3)	32 recurrent	28%	14%~47%	6 mos		Oliver 1984
4)	21 metastatic	43%	22%~66%	6 mos		
5) CDDP ADM CTX	28 bidimensional	46%	28%~66%	8 mos	responder:91 wks non-responder: 38 wks	Schwartz 1983
6) CDDP ADM CTX	96 bidimensional	17%	9.8%~26%	16 wks	responder:45 wks MR+Stab:39 wks PD:19 wks overall:29 wks	Maru 1987
7) MTX ADM CDDP	38 measurable	39%	24%~57%	6 mos	responder:54 wks non-responder: 24 wks	Tannock 1983

(Table 1. continued)

8) MTX } VBL }	47 bidimensional	40%	26%~56%	8 mos	responder:14 mos non-responder: 8 mos	Ahmed 1985
9) CDDP } MTX } VBL }	50 metastatic evaluable	56% (CR:14 cases)	42%~70%	CR:9 mos	CR:11 mos PR: 7 mos non-responder: 6 mos	Harker 1985
10) MTX } VBL } ADM } CDDP }	24 bidimensional	71% (CR:12 cases)	CR+PR:49%~87% CR:30%~70%	CR:9.5 mos (+)		Sternberg 1985
11) 5Fu } ADM } CDDP } VM26 }	36 evaluable	53% (CR:4 cases)	35%~70%	26 wks	overall:44 wks	Veronesi 1986

* 1 vs. 2, 4, 5, 7, 8 $P < 0.05$,   2 vs. 6 $P < 0.05$,   3 vs. 9 $P < 0.05$
  1 vs. 9, 10, 11 $P < 0.01$,   3 vs. 10, 11 $P < 0.01$,   4 vs. 6 $P < 0.05$
  5 vs. 6 $P < 0.01$,   6 vs. 7, 8, 9, 10, 11 $P < 0.05$,   7 vs. 10 $P < 0.05$
  8 vs. 10 $P < 0.05$

chemotherapy study, which showed the lowest response rate, the median survival length was the longest: 21 months for the total cases when excluding only the progressive disease (PD) cases. Similarly, the median survival rates for the responders in the other clinical studies ranged from 10 months to 20 months. There was thus no great difference detected between these studies in terms of the median survival length. This fact probably indicates the limits of present-day chemotherapy of advanced unresectable and/or metastatic bladder cancer.

There is an opinion (Van Oosterom, 1986) that it is necessary to compare the overall survival rate if one desires to investigate the life-prolonging efficacy of chemotherapies. This is because, even if the survival rate for only responder cases is higher than the survival rate for the nonresponder cases, this is merely equivalent to separating the treated subjects into the patients with a good prognosis and the patients with a poor prognosis. In fact, however, the efficacy of the chemotherapy is perhaps not very strongly involved in the survival rate. There have been very few reports which clearly recorded the overall survival rate, and moreover it is no exaggeration to say that at present, at least with regard to progressive metastatic bladder cancer, there are absolutely no reports of studies that were carried out as a well-controlled randomized trial including untreated patients.

Among the reports selected and reviewed here by the author, only two provided data on the overall median survival length. One was a study employing CDDP + ADM + CTX (Maru, 1987) and the other dealt with 5Fu + ADM + CDDP + VM26 (Veronesi, 1986). The overall median survival lengths in these two studies were 29 weeks and 44 weeks. It is interesting that, although there was a big difference in the response rates in these two studies (17% vs. 53%, $P < 0.05$), the difference in their overall survival lengths was not statistically significant (Cox-Mantel $P \doteq 0.127$, generalized-Wilcoxson $P \doteq 0.313$).

A more detailed analysis was made of the results reported (Maru, 1987) by The Japanese Urological Cancer Research Group for Adriamycin (Chairman: T. Niijima). Figure 1 shows the actual survival curves for the total evaluated cases and for each type of response. The generalized Wilcoxon test found statistically significant differences between CR and minor response (MR), and for PD versus the sum of CR, PR and no change (NC). However, the overall survival curve showed no significant improvement compared with a historical control (Akaza, 1985).

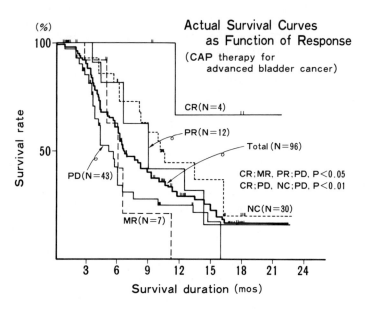

Figure 1. Survival of 96 patients with advanced bladder cancer according to response to CAP treatment.

In the comparison carried out here, the differences in the background factors of the subject patients and the differences in the evaluation methods between the various clinical studies were ignored. Therefore, it is obvious that the differences in the patient populations have greatly influenced the data for the response rates and the survival length, and the comparison of the relative merits of the therapeutic methods themselves was accompanied by great difficulty. For example, even in the case of clinical trials carried out separately by the same regimen (i.e., Maru, 1987, and Schwartz, 1983), it was not unusual for the response rates to be completely different (17% vs. 46%, P < 0.01). However, the antitumor efficacy of combination chemotherapy in recent years has also seemed to be showing steady improvement even in the treatment of advanced unresectable and/or metastatic bladder cancer. This impression is supported by the increased number of CR cases that have been reported by Harker et al. (1985) and Sternberg et al. (1985). Especially in the case of M-VAC therapy (Sternberg, 1985), a CR rate of 50% was achieved. If it can be confirmed by the results of subsequent long-term follow-up that both the disease-free interval and the survival duration are also prolonged, then it will probably mean that even in this field the progress achieved in chemotherapy has been epoch-making.

THE CENTRAL NERVOUS SYSTEM (CNS) AS THE MOST-FORWARD BATTLE-LINE BETWEEN CANCER AND CHEMOTHERAPY

In recent years, it has been recognized that there is CNS involvement in some cases of relapse after attaining CR or PR by means of chemotherapy of cancer. In the clinical reports that have been surveyed here, as well, a new brain metastasis was detected in 1 of 2 CR cases by Schwartz et al. (1983), 4 of 19 responders by Ahmed (1985), 1 of 14 CR cases by Harker et al. (1985), and 2 of 12 CR cases and 1 of 5 PR cases by Sternberg et al. (1985). This fact of CNS metastatic relapse indicates (1) that the survival period of patients with advanced unresectable and/or metastatic bladder cancer has been extended to some degree by chemotherapy (Yagoda, 1985) and, at the same time, (2) the need to declare war in an unavoidable battle at the blood-brain barrier if we desire to achieve further improvement in the efficacy of chemo-therapy. To date, it has been common for the drug dosage, administration method, duration of administration, con-comitant drugs, etc., of chemotherapeutic regimens to be decided on the basis of experience. Therefore, it is logical that it should be possible to develop much more potent chemotherapeutic regimens by the application of proven scientific research and development techniques.

PROSPECTS

It is thought that there are two factors resulting in the failure of chemotherapy of cancers. One is that the cancer cells have temporary resistance to the chemo-therapeutic agent, while the second is that the cancer cells have developed permanent resistance to the drug. Temporary resistance is considered to arise from the existence of pharmacologic sanctuaries, which make it impossible for the drug to make actual contact with the cancer cells, or altered cell kinetics, a state in which the anticancer drug is unable to express its activity. Permanent resistance, on the other hand, means that the cancer is comprised of a cell line which has native resistance to the anticancer agent. DeVita (1983) wrote of the prospects of giving the cancer cell a series of impossible choices (Table 2). In fact, one group reported designing a therapeutic study on the basis of this theory (Natale, 1985), and good results were obtained. This theory can thus be thought to be a very good criterion for establishing chemotherapy as a truly useful method of treatment of cancer.

Table 2. <u>Presenting the Cancer Cell a Series of Impossible Choices (DeVita, 1983)</u>

I. Expose it to alternating cycles of non-cross-resistant drug combinations

   RESULTS: Cure of some fraction of patients
   - Remaining fraction of patients have residual "resistant" cell lines
   - Resistant cell lines may be
     —Permanently resistant
     —"Temporarily" resistant
     —In sanctuaries
   - Resistant lines may have developed collateral sensitivity to drugs previously ineffective

II. Attack mechanism of resistance
   - Pleiotropic transport resistance due to P-glycoprotein
     —Monoclonal antibodies directed at cells containing protein
     —Other
   - Single drug specific resistance
     —Eliminate drug
     —Manipulate drug dose or structure

III. Exploit collateral sensitivity
   - Identify direction of development of collateral sensitivity
   - Intersperse combinations of drugs made collaterally effective

The use of an accurate and objective evaluation method to conduct well-controlled randomized studies and develop combination chemotherapy regimens in line with this theory is thought to be the quickest way to elevate the position of chemotherapy for treatment of advanced unresectable and/or metastatic bladder cancer to a position comparable to that held by chemotherapy in the treatment of testicular cancer.

REFERENCES

Ahmed T, Yagoda A, Needles B, Scher HI, Watson RC, Geller N (1985). Vinblastine and methotrexate for advanced bladder cancer. J Urol 133:602-604.

Akaza H, Koseki K, Kishi H, Umeda T, Isurugi K, Niijima T (1986). Multidisciplinary treatment of invasive bladder cancer. Jpn J Urol 77:716-721.

Chabner BA, Fine RL, Allegra CJ, Yeh GW, Curt GA (1984). Cancer chemotherapy, Progress and expectations, 1984. Cancer 54:2599-2608.

deKernion JB (1977). The chemotherapy of advanced bladder carcinoma. Cancer Res 37:2771-2774.

DeVita VT, Jr (1982). Cancer-principles and practice of oncology. DeVita VT, Jr, Hellman S, Rosenberg SA (eds): Philadelphia, Tronto, Lippincott JB.

DeVita VT, Jr (1983). The James Ewing lecture, The relationship between tumor mass and resistance to chemotherapy, Implications for surgical adjuvant treatment of cancer. Cancer 51:1209-1220.

Harker WG, Meyers FJ, Freiha FS, Palmer JM, Shortliffe LD, Hannigan JF, McWhirter KM, Torti FM (1985). Cisplatin, Methotrexate, and Vinblastine (CMV): An effective chemotherapy regimen for metastatic transitional cell carcinoma of the urinary tract, A Northern California Oncology Group study. J Clin Oncol 3:1463-1470.

Herr HW (1980). Cis-diamminedichloride platinum II in the treatment of advanced bladder cancer. J Urol 123:853-855.

Maru A, Akaza H, Isaka S, et al (1987). Phase III trial of the Japanese urological cancer research group for adriamycin: Cyclophosphamide, adriamycin, and cis-platinum versus cyclophosphamide, adriamycin and 5-fluorouracil in patients with advanced transitional cell carcinoma of the urinary bladder. Cancer Chemother Pharmacol (in press).

Natale RB, Wittes RE (1985). Alternating combination chemotherapy regimens in small-cell lung cancer. Seminars in Oncol 1(suppl 2):7-13.

Oliver RTD, England HR, Risdon RA, Blandy JP (1984). Methotrexate in the treatment of metastatic and recurrent primary transitional cell carcinoma. J Urol 131: 483-485.

Schwartz S, Yagoda A, Natale RB, Watson RC, Whitmore WF, Lesser M (1983). Phase II trial of sequentially administered cisplatin, cyclophosphamide and doxorubicin for urothelial tract tumors. J Urol 130:681-684.

Sternberg CN, Yagoda A, Scher HI, et al (1985). Preliminary results of M-VAC (methotrexate, vinblastine, doxorubicin and cisplatin) for transitional cell carcinoma of the urothelium. J Urol 133:403-407.

Stoter G (1985). Chemotherapy for metastatic bladder carcinoma. World J Urol 3:110-114.

Tannock IF, Gospodarowicz M, Evans WK (1983). Chemotherapy for metastatic transitional carcinoma of the urinary tract, A prospective trial of methotrexate, adriamycin, and cyclophosphamide (MAC) with cis-platinum for failure. Cancer 51:216-219.

Van Oosterom AT, Akaza H, Hall R, Hirao Y, Jones WG, Matsumura Y, Raghaven D, Tannock IF, Yagoda A (1986). Response criteria phase II/phase III invasive bladder cancer. In; Denis L, Niijima T, Prout G, Jr, Schröder FH (eds): Developments in bladder cancer, New York, Alan R Liss, pp 301-310.

Veronesi A, Galligioni E, Lore G, Sorio R, Saracchini S, Francini M, Merlo A, Dalbo V, Monfardini S (1986). Combination chemotherapy with fluorouracil, adriamycin, cis-platinum and VM-26 in advanced transitional cell carcinoma of the urinary tract. Eur J Cancer Clin Oncol 22:1457-1460.

Yagoda A, Watson RC, Whitmore WF, Grabstald H, Middleman MP, Krakoff IH (1977). Adriamycin in advanced urinary tract cancer, Experience in 42 patients and review of the literature. Cancer 39:279-285.

Yagoda A (1983). Chemotherapy for advanced urothelial cancer. Seminars in Urol 1:60-74.

Yagoda A (1985). Progress in treatment of advanced urothelial tract tumors. J Clin Oncol 3:1448-1450.

EORTC Genitourinary Group Monograph 5: Progress
and Controversies in Oncological Urology II, page 549
© 1988 Alan R. Liss, Inc.

Discussion: Progress and Controversies in Chemotherapy of
Advanced Unresectable and/or Metastatic Carcinoma of the
Bladder

Gerrit Stoter, Rotterdam, The Netherlands

Van Oosterom: Thank you, Professor Akaza. The paper is open
for discussion.

N.N.: Much of your discussion was centered around survival.
I understand that most of the data you showed were from
phase II studies. Phase II studies are aimed at reporting
responses. How can it be that you discussed all this
survival business on the basis of only phase II studies. In
my opinion it cannot be used for anything at all.

Akaza: You got a good point. However, in my opinion phase II
and phase III studies should all be used to determine survival. That is why I made this analysis.

N.N.: You showed that patients with CR survived significantly longer than patients who did not achieve CR. On the
other hand, the total group of patients survived exactly as
long as the historical controls. Can you explain that to me?
I think this indicates that the comparison of survival with
historical controls is very dubious indeed.

Gad el Mawla: Have you noticed that the responses in distant
metastases are better than in locally advanced cases? We
noticed that in our experience in Egypt.

Akaza: I did not analyze that.

EORTC Genitourinary Group Monograph 5: Progress
and Controversies in Oncological Urology II, pages 551–565
© 1988 Alan R. Liss, Inc.

INTRA-ARTERIAL CHEMOTHERAPY FOR BLADDER CANCER:
ITS RESULTS AND FUTURE ROLE

Tetsuro Kato, Kazunari Sato, Ryoetsu Abe and
Masatsugu Moriyama

Department of Urology
Akita University School of Medicine
Akita 010, Japan

INTRODUCTION

Since the early 1950's, intra-arterial (IA) chemotherapy has been frequently used for the treatment of localized malignancies, with an attempt to enhance the therapeutic effects of anticancer drugs (Bierman et al, 1950; Klopp
et al, 1950). Advance in the percutaneous catheterization
technique has also made this treatment modality readily
applicable to a variety of tumor-bearing organs such as the
liver, kidney, lung, head and neck, bone and intrapelvic
organs including the bladder. Theoretically IA chemotherapy
may deliver a high drug concentration into the targeted area
and at the same time reduce the drug levels in the systemic
circulation, thus increasing the therapeutic index of the
cytotoxic agents. If this commonly occurs, invasive bladder
cancer of which prognosis is still unsatisfactory (Klimberg
and Wajsman, 1986) will be one of the best candidates for IA
chemotherapy. However, "we really do not know if IA chemotherapy is better for local disease than intravenous (IV)
chemotherapy, if there is a systemic effect comparable to IV
chemotherapy, if the over-all toxicity is truly less than IV
chemotherapy, which drugs are pharmacologically best suited
for IA chemotherapy, what doses or schedule can be tolerated
or if adding other modifications is valuable" (Montie, 1986).

EXPERIMENTAL BASIS

Takai et al (1960), by infusing 32P solution into the
inferior vena cava, abdominal aorta and hypogastric artery,

reported a ratio of 32P concentration in the bladder tissues of each group of 1:3:6 during the observed period of 30 minutes, suggesting an advantage of selective IA chemotherapy. In the same experiment, they showed that there was no difference in systemic blood levels of 32P among the 3 experimental groups. Comparing IA and IV administration of cisplatin (CDDP) in cancer patients, Stewart et al (1983) found that pharmacokinetic parameters in plasma and urine after IA infusion were similar to those after IV infusion, and concluded that IA administration of CDDP results in increased drug exposure of tumor in the infused area without substantially decreasing exposure of systemic tumor.

A linear,physiologically based pharmacokinetic model was used by Chen and Gross (1980) to study drug delivery characteristics of anticancer drugs after both IV and IA chemotherapy. It confirmed the general belief that IA infusion produces an increase in local tissue levels and a reduction in systemic drug availability. The increase in local drug concentration depends largely on the blood flow rate of the infusing artery and the rate of drug elimination by the rest of the body; a low arterial blood flow rate and a high drug elimination rate will ensure a high local drug level. On the other hand, lower systemic availability will be obtained if a substantial amount of the drug is removed during the first pass through the infused region. Anderson et al (1981), by combining IA infusion of 14C-labeled 5-fluorouracil (5-FU) with temporary vascular occlusion using double lumen balloon catheter in the external iliac artery of dogs, increased the local 5-FU concentration 7 to 9 times compared with that produced by IA infusion alone.

Reviewing the biophysical targeting of anticancer drug, Widder et al (1979) identified three stages of targeting. First-order targeting involves the restricted distribution to the predetermined vascular beds and the transendothelial migration of the drug or drug-carrier complex. Second-order targeting refers to the selective direction of the drug to tumor cells within the tissue parenchyma. Third-order targeting involves the enhanced interaction between the drug and tumor cells. The first-order targeting may be well consistent with the first-pass effect described by Chen and Gross (1980). To design a strategy for drug targeting, it appears most essential to achieve the first-order targeting (Kato, 1983).

The authors and associates developed ethylcellulose microencapsulation of anticancer drugs for IA chemotherapy, introducing a new therapeutic concept of chemoembolization to achieve the first-order targeting (Kato and Nemoto, 1978; Kato et al, 1981; Kato, 1983). When the microcapsules (mc) are infused intra-arterially, they are entrapped by the target arteriolar beds, make hemostasis and then gradually release the encased drug. Animal experiments demonstrated a sustained drug activity in the target tissues such as the kidney, bladder, prostate and regional lymph nodes, and a decrease in systemic blood levels of the drug as compared with those by IA drug infusion either alone or in combination with embolization. Clinical pharmacokinetic studies and findings of antitumor effects confirmed these experimental results, indicating an enhanced therapeutic effect on target tumors with a decrease in systemic drug toxicity (Kato, 1983; Nemoto and Kato, 1981; Okamoto et al, 1986). Microcapsules of mitomycin C (MMC-mc), peplomycin (PEP-mc) and cisplatin (CDDP-mc) with a mean particle size of approximately 200 μm and with various release rates have been developed as a prototype of targeting drug delivery systems (Kato et al, (1985).Magnetic control of the microcapsules has also been investigated to facilitate the drug targeting (Kato et al, 1984).

CLINICAL EXPERIENCES IN LITERATURE

Bonner et al (1952) treated 16 patients with inoperable cancer in various sites with IA infusion of nitrogen mustard. Two patients with bladder cancer obtained pain relief. Though they observed subjective or objective improvement in 44 % of the patients, they encountered certain technical difficulties requiring great caution. Takai et al (1960) treated 15 patients with stages A-D bladder cancer by IA infusion of nitromin and/or chromomycin A either alone in 3 patients or in combination with radiation and/or surgery in 12. Posttreatment histological examination revealed a rest of tumor cells in the 3 patients treated with IA chemotherapy alone, but no tumor cells in 10 of the 12 patients combined with radiation, indicating the need of combination therapy.

Ogata et al (1973) reported 33 patients with T1-4 disease treated with continuous IA infusion of MMC. Cystoscopically partial response (PR) was found in 12 patients and complete response (CR) in 5, thus making the response rate

Table 1. Intra-arterial Chemotherapy in Bladder Cancer

References	No.Pts.	Drugs[@]	Concurrent Treatments	Responses (CR+PR)
Takai et al (1960)	15	NTM,CMA	Radiation	#67%
Ogata et al (1973)	33	MMC	-	52%(5CR)
Nevin et al (1974)	15	5FU /BLM,ADR	Radiation	93%(9CR)
Nakazono & Iwata(1981)	13	ADR	-	69%(3CR)
Wallace et al (1982)	15	CDDP	-	60%
Jacobs & Lawson(1982)	9	ADR	Hyper- thermia	#11%
Logothetis et al(1982)	29	5FU	ADR,MMC(iv)	58%
Kanoh et al (1983)	13	ADR	-	70%
Uyama et al (1983)	20	ADR	-	89%(13CR) #31%
Kato (1984)	49	MMC-/PEP- /CDDP-mc	-	63%(24/38)
Jacobs et al (1984)	6	CDDP	Hyper- thermia	#33%
Stewart et al (1984)	7	CDDP	-	100%(4/4, 3CR)
Logothetis et al(1985)	29	CP,ADR, CDDP	CP,ADR, CDDP(iv)	64%(11CR)
Maatman et al (1986)	25	CDDP /ADR	CP(iv)	75%(6CR) #19%
Mitsuhata et al(1986)	20	CDDP,ADR	Angiotensin	85%(9CR) #27%
Ozono et al (1987)	22	MMC-mc	Embolization	41%
Kato et al (1987)	99	MMC-/PEP- /CDDP-mc	-	57%(35/61)

@;ADR-adriamycin,BLM-bleomycin,CDDP-cisplatin,CMA-chromomy-
cin A,CP-cyclophosphamide,5FU-5fluorouracil,MMC-mitomycin
C,NTM-nitromin,PEP-peplomycin,mc-microcapsule.
#;pathological CR(pTo).

(CR+PR) 52%. These patients were followed by transurethral resection (TUR) or partial cystectomy. Five years later, 22 patients were alive with (6) or without (16) tumors, 5 were dead of cancer (one in T3 and 4 in T4), and 6 were dead of other disease (Sakamoto et al, 1981). Nevin et al (1974) reported 15 patients with inoperable stages C-D cancer, who received IA infusion of 5-FU with or without bleomycin (BLM) or adriamycin (ADR). Radiation was also combined in 14 patients. They achieved 93% response rate (9 CR), and 12 patients were reported to be alive without disease for 6 to 66 months (median survival, 42 months).

In the 1980's, there is an increasing number of clinical reports on IA chemotherapy in the treatment of bladder cancer (Table 1). ADR, 5FU, cyclophosphamide (CP), CDDP and microcapsules (MMC-mc, PEP-mc, CDDP-mc) have been used as a single agent or in combination. CDDP seems to be a current choice. In half of these trials, other treatments such as hyperthermia or IV chemotherapy have been combined with an attempt to enhance the topical or systemic effect of IA chemotherapy. Despite the considerably high dose schedules as compared with IV chemotherapy, the majority of the patients have been reported to tolerate well the treatment employed. With the response rate (CR+PR) ranging from 41 to 100%, the investigators have suggested or claimed the superiority of IA chemotherapy in the management of locally advanced bladder cancer.

Response to the treatment will depend on: first, drugs and dose schedules; second, situations of the tumor such as grade, stage, vascularity and chemosensitivity; third, catheter technique (selectivity of drug delivery); and fourth, modifications of infusion technique or dosage form and conbination of other treatments. Also the response rate will be influenced by the number of subjects investigated. There are large variations of these factors among the individual series reviewed, which makes it difficult to evaluate each treatment protocol. On the other hand, there still are only a small number of reports on histological evaluation. Histologically tumor-free rates in the biopsy or surgical specimens have been reported as 67% (10/15; Takai et al, 1960), 11% (1/9; Jacobs and Lawson, 1982), 31% (5/16; Uyama et al, 1983), 33% (2/6; Jacobs et al, 1984), 19% (3/16; Maatman et al, 1986) and 27% (4/15; Mitsuhata et al, 1986), respectively. Maatman et al (1986), by studying 16 cystectomy specimens of T3 disease which clinically responded (CR in 6 and PR in 10), found pT0 in 3 cases, pT1 in 1, pT3 in 11 and pT4 in 1. Of the 6 cases with clinical CR, 3 had pT0, 1 had pT1 and 2 had pT3. Of the 10 cases with clinical PR, 9 had pT3 (no change) and 1 had pT4 (up staged). This means that, although IA chemotherapy with or without other therapy often provides a remarkable tumor response clinically, it does not always eradicate the tumor cells within the bladder muscle layer. The same findings were described by others (Jacobs and Lawson, 1982; Jacobs et al, 1984).

IA chemotherapy has been often used as a palliative measure for inoperable, advanced tumor with or without distant metastasis. It often relieves the patient from intractable life-threatening symptoms such as pain and hematuria (Wallace et al, 1982; Abe et al, 1982; Stewart et al, 1984). Furthermore, it seems likely to prolong the survival of the select patients with unresectable stages C-D disease. Twelve of 15 patients treated with IA-5FU and radiation (Nevin et al, 1974) were alive without tumor for a median survival of 42 months. Nine responders in 15 patients treated with IA-CDDP (Wallace et al, 1982) survived for a median period of 52 weeks. Median survivals of 17 responders and 12 nonresponders to IA-5FU combined with IV-ADR and MMC (Logothetis et al, 1982) were 52 and 28 weeks respectively. Median survival of 11 patient with CR to IA-CISCA combined with IV-CISCA (Logothetis et al, 1985) was 62 weeks, while those of 17 patients with PR and no response were 29 and 25 weeks.

Some investigators have employed IA chemotherapy as a preoperative measure with an attempt to prevent local recurrence and even the distant metastasis after operation. This approach can be used as an adjuvant to bladder preserving operation for T2-3 tumors. Ogata et al (1973) treated 12 patients with TUR or partial cystectomy following IA-MMC; 6 patients were alive without recurrence, 2 had recurrence but alive, 3 died of other disease and 1 died of cancer within five years. Sato et al (1986) analyzed 29 patients treated by TUR or partial cystectomy with preoperative microcapsule therapy (15 patients) or without the adjuvant (14 patients); both the disease-free and actuarial survivals of the adjuvant group were significantly superior to the non-adjuvant group. On the other hand, IA chemotherapy has also been used as a preoperative measure for total cystectomy. Kanoh et al (1983) performed total cystectomy in 7 patients with T3-4 disease after IA-ADR; 5 patients were alive without tumor for 6 to 31 months, 1 died of sepsis and 1 died of cancer.

Maatman et al (1986) cystectomized 18 patients with T3 disease after IA-CDDP either alone or in combination with IA-ADR or IV CP; 16 patients were alive for 1 to 28 months, 1 died of cancer and 1 died of unrelated disease.

Systemic side effects related to the drugs used have been frequently experienced at various degrees. These include bone marrow suppression, gastrointestinal discomfort, alopecia, and/or neurologic disturbance. Though most investigators including us believe that a much higher dose can be tolerated in IA chemotherapy, there is no proof to support the general concept that systemic toxicity is reduced in IA chemotherapy compared with IV chemotherapy (Chen and Gross, 1980; Haskell et al, 1975). Intractable complication characteristic of IA chemotherapy is the buttock skin reaction such as eruption, erosion or ulcer. It is caused by drug migration into the non-target vascular branches such as the superior and inferior gluteal arteries. When selective catheterization fails, temporary occlusion of the non-target arteries by balloon or embolic materials is recommended. Drugs highly toxic to normal tissues, such as 5FU, MMC and ADR, are responsible for this complication, but CDDP, BLM and PEP do not cause such a skin reaction.

RECENT RESULT OF INTRA-ARTERIAL MICROCAPSULE THERAPY

During the past 8 years, 99 patients with bladder tumor have been subjected to percutaneous IA infusion of microencapsulated anticancer drugs (chemoembolization). Mean patient's age was 67 years (34-83 years), and male and female ratio was 75:25. Clinical stages were A in 16 patients, B in 31, C in 20 and D in 32, and 67 patients underwent operation after microcapsule therapy (Table 2). MMC-mc, PEP-mc and CDDP-mc were used as a single agent or their combination with a mean number of treatment of 1.5 (1-3) and a mean interval of treatment was 30 days (Table 3).

Of 61 evaluable cases, 35 (57%) had an objective response (CR and PR), 8 had a minor response of less than 50%, 15 had no change and 3 had progressive disease. Side effects were experienced as follows: fever in 41% of the patients (6%, need for medical cares), pain in 39% (11%), gastro-intestinal discomfort in 23% (6%), myelosuppression in 22% (4%), and skin erosion in 13% (6%). No patient experienced any symptom related to distant migration of microcapsules except for the buttock erosion, and all patients tolerated the IA microcapsule chemoembolization.

Fifty-three patients are, thus far, alive, 28 died of cancer and 18 died of other disease. Five-year Kaplan-Meier survival rate was 92% for stage A disease, 59% for stage B-C disease and 5.6% for stage D disease (Fig. 1). When these patients were compared with the patients treated without microcapsule therapy during the same period in our hospital, there was no statistical difference in the prognosis for each of stage A and D diseases. For stages B-C disease, however, significant improvement of prognosis was found in the patients with microcapsule therapy (MC-group) compared with the control patients. Details of the analysis will be described below.

The MC-group consisted of 47 patients with T2 tumor in 18 and T3 in 29, of whom 41 were followed by surgery (TUR in 17

Table 2. Patients Subjected to Microcapsule Therapy

Stages	No.Pts.	Surgery	TUR	PCX	TCX
A	16	12 (75%)	7	2	3
B	31	29 (94%)	15	4	10
C	20	14 (70%)	2	2	10
D	32	12 (38%)	2	0	10
Totals	99	67 (68%)	26	8	33

Table 3. Microcapsule Therapy in Bladder Cancer

Microcapsules	No.Pts	Total Dose#	No.Treatment#
MMC	41	27 mg	1.4
PEP	19	69 mg	1.4
CDDP	13	109 mg	1.4
MMC + PEP	5	60 mg	1.6
MMC + CDDP	21	113 mg	1.6

mean value

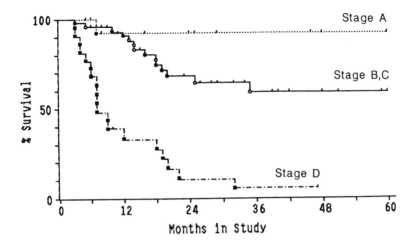

Figure 1. Actuarial survival curves of 99 patients with bladder cancer subjected to intra-arterial microcapsule therapy (1978 - 1986).

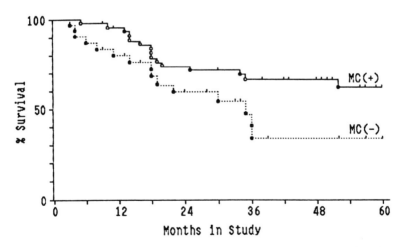

Figure 2. Actuarial survival curves of T2-3(MO) bladder cancer with (MC+, n=47) or without (MC-, n=32) microcapsule therapy (1978 - 1986). Difference between the two groups is significant (p < 0.05).

and cystectomy in 24). The control-group included 32 patients with T2 tumor in 19 and T3 in 13, of whom 30 underwent surgery (TUR in 17 and cystectomy in 13). The age distribution was the same between both groups, but the male population was predominant in the MC-group. Patients who died within 3 months after the onset of treatment were excluded from the study. In the MC-group, 24 patients are alive without disease so far, 4 are alive with tumor, 10 died of cancer and 8 died of other disease. In the control-group, 16 patients are alive without tumor, 1 is alive with tumor, 10 died of cancer and 5 died of other causes. A five-year survival rate of 62% in the MC-group was well contrasted with that of 34% in the control-group (p< 0.05, generalized Wilcoxon test)(Fig. 2). Of these groups, 36 patients in the MC-group and 27 in the control-group were evaluated to be curatively operated; the five-year survival rate was 75% in the MC-group while 43% in the control-group. Possibly due to the follow-up period and patient number, the difference in prognosis between the two groups remained insignificant (p < 0.1). However, these findings may indicate the beneficial effect of the preoperative IA chemotherapy in the treatment of invasive bladder cancer.

COMMENT

At present several treatment options are available in the treatment of bladder cancer. These include surgical resection with or without bladder preservation, topical or systemic chemotherapy and radiotherapy. But the place of the individual treatment modalities still remains controversial mainly because of the lack of a randomized study as well as an experimental study. Regardless of aggressive therapy, more than half of the patients with locally invasive bladder cancer have died of this disease within 5 years. Death will be caused by clinically undetectable (microscopic) distant metastasis, regional lymph node metastasis beyond the limitation of surgical or radiological treatment, tumor dissemination or implantation during surgery and/or tumor rest escaped from the treatments. Optimal treatment protocols are desired to be established earlier.

Although there has not yet been a controlled study, previous investigations reviewed in this article will indicate that IA chemotherapy in general exerts an enhanced effect on the targeted tumor. The response rates appear to be far superior to those by IV chemotherapy, indicating the benefit of IA chemotherapy for locally invasive tumors. But, even when the tumors disappeared clinically, some tumor cells will remain viable within the bladder wall (Maatman et al, 1986). In this respect, IA chemotherapy should be effectively combined with surgery to cure the patients. The authors have achieved an improved prognosis in T2-3 disease by combination with preoperative microcapsule therapy and surgery. The most effective use of IA chemotherapy must be as the adjuvant prior to TUR and cystectomy.

Systemic toxicity by IA chemotherapy, in another way, may reflect a systemic therapeutic effect. This will be the case for CDDP (Stewart et al, 1983). But there is no proof if IA chemotherapy has a systemic effect comparable to IV chemotherapy. Most urologists consider IA chemotherapy as having a lower systemic toxicity, and combine it with IV chemotherapy in the treatment of disseminated diseases (Logothetis et al, 1982). Another problem in IA chemotherapy is if it has any effect on the regional lymphatics. Nemoto and Kato (1981) demonstrated a sustained but low drug activity in lymph nodes of dogs after IA infusion of MMC-mc, while they failed to detect the drug after nonencapsulated MMC infusion. Further information is needed in respect to lymphatic drug delivery.

Despite the long experience for more than 30 years, the place of IA chemotherapy is still dubious. It is needed for IA chemotherapy to establish its own province as a targeted drug delivery. Recent advances in pharmaceutical technology will provide various drug-carrier systems, other than the microcapsules, suitable to IA chemotherapy. Integration with biotechnology may, in part, lead us to know the real role of IA chemotherapy in cancer treatment.

ACKNOWLEDGMENTS

The authors appreciate the co-operation of Dr. Y. Tamakawa in the microcapsule therapy, of Mr. A. Goto for the preparation of microcapsules and of Miss H. Kato for the preparation of the manuscript.
This work was supported in part by a Grant-in-Aid for Cancer Research from the Ministry of Education, Science and Culture of Japan.

REFERENCES

Abe R, Kato T, Mori H, Etori K, Shindo M, Nemoto R, Miura K, Shimizu S (1982). Hemostatic effects of chemoembolization using encapsulated anticancer drugs on intractable bleeding from intrapelvic cancers. Jpn J Clin Urol 36:637-641.

Anderson JH, Gianturco C, Wallace S (1981). Experimental transcatheter intra-arterial infusion-occlusion chemotherapy. Invest Radiol 16:496-500.

Bierman HR, Byron RL, Miller ER, et al (1950). Effect of intra-arterial administration of nitrogen mustard. Am J Med 8:535.

Bonner C, Thurman A, Honberger F (1952). A critical study of regional intra-arterial nitrogen mustard therapy in cancer. Ann Surg 136:912-918.

Chen HSG, Gross JF (1980). Intra-arterial infusion of anticancer drugs; theoretic aspects of drug delivery and review of responses. Cancer Treat Rep 64:31-40.

Haskell CM, Eilber FR, Morton DL (1975). Adriamycin (NSC-123127) by arterial infusion. Cancer Treat Rep 6:187-189.

Jacobs SC, Lawson RK (1982). Pathologic effects of pre-cystectomy therapy with combination intra-arterial doxorubicin hydrochloride and local bladder hyperthermia for bladder cancer. J Urol 127:43-47.

Jacobs SC, McCellan SL, Maher C, Lawson RK (1984). Pre-cystectomy intra-arterial cis-diamminedichloroplatinum II with local bladder hyperthermia for bladder cancer. J Urol 131:473-476.

Kanoh S, Umeyama T, Nemoto S, Ishikawa S, Nemoto R, Rinsho K, Yazaki T, Koiso K, Takahashi S, Kitagawa R (1983). Long-term intra-arterial infusion chemotherapy with adriamycin for advanced bladder cancer. Cancer Chemother Pharmacol 11:S51-58.

Kato T (1983). Encapsulated drugs in targeted cancer therapy. In Bruck SD (ed):"Controlled Drug Delivery, Vol.II," Boca Raton: CRC Press, pp 189-240.

Kato T (1984). Microcapsule chemoembolization therapy; a new approach to bladder cancer. In Küss R, Khoury S, Denis LJ, Murphy GP, Karr JP (eds): "Bladder Cancer, Part B; Radiation, Local and Systemic Chemotherapy, and New Treatment Modalities," New York: Alan R. Liss, pp 359-363.

Kato T, Nemoto R (1978). Microencapsulation of mitomycin C for intra-arterial infusion chemotherapy. Proc Jpn Acad 54B:413-417.

Kato T, Nemoto R, Mori H, Abe R, Unno K, Goto A, Murota H, Harada M (1984). Magnetic microcapsules for targeted delivery of anticancer drugs. Appl Biochem Biotechnol 10:199-211.

Kato T, Nemoto R, Mori H, Takahashi M, Tamakawa Y, Harada M (1981). Arterial chemoembolization with microencapsulated anticancer drug; an approach to selective cancer chemotherapy with sustained effects. JAMA 245:1123-1127.

Kato T, Unno K, Goto A (1985). Ethylcellulose microcapsules for selective drug delivery. In Widder KJ, Green R (ed): "Drug and Enzyme targeting, Methods in Enzymology, Vol. 112, Part A," New York: Acadmic Press, pp 139-150.

Klimberg IW, Wajsman Z (1986). Treatment for muscle invasive carcinoma of the bladder. J Urol 136:1169-1175.

Klopp CT, Alford TC, Bateman J (1950). Fractionated intra-arterial cancer chemotherapy with methly bis amine hydrochloride; a preliminary report. Ann Surg 132:811-832.

Logothetis CJ, Samuels ML, Selig DE, Wallace S, Johnson DE (1985). Combined intravenous and intra-arterial cyclophosphamide, doxorubicin, and cisplatin (CISCA) in the management of select patients with invasive urothelial tumors. Cancer Treat Rep 69:33-38.

Logothetis CJ, Samuels ML, Wallace S, Chuang V, Trindade A, Grant C, Haynie TP, Johnson DE (1982). Management of pelvic complications of malignant urothelial tumors with combined intra-arterial and IV chemotherapy. Cancer Treat Rep 66:1501-1507.

Maatman TJ, Montie JE, Bukowski RM, Risius B, Geisinger M (1986). Intra-arterial chemotherapy as an adjuvant to surgery in transitional cell carcinoma of the bladder. J Urol 135:256-260.

Mitsuhata N, Seki M, Matsumura Y, Ohmori H (1986). Intra-arterial infusion chemotherapy in combination with angiotension II for advanced bladder cancer. J Urol 136:580-585.

Montie JE (1986). Editorial comment. J Urol 136:585.

Nakazono M, Iwata S (1981). Preoperative intra-arterial chemotherapy for bladder cancer. Urol Res 9:289-295.

Nemoto R, Kato T (1981). Experimental intra-arterial infusion of microencapsulated mitomycin C into pelvic organs. Brit J Urol 53:225-227.

Nevin JE, Melnick I, Baggerly JT, Easley CA, Landes R (1974). Advanced carcinoma of bladder; treatment using hypogastric artery infusion with 5-fluorouracil, either as a single agent or in combination with bleomycin or adriamycin and supervoltage radiation. J Urol 112:752-758.

Oberfield RA, McCaffery JA, Polio J, et al (1979). Intra-arterial hepatic infusion chemotherapy in advanced metastatic adenocarcinoma from colorectal primary. Cancer 44: 414-423.

Ogata J, Migita N, Nakamura T (1973). Treatment of carcinoma of the bladder by infusion of the anticancer agent (mitomycin C) via the internal iliac artery. J Urol 110:667-670.

Okamoto Y, Konno A, Togawa K, Kato T (1986). Arterial chemo-embolization with cisplatin microcapsules. Brit J Cancer 53:369-375.

Ozono S, Okajima E, Hirao Y, Matsuki H, Takahashi S, Ohishi H (1987). Transcatheter arterial embolization of vesical artery in the treatment of bladder cancer. J Urol, submitted for publication.

Sakamoto S, Ogata J, Maeta H (1981): Chemotherapy of bladder cancer; effects of continuous infusion of mitomycin C via internal iliac artery and systemic administration of neocarzinostatin. Nishi-nihon Hinyoukika 43:223-234.

Sato K, Kato T, Mori H, Abe R, Moriyama M, Tamakawa Y, Kato T (1986). Adjuvant chemotherapeutic effects of microcapsules on organ-preserving operation for invasive bladder carcinoma. Jpn J Urol 77:474-481.

Seldinger SI (1953). Catheter replacement of needle in percutaneous angiography; new technique. Acta Radiol 39 368-376.

Stewart DJ, Benjamin RS, Zimmerman S, Capriolo RM, Wallace S, Chuang V, Calvo D, Samuels M, Bonura J, Loo TL (1983). Clinical pharmacology of intraarterial cis-diamminedichloroplatinum (II). Cancer Res 43:917-920.

Stewart DJ, Futter N, Maroun JA, Murphy P, McKay D, Rasuli P (1984). Intra-arterial cisplatin treatment of unresectable or medically inoperable invasive carcinoma of the bladder. J Urol 131:258-261.

Takai S, Oyama T, Yamashita G, Igawa K (1960). Treatment of bladder tumor by regional intra-arterial injection of nitromin and chromomycin A. Jpn J Urol 51:1317-1323.

Uyama T, Moriwaki S, Yonezawa M, Fujita J (1983). Intra-arterial adriamycin chemotherapy for bladder cancer; semi-selective intra-arterial chemotherapy with compression of the femoral arteries at the time of injection. Cancer Chemother Pharmacol 11:S59-63.

Wallace S, Chuang VP, Carrasco H, Charnsangavej C, Bechtel W, Wright KC, Gianturco C (1984). Physioanatomic concepts and radiologic techniques for intra-arterial delivery of therapeutic agents. Cancer Bull 36:6-14.

Wallace S, Chuang VP, Samuels M, Johnson D (1982). Transcatheter intraarterial infusion of chemotherapy in advanced bladder cancer. Cancer 49:640-645.

Widder KJ, Senyei AE, Ranney DF (1979). Magnetically responsive microspheres and other carriers for the biophysical targeting of antitumor agents. Adv Pharmacol Chemother 16:212-271.

EORTC Genitourinary Group Monograph 5: Progress and Controversies in Oncological Urology II, page 567
© 1988 Alan R. Liss, Inc.

Discussion: Intra-Arterial Chemotherapy for Bladder Cancer: Its Results and Future Role

Gerrit Stoter, Rotterdam, The Netherlands

Kurth: Dr. Kato, may I ask you with regard to the microcapsule technique, do you have pharmacokinetic data on what happens with the drug once the bladder has been embolised with the capsules. Are there differences in tissue concentration and intravascular concentration compared with systemic chemotherapy?

Kato: I have never compared the intra-arterial encapsulated chemotherapy with systemic chemotherapy, but I have compared the micro-encapsulated chemotherapy with intra-arterial chemotherapy. When you determine tissue concentration three hours after embolisation you find much higher concentrations as compared to intra-arterial chemotherapy. Three hours after the administration of intra-arterial Mitomycin-C there is no detectable tissue concentration at all, whereas at that time point following micro-encapsulated Mitomycin-C the tissue concentration still is 0.1 microgram per gram of tissue. This kind of activity is also demonstrated in locoregional lymph nodes.

Schröder: I understand that you treated 41 patients, half of them with TUR and half of them with cystectomy following micro-encapsulated Mitomycin-C neo-adjuvant chemotherapy. I also observed that you have T2 as well as T3 bladder cancer patients in the study group. All patients were diagnosed by TUR. Do you not think you should focus on a group of patients of whom you know for sure that you cannot resect the whole tumor by TUR only, such as T3b lesions. That would enable you to focus more clearly on the question how effective your neo-adjuvant micro-encapsulated Mitomycin-C treatment really is.

Kato: Thank you very much.

EORTC Genitourinary Group Monograph 5: Progress
and Controversies in Oncological Urology II, pages 569–575
© 1988 Alan R. Liss, Inc.

SURVIVAL AND NEO-ADJUVANT CHEMOTHERAPY IN INVASIVE BLADDER
CANCER

R. R. Hall

Department of Urology, Freeman Hospital,
Freeman Road, Newcastle upon Tyne, U.K.

The advent of neo-adjuvant chemotherapy for invasive
bladder cancer has changed the criteria for judging the
success of treatment so that "survival" may be considered
from three points of view.

SURVIVAL

When reviewed several years after treatment patients with
bladder cancer are glad to be alive whether they are cured
permanently or not and whatever the cost or side effects
of treatment. For this reason overall survival, although a
crude measure, is still an important measure of the
success of treatment. For muscle invading bladder cancer
this crude survival statistic has remained remarkably
unchanged for several years. Considering the best
published data for the different treatments available, be
this radical cystectomy, radiotherapy or combinations of
both, the chance of survival is the same and the 40%
chance of dying of metastases has remained unaltered.

The addition of adjuvant chemotherapy has not improved
this situation so far. Reviewing the impact of adjuvant
chemotherapy Torti et al (1986) concluded that it has had
no demonstrable benefit and the overall cancer related
death rate has not improved.

DISEASE FREE SURVIVAL

For several years the more strict criterion of disease
free survival has received occasional consideration but
has not been accepted as the prime measure of treatment
success.

One of the main reasons for advocating pre-cystectomy
radiotherapy 15 years ago was that it reduced the
incidence of pelvic recurrence: although the overall
survival might not be improved, the absence of recurrent
disease in the pelvis would improve the quality of
survival. Others argue that the more recent results of
radical cystectomy suggest that the same control of
regional disease can be obtained without the use of
additional radiation.

By this discussion urologists have shown their concern not
only for the length of survival but the quality of
survival. The same proportion of patients may still die
from metastases but the patient has been spared the misery
of tumour persisting in the bladder and the pain of
regional recurrence.

This attention to the quality of survival was ignored by
those who treated with radiotherapy alone but has been
recognised by the more recent practice of planned, early
salvage cystectomy when tumour persists after full dose
radiation.

Unfortunately this leads back to the situation that
existed before the debate began between radiotherapy and
cystectomy for T3 bladder cancer: to achieve survival of a
reasonable quality the bladder has to be removed in the
majority of patients. This dilemma leads to a third and
new aspect of survival to which neo-adjuvant therapy may
be relevant.

BLADDER CONSERVING SURVIVAL

As surgeons, urologists are attracted by the operation of
cystectomy for several reasons. For the same reasons the
disadvantages of cystectomy tend to be minimised or
overlooked.

Patients with urinary diversion cope remarkably well with a urinary conduit and stoma but the development of continent pouches reflects the inherent distaste for external appliances. Similarly the growing interest in nerve sparing cystectomy and bladder replacement rather than urinary diversion recognises the increasing dissatisfaction with the side effects of cystectomy and a desire for a better quality of survival.

The development of neo-adjuvant chemotherapy has coincided fortuitously with the introduction of Cisplatinum and Cisplatin-based chemotherapy combinations which appear to be more effective than other drugs or combinations used in the past. It is not possible to discuss long term survival following this new type of adjuvant chemotherapy because no such data are available yet. Nonetheless, the short term results are interesting for two reasons.

1. The survival of patients who respond in Phase II trials, especially with the M-VAC regime (Sternberg et al 1986) is longer than reported before and the proportion of complete remissions is greater. In 64 patients with metastatic and node positive transitional cell carcinoma 25 (39%) clinical complete remissions were observed and the median duration of complete remission has not been reached after 26 months mean follow up. As a result of this increased survival of patients with metastatic bladder cancer a new factor has emerged, namely, the appearance of brain metastases in 11% of patients treated.

If the mathematics of adjuvant chemotherapy are considered it is clear why it has failed in the past. In Phase II studies the best single agent or combination treatment produced a complete response rate of 10%. If it is assumed that adjuvant chemotherapy has the same effect on the micrometastases it seeks to eliminate, a 10% improvement will increase 5 year survival from 40-44%. Similarly, the 20% complete response rate observed with Cisplatin and Methotrexate will improve five year survival from 40-48%. The complete response rate reported for the M-VAC regime would yield a 16% improvement in survival which would be beneficial from the clinical point of view but would still require a very large randomised trial to prove. Whether such treatment will increase long term survival or only delay the appearance of metastases

remains to be seen but the previously unknown high
risk of brain metastases observed by Sternberg et al
(1986) is worrying.

2. More interesting than the systemic effect of
Cisplatin-based chemotherapy has been the finding that its
neo-adjuvant use has a demonstrable effect on the primary
invasive tumour in the bladder and that drugs alone can
induce complete remissions of T3 bladder cancers. The
collective data from several Phase II studies that have
used the primary tumour as the indicator lesion confirm
that chemotherapy alone may achieve complete remission in
up to 50% of tumours (Calais Da Silva 1986; Francini 1986;
Ingargiola 1986; Sternberg 1986). This complete remission
rate is encouraging because it is greater than that seen
with metastases but, by itself, is not greater than that
obtained by radiotherapy. A few patients may become tumour
free permanently with chemotherapy alone but, like
radiotherapy or endoscopic resection as sole treatment it
is inadequate for the majority of patients.

Despite this the activity of neoadjuvant chemotherapy that
is now obvious in the primary tumour may be exploited in
two ways.

(i) The partial remission of a T4b tumour may convert an
inoperable cancer into one that is amenable to cystectomy.
Evidence to support this is only anecdotal but the number
of encouraging anecdotes is growing.

(ii) Of greater relevance for T3 bladder cancer is the
combination of neoadjuvant chemotherapy with radiotherapy
or TUR to achieve the same or, possibly greater, long term
survival of better quality by allowing preservation of
normal bladder function without local recurrence.

Socquet's use of high dose Methotrexate with partial
cystectomy (Socquet 1981) did not improve three year
survival but it did preserve normal bladder function
without local recurrence. In a trial of primary TUR with
high dose Methotrexate (Hall et al 1984) long term
survival was not improved either: 4 year crude survival
was 37% (cancer related deaths 55%). Metastasis was still
the commonest cause of death but 59% of patients remained
tumour free in the bladder with normal bladder function

when they died or at last follow up, after an average follow up of 42 months.

In view of the foregoing discussion the failure of these two treatments to improve survival is not surprising and in this respect both studies are obsolete having been conducted in the pre-cisplatin era. Nonetheless the demonstration that bladder function could be preserved is important and worthy of further consideration.

Is there any evidence that newer chemotherapy can help with bladder preservation and increase survival? Data is limited but two pilot studies may point the way.

A recent pilot study of radical TUR with three cycles of Cisplatin and Methotrexate (Hall et al 1986) has reported 16/18 patients tumour free at the completion of treatment and 17/18 (94%) alive without recurrence at a mean follow up of 22 months. Of the 18 patients, 2 had persisting invasive tumour at the completion of treatment and another recurred after one year. All three received full dose radiotherapy and are tumour free. One patient developed recurrent tumour in the bladder and metastases at 10 months and died subsequently. None have required cystectomy.

More recently Shipley et al (1986) and Jakse et al (1987) have used Cisplatin or Cisplatin and Adriamycin integrated with radiotherapy for T3 bladder cancer and have achieved 80% complete response rates at the completion of treatment. This is almost double the complete response rate observed for radiotherapy alone. Furthermore, in 25 patients with T3 bladder tumour Jakse reports 17/25 (68%) bladder tumour free after a mean follow up of 16 months and an actuarial 2 year survival of 80%.

With mean follow up less than two years in both these trials no conclusions can be made concerning long term survival but if the response of the primary tumour is related to subsequent survival these results are encouraging. Furthermore, the combined results of these bladder preserving treatments incorporating primary chemotherapy reveal that 72% of 129 patients were alive without tumour in the bladder at the time of last follow up or had died with a disease free bladder.

CONCLUSION

For a variety of reasons all bladder tumours invading
muscle, especially those of moderate or poor
differentiation have been regarded by urologists and
radiotherapists as a single type of cancer that can be
treated best by one form of treatment. In one institution
T2, T3a, T3b and possibly T4a bladder tumours will all be
treated by the same method.

It is becoming increasingly apparent that this is no
longer appropriate. Within the generality of muscle
invading bladder cancer there is at least a subgroup for
whom neoadjuvant chemotherapy is already improving
survival and obviates the need for cystectomy and
possibly radiotherapy. In addition a second subgroup
T4b bladder tumours may become treatable by the use of
similar primary systemic chemotherapy.

REFERENCES

Calais Da Silva, Denis L (1986). Preoperative
    chemotherapy and cystectomy in invasive bladder cancer.
    Presented at International School of Urology and
    Nephrology. Treatment of advanced bladder cancer. Erice,
    Italy 1986. Proceedings to be published, Alan R. Liss,
    New York.
Francini M, Dal Bo V (1986). Neoadjuvant chemotherapy in
    local advanced bladder cancer. Presented at
    International School of Urology and Nephrology.
    Treatment of advanced bladder cancer. Erice, Italy
    1986. Proceedings to be published, Alan R. Liss, New
    York.
Hall RR, Newling DWW, Ramsden PR, Richards B, Robinson
    MRG, Smith PH (1984). Treatment of invasive bladder
    cancer by local resection and high dose methotrexate.
    Brit J Urol 56: 668-672.
Hall RR, Roberts T, Powell PH, Marsh MM (1986). TUR and
    chemotherapy or radiotherapy for invasive bladder
    cancer. Presented at International School of Urology
    and Nephrology. Treatment of advanced bladder cancer.
    Erice, Italy 1986. Proceedings to be published, Alan
    R Liss, New York.

Ingargiola GB, Lamartina M, Cassata G, Coselli G,
    Serretta V, Caramia G, Rizzo FP, Pavone-Macaluso M
    (1986). The methotrexate cisplatin neoadjuvant therapy
    protocol; present experience in Palermo. Presented at
    at International School of Urology and Nephrology.
    Treatment of advanced bladder cancer. Erice, Italy
    1986. Proceedings to be published by Alan R. Liss, New
    York.
Jakse G, Fritsch E, Frommhold H (1987). Treatment of
    locally advanced bladder cancer by combined
    chemotherapy and irradiation. Proceedings of 10th
    International Symposium, Ludwig-Boltzmann-Institut
    Zur Erforschung der Infektionen und Geschwulste des
    Harntraktes, Vienna February 1987. Hubner W,
    Porpaczy P, Schramek P, Studler G (eds). Gisteldruck,
    Vienna.
Shipley WU, Kaufman SD, Prout GR (1986). Combined
    chemotherapy and full dose irradiation in the treatment
    of patients with locally advanced bladder carcinoma.
    Presented at International School of Urology and
    Nephrology. Treatment of advanced bladder cancer. Erice,
    Italy 1986. Proceedings to be published by Alan R. Liss,
    New York.
Socquet Y (1981). Combined surgery and adjuvant
    chemotherapy with high dose methotrexate and folinic
    acid rescue (HDMTX-CF) for infiltrating tumours of the
    bladder. Brit J Urol 53: 439-443.
Sternberg CN, Yagoda A, Scher HI, Whitmore WF, Herr HW,
    Morse MJ, Sogani PC, Watson RC, Hollander PS, Fair WR
    (1986). Neoadjuvant M-VAC chemotherapy trials in
    transitional cell carcinoma: perspectives for first line
    chemotherapy. Presented at International School of
    Urology and Nephrology. Treatment of advanced bladder
    cancer. Erice, Italy 1986. Proceedings to be published
    by Alan R. Liss, New York.
Torti FM, Lum BL (1986). Adjuvant or neoadjuvant CMV
    chemotherapy for bladder cancer: practical and
    theoretical considerations. In Yagoda A (ed): "Bladder
    Cancer: Future Directions for Treatment," New York:
    Park Row Publishers, pp 107-110.

EORTC Genitourinary Group Monograph 5: Progress
and Controversies in Oncological Urology II, page 577
© 1988 Alan R. Liss, Inc.

Discussion: Survival and Neo-Adjuvant Chemotherapy in
Invasive Bladder Cancer

Gerrit Stoter, Rotterdam, The Netherlands

Schröder: Dr. Hall, we are conducting a similar pilot study
of neo-adjuvant Cisplatin and Methotrexate chemotherapy. We
have evaluated the antitumor response after 2 and 4 cycles
of chemotherapy by palpation and TUR. We have demonstrated
that there is no good correlation between these findings and
the histological examination of the cystectomy specimens. In
your study no cystectomy is performed. Would you like to
comment on that?

Hall: I certainly will. If you biopsy from a previously
biopsy diagnosed bladder lesion, it may be difficult to
assess the antitumor response. However, we perform radical
TUR at the time of diagnosis, such that no residual tumor is
left behind in our opinion. If you then treat with chemotherapy and follow with extensive reresection of the full
thickness of the bladder wall into the fat by TUR and still
find no viable tumor cells, we believe this is a valuable
finding. Anyway you will detect residual cancer with further
cystoscopies since these patients will progress either in
the bladder or in the locoregional lymph nodes.

Schröder: I see, but would you not be worried that some of
these patients miss the chance for cure?

Hall: Yes, I was worried in the beginning. From the data
that I have shown you today I am no longer concerned. Seventeen out of 18 patients are still without evidence of
disease. Are you worried?

Schröder: I am neither convinced nor reassured.

Hall: I agree. I am terrified by these data. I still have
the feeling that there ought to be something wrong with
these data. At the present time I still offer my patients a
chance of TUR and some chemotherapy, radical radiotherapy or
cystectomy and I yet have to meet a patient who wants to
have his bladder removed.

EORTC Genitourinary Group Monograph 5: Progress
and Controversies in Oncological Urology II, pages 579–587
© 1988 Alan R. Liss, Inc.

NEOADJUVANT CHEMOTHERAPY IN T_{3-4} N_{0-X} M_0 TRANSITIONAL CELL
CARCINOMA OF THE BLADDER.

Problems of clinical and pathological evaluation of response

T.A.W. Splinter[1], F.J.W. ten Kate[1], F.H. Schröder[1], L. Denis[2], D. Newling[3], W.G. Jones[4], D.
Jacqmin[5], C.G.G. Boeken Kruger[6], G. Stoter[7], H.J.
de Voogt[8], M. de Pauw[9]

1. University Hospital Dijkzigt, Rotterdam,
2. University Hospital Middelheim, Antwerp,
3. Princess Royal Hospital, Hull, 4. Cookridge
Hospital, Leeds, 5. Hospices Civils de Strasbourg,
Strasbourg 6. Zuiderziekenhuis, Rotterdam, 7.
R.R.T.I., Rotterdam, 8. Free University Hospital,
Amsterdam, 9. EORTC Data Center, Brussels

INTRODUCTION

Despite aggressive locoregional treatment with preoperative radiotherapy and radical cystectomy, 50 - 60% patients
with T_3 bladder cancer and 90% of patients with T_4 bladder
cancer will die of their disease. The majority will die from
distant metastases.
Recently it has been shown that several Cisplatin-based
chemotherapy regimes can induce major responses in 50% or
more of patients with advanced transitional cell carcinoma
of the bladder (Shapiro et al 1984; Harker et al, 1985;
Sternberg et al, 1985; Stoter et al, 1985; Carmichael et al,
1985). So the time had come to start trials of adjuvant
chemotherapy in locally advanced bladder cancer. Surprisingly, as a silent international consensus neoadjuvant chemotherapy was the investigational method of choice in several
centres all over the world, including the EORTC-GU group.
Recent reports have shown that pathological complete
remissions of the primary tumor can be obtained by chemotherapy (Veronesi et al, 1986; Meyers et al, 1985; Simon et al,
1986; Scher et al, 1986; Denis et al, 1986).
The main impetus for neoadjuvant chemotherapy has come from

the studies in osteosarcoma by Rosen (1986) who showed in a non-randomized way that the cure rate could be increased from 20% (historical controls) up to 85% by using neoadjuvant chemotherapy and that the amount of chemotherapy induced necrosis or viable tumor left in the primary tumor was predictive of the increased survival. Recently Eilber et al (1987) confirmed the increased survival in a randomised trial. Remarkably, the chemotherapy-regime used in the neoadjuvant setting can only produce 40-50% major responses, mostly PR´s and no cures in patients with metastatic disease. In contrast, neoadjuvant studies in head and neck cancer have shown very little or no benefit in terms of survival (Taylor, 1987), while the chemotherapy, used in the neoadjuvant setting, produces high response rates of 70-80% with approximately 30% CR´s. The majority of failures occur locoregional. These two examples show that the efficacy of chemotherapy in metastatic disease is not predictive for its effect on micrometastases. At the same time micrometastases may be killed by the same chemotherapy, which still leaves behind viable tumor cells at the primary site. Since both in the osteosarcoma and head/neck cancer studies no benefit was seen of neoadjuvant chemotherapy in non-responding patients, we have evaluated the clinical and pathological response criteria, which are used in an ongoing EORTC phase II study of preoperative chemotherapy in T_{3-4} N_{0-X} M_0 transitional cell carcinoma of the bladder. The results are reported in this paper.

MATERIALS AND METHODS

Twenty patients with T_{3-4} N_{0-X} M_0 transitional cell cancer of the bladder were selected from a group of 60 patients, because 10 had been evaluated as responders and 10 as non-responders and enough data were available of all 20 patients to evaluate both the clinical response and pathological response after chemotherapy. Thirteen of these patients were entered into the EORTC study 30851 and 7 were treated accordingly but outside the study, because it had not been activated yet. The 10 responders and 10 non-responders are not representative for the overall response rate.

SELECTION CRITERIA

The selection criteria for entry into the neoadjuvant study included histologically proven transitional cell carcinoma of the bladder, stage T_{3-4} N_{0-X} M_0, age lower than 76 years, performance status lower than 3 according to the WHO, serum creatinine lower than 140 micromol/l or a creatinine clearance higher than 60 ml/min, no previous treatment with Cisplatin, Methotrexate or radiotherapy to the bladder and the presence of a measurable primary tumor after TUR-biopsy.

STAGING AND RESTAGING PROCEDURES

Before entry into the study the following staging procedures had to be performed: physical examination, chest X-ray, CT-scan of the abdomen, IVU, cystoscopy plus biopsy followed by bimanual palpation under general anaesthesia, measurement of the residual primary tumor by bimanual palpation and/or CT-scan and/or ultrasound (intravesical or transrectal).
Radionuclide bone-scanning was optional. At restaging all investigations except IVU were repeated.

STUDY DESIGN

After fulfilling the selection criteria the patients were treated with 2 courses of chemotherapy, followed by restaging. In case of clinical stable disease (SD) or progressive disease (PD) the patient went off protocol. Further treatment was left to the judgement of the responsible physician. In case of a clinical major response (CR or PR) another 2 courses of chemotherapy were given followed by restaging. After the second evaluation, treatment was again left to the judgement of the responsible physician.

CRITERIA FOR RESPONSE

The following criteria for the assessment of response of the primary tumour were used:

cCR: complete disappearance of all clinical evidence of bladder cancer, including tumor-negative biopsies.

cPR: clinical PR according to the WHO criteria independent of histological evidence of bladder cancer or clinical CR plus histological evidence of bladder cancer.

cPD: clinical PD according to the WHO criteria independent of histological evidence of bladder cancer.

cSD: any other clinical response independent of histological evidence of bladder cancer.

pCR: complete disappearance of all histological evidence of bladder cancer in specimens obtained by extended TUR, partial or total cystectomy independent of the clinical response.

CHEMOTHERAPY REGIME

Cisplatin 70 mg/m^2 i.v. day 1 and Methotrexate 40 mg/m^2 day 8 and 15 every 3 weeks. Leucovorin-rescue (4 x 15 mg orally 24 hrs after MTX-administration) was advised.

RESULTS

The results of the clinical and pathological evaluation of the 10 non-responders and the 10 responders are depicted in tables 1 and 2 respectively. The columns from the left to the right represent the clinical T-staging before, after 2 and after 4 courses of chemotherapy based on biopsies; the clinical evaluation after 2 and 4 courses of chemotherapy, based on the sum of the measurements obtained by CT-scan, ultrasound and bimanual palpation; the definitive response, based on the pathological investigation of extended TUR biopsies or the bladder specimen and the clinical response; in the last column some details are given. The exclamation marks indicate discrepancies between the definitive response and the clinical response.

Concerning the non-responders (table 1) all patients underwent a total cystectomy, except patient n° 7, who was treated by a partial cystectomy. Only patients n° 4 and 9 did not receive anymore chemotherapy after the first 2 courses. In patients n° 3 and 10 false-negative biopsies were obtained after 4 courses. Patient n° 7 developed a new invasive lesion, which was completely resected. Therefore after 4 courses a pseudo CR was found. It is clear from these data that all patients who were `definitive non-responders´, were clinically non-responders after 2 courses. Five of the 10 patients have died of metastases and one of a local relapse (n° 7), 2 patients are without evidence of disease and 2 have only very recently undergone surgery.

Concerning the responders (table 2) all patients except n° 14 and 15 underwent a total cystectomy, because of the

Table 1

Evaluation of response after 2 and/or 4 courses of chemotherapy

	pre	T eval. 1	T eval. 2	clin. eval. 1	clin. eval. 2	defin. resp.	remarks
1	T_3a	T_2	T_3a	SD	SD	SD	NED
2	T_3a	T_3a	T_3a	SD	SD	SD	NED
3	T_3b	T_3b	T_0	SD	SD	SD!	DEAD
4	T_3	–		SD	–	SD	T_3N_1
5	T_4a	T_3	T_3	SD	SD	SD	DEAD
6	T_3	–	–	PD	SD	SD	DEAD
7	T_3	T_3	–	PD	CR	CR!	DEAD
8	T_3	–	–	PD	–	PD	DEAD
9	T_3	T_3	–	PD	–	PD	T_3N_1
10	T_3a	T_3a	T_0	PD	–	PD!	NED

Table 2

Evaluation of response after 2 and/or 4 courses of chemotherapy

	pre	T eval. 1	T eval. 2	clin. eval. 1	clin. eval. 2	defin. resp.	remarks
11	T_3a	T_2	T_0	SD	PR	CR!	NED
12	T_3b	T_1	T_1	PR	PR	PR	NED
13	T_3b	T_0	T_0	SD	PR	CR!	NED
14	T_3a	T_0	T_0	PR	PR	CR	relapse
15	T_3b	T_0	T_0	CR	CR	CR	NED
16	T_3	–	–	PR	PR	CR	NED
17	T_3	T_3	T_0	PR	PR	PR	$T_0 N_1$
18	T_4	–	–	PR	CR	PR	NED
19	T_3	–	–	SD	PR	CR!	NED
20	T_3	T_0	T_0	–	–	CR	NED

presence of a second primary lung tumor in the former and a pCR, determined by extended TUR, in the latter. Patients 11, 13 and 19 did not show a clinical response after 2 courses according to our definition, but two of them (n° 11 and 13) had a pathological down-staging and from patient n° 19 no biopsies were taken. All remaining patients showed a major clinical response after 2 courses. Patients n° 11 and 17 show that at least 4 courses of chemotherapy are needed for a maximal response of the primary tumor. None of the patients have died; 9 patients are clinically without evidence of bladder cancer (NED); patient n° 14 has developed a local relapse; in patients n° 11 and 14 a second primary cancer in the lung has been detected. Finally, very interestingly patient n° 17 had a pT_0 together with viable tumor in 3 regional lymph nodes, which raises the question whether the primary tumor is a good parameter for the effect of chemotherapy on distant metastases.

So, in only 3 out of 20 patients (15%) the evaluation of the clinical response after 2 courses differed from the definitive evaluation after 4 courses.

The pathology of all available specimens from 7 patients have been reviewed by F.J.W. ten Kate and myself. Two important items have been observed. Firstly, in case of chemotherapy-induced tumor kill intact interstitial tissue is found with necrosis and/or fibrosis and/or inflammation with a foreign body giant cell reaction in between (figure I). In non-responding patients only viable tumors without such changes were observed. In several patients ischemic necrosis was seen (figure 2), which differed from chemotherapy-induced necrosis by the absence of intact interstitial tissue. Finally in two patients with a pCR carcinoma in situ grade III was found in the bladder (figure 3), which means that the organ was still at risk of developing a second primary bladder cancer after systemic chemotherapy.

DISCUSSION AND CONCLUSIONS

This analysis of 20 selected patients with T_{3-4} bladder cancer, who have been treated with Cisplatin and Methotrexate before surgery shows:

I. The distinction between responders and non-responders after 2 courses of chemotherapy is correct in 85% of the patients. It seems that both tumor measurements and multiple biopsies are needed to achieve an accurate evaluation. It is important to evaluate the response after 2 courses in order

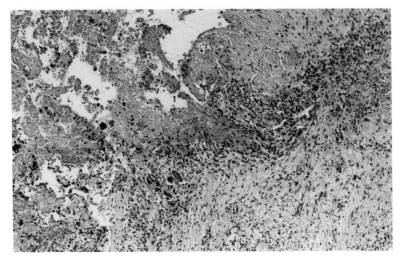

Fig. 1

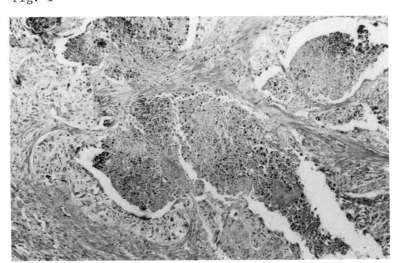

Fig. 2

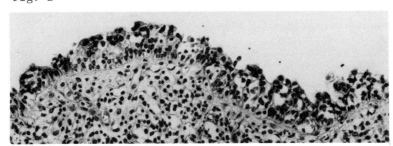

Fig. 3

Legends to Figs. 1 - 3:
(top) Area of chemotherapy-induced necrosis, fibrosis and foreign giant cell reaction. (middle) Area of ischemic necrosis including interstitial tissue and surrounded by viable tumor. (bottom) Marked atypia of the bladder epithelium with focally Cis G3. All three specimens are from the same patient n° 19 (table 2).

to save the non-responders useless and toxic chemotherapy. In case of doubt it is advisable to give the patient the possible benefit of 2 more courses.
In view of the histological changes such as necrosis, fibrosis and inflammatory reaction with foreign body giant cells, which were seen only in responding patients, it seems worthwhile to add pathological criteria such as pPR and pSD, based on the presence or absence of the above mentioned histological features next to viable tumor, to the criteria for response, which have been used. Such an addition is analogous to the scoring of the amount of necrosis in neo-adjuvant studies of osteosarcoma (Rosen, 1986).

II. The presence of Cis-G3 and the local relapse in one of the patients after a CR had been reached, are a serious warning against the wishful thinking that chemotherapy may replace surgery in complete responders. I would not be surprised if after careful analysis of all data from the EORTC-study 30851 this wishful thinking will be turned around 180°, i.e. all responders should receive aggressive local treatment and non-responders should be treated palliatively, because it will be shown that a response of the primary tumor is a very strong prognostic factor for survival but insufficient to assure the real absence of local tumor.
Last but certainly not least, the value of neoadjuvant chemotherapy in terms of survival and cure can only be proven in a randomized phase III trial.

REFERENCES.

Carmichael J, Cornbleet MA, MacDougall RM, et al (1985). Cis-platin and Methotrexate in the treatment of transitional cell carcinoma of the urinary tract. Br J Urol 57: 299-30.
Denis L, Hendrickx G, and Keuppens F (1986). Preoperative chemotherapy in T_3 T_4-N_X-M0 bladder cancer. J Urol 135:

222a.

Eilber F, Giuliano A, Eckhardt J, Patterson K, Moseley S, and Goodnight J (1987). Adjuvant chemotherapy for osteo-sarcoma: A randomized prospective trial. J Clin Oncol 5: 21-26.

Harker WG, Meyers FJ, Freiha FS et al (1985). Cisplatin, Methotrexate and Vinblastine (CMV): an effective chemothe-rapy regimen for metastatic transitional cell carcinoma of the urinary tract. A Northern California Oncology Group Study. J Clin Oncol 3: 1463-1470.

Meyers FJ, Palmer JM, Freiha FS, Harker EG, Shortliffe LD, Hannigan J, McWhirter K and Torti FM (1985). The fate of the bladder in patients with metastatic bladder cancer treated with Cisplatin, Methotrexate and Vinblastine: A Northern California Oncology Group Study. J Urol 134: 1118-112

Rosen G (1986). Neo-adjuvant chemotherapy for bone and soft tissue sarcomas. In: Neo-adjuvant chemotherapy: 359-556. Eds. Jacquillat C, Weil M, Khayat D, John Libbey, London.

Scher HI, Yagoda A, Sternberg CN, Whitmore Jr. WF, Watson R C, Hollander PS, Morse MJ, Herr W, Sogani PC and Fair WR (1986). Neo-adjuvant M-VAC for transitional cell carcinoma of the urothelium. ASCO Proceedings 5: 419.

Shapiro GR et al (1984) Cisplatin, Doxorubicin therapy: a highly effective combination for transitional cell carci-noma of the bladder (TCCB). ASCO Proceedings 3: 154.

Simon SD and Srougi M (1986). Systemic M-VAC chemotherapy for primary treatment of locally invasive transitional cell carcinoma of the bladder (TCCB): A pilot study. ASCO Proceedings 5: 432.

Sternberg CN, Yagoda A, Scherr HI, et al(1985).Preliminary results of MVAC (Methotrexate, Vinblastine, Doxorubicin and Cisplatin) for transitional cell carcinoma of the urothelium. J Urol 133: 403-407.

Stoter G, Fossa SD, Klijn JGM et al (1985). Combination chemotherapy with Cisplatin and Methotrexate in advanced bladder cancer. An EORTC phase II study. ASCO Proceedings 4: 106.

Taylor IV SG (1987). Why has so much chemotherapy done so little in head and neck cancer? J Clin Oncol 5: 1-3.

Veronesi A, Galligioni E, Lo Re G, Sorio R, Saracchini S, Francini M, Merlo A, Dal Bo V, Monfardini S, (1986). Combination Chemotherapy with Fluorouracil, Adriamycin, cis-Platinum and VM-26 in advanced transitional cell carcinoma of the urinary tract. Eur J Cancer Clin Oncol 22: 1457-1460.

EORTC Genitourinary Group Monograph 5: Progress
and Controversies in Oncological Urology II, pages 589–590
© 1988 Alan R. Liss, Inc.

Discussion: Neoadjuvant Chemotherapy in $T_{3-4} N_{0-x} M_0$
Transitional Cell Carcinoma of the Bladder: Problems of
Clinical and Pathological Evaluation of Response

Gerrit Stoter, Rotterdam, The Netherlands

Gad el Mawla: Dr. Splinter, we noticed in our studies that
patients must receive 4 cycles of chemotherapy in the neo-
adjuvant situation before the maximum result can be
achieved. I think 2 cycles are not enough to permit the
assessment of response.

Splinter: Thank you.

Lachand: We used in a similar group of patients chemotherapy
consisting of Cisplatin, Adriamycin and Cyclophosphamide. In
half of the patients the chemotherapy was not effective, in
the other half complete and partial responses were observed.
We are not very happy with these results, because yet another problem remains. Since the diagnosis has been made by
radical TUR in many patients, not leaving any tumor behind,
what is the meaning of the evaluation of antitumor response
to chemotherapy after 2 or 4 cycles.

Splinter: I agree with your statement. We have solved this
problem by the requirement in the protocol that each patient
should have a residual measurable bladder lesion after TUR,
measurable by either CT-scan, ultrasound or cystoscopy.

Lachand: Yes, but you come across some patients in whom you
can and should remove the whole bladder lesion. How should
you go about these patients?

Splinter: In that case a patient should be treated optimally
in the way you state, but he would not be eligible for the
kind of protocol we currently have. In addition I would like
to make the statement that at the present time some 15 phase
II studies have been performed or are ongoing throughout the
world without any randomized study being performed. If this
situation does not change, the discussion will remain to be
limited to response rates and the difficulties involved in
the assessment of response. What we need is a randomized

controlled phase III trial to assess the value of this type of neo-adjuvant chemotherapy in muscle invasive bladder cancer.

Schröder: Dr. Splinter, what type of result would make you think that you have made a major step forward and that you would like to continue neo-adjuvant chemotherapy?

Splinter: My personal opinion is that we should require an overall response of at least 50% of the cases. I do not agree with the opinion of Dr. Hall that only complete responders will benefit from the treatment. For example in metastatic osteosarcoma the percentage of response to chemotherapy is limited and usually partial in nature. Despite this fact the cure rate with neo-adjuvant chemotherapy is surprisingly high. Therefore, I think that we take the right view in requiring 50% major responses, not necessarily complete.

De Voogt: Is it conceivable that this type of adjuvant or neo-adjuvant chemotherapy would lead us to more conservative forms of surgery or no surgery at all in the future? I noticed that in your present study approach the patients not only have to undergo cystectomy but also suffer from quite toxic chemotherapy.

Splinter: As I said previously, this protocol is a phase II study with all its limitations. We should do a randomized phase III study to demonstrate and improve disease free and overall survival in order to show that the addition of chemotherapy will benefit the patients. Once that has been established the next question is how can we achieve the same results with less radical therapies, including the omission of cystectomy.

EORTC Genitourinary Group Monograph 5: Progress
and Controversies in Oncological Urology II, pages 591–597
© 1988 Alan R. Liss, Inc.

COMBINED RADIOTHERAPY, CHEMOTHERAPY AND SURGERY IN THE
MANAGEMENT OF INVASIVE BLADDER CANCER

Gerhard Jakse, M.D. and Hermann Frommhold, M.D.

Department of Urology and Radiotherapy, University
of Innsbruck, A-6020 Innsbruck, Austria

T3 bladder cancer can be controlled locally by definitive
irradiation in some 40% of the patients (Hope-Stone et al,
1981; Wallace and Bloom, 1976). It is suggested that the addition of systemic chemotherapy increases the local tumor
control rate. There are essentially three modes to deliver
chemotherapy: one is before, the other one is simultaneously
and the third is after irradiation. All three ways have been
used so far (Jakse et al, 1985; Lundbeck and Christophersen,
1979; Rhagavan et al, 1985; Richards et al, 1983). We chose
simultaneous chemotherapy and irradiation because there
should be at least three advantages over the other modalities:
there is immediate treatment of micrometastases while you are
already treating the tumor bulk with both modalities, radio-
sensitisation can be achieved in case of specific drugs such
as adriamycin and finally there is an immediate attack to the
tumor bulk by both treatment modalities at the same time. The
major disadvantage may be the increased local toxicity.

Since 1980 we used simultaneous irradiation and chemotherapy in locally advanced bladder cancer. We treated more
than 60 patients and used 2 protocols consecutively.
A) TUR plus cisplatinum and irradiation (Jakse et al, 1985).
Cisplatinum was given 4 times at a dosage of 70 mg/m^2. Irradiation was delivered as a split course with a total dose of
60 Gy.
B) TUR plus cisplatinum, adriamycin and hyperfractionated,
accelerated irradiation (Jakse et al, 1987). Besides cisplatinum we used adriamycin 10 mg/m^2 and hyperfractionated irradiation with 2 daily fractions of 1.6 Gy on 3 consecutive
days a week.

In case of a new therapeutic approach we should always compare this new modality with a standard one which ought to give optimal results in terms of local tumor control. We are well aware of the limitations of such a comparison, but still then it is of some value for those who want to know the role of the new treatment modality in the therapy of a given tumor. In the following we compare our results with those reported in the literature for cystectomy. We will only deal with T3 bladder cancer since we believe that this is the most applicable one for both treatment modalities. As special points of interest we will consider the following aspects: local tumor control, morbidity and mortality, local tumor recurrence, distant metastases and survival.

Patients

TABLE 1.

	cRT + CHT*	hRT + CHT**
patients	29	27
men	23	20
women	6	7
age	42 - 85	48 - 85
T2	–	2
T3	24	18
T4	5	7
grade III	8	2
grade IV	20	25

* conventional irradiation plus cisplatinum
**hyperfractionated irradiation plus cisplatinum
  and adriamycin

Local Tumor Control

In patients who undergo cystectomy for T3 bladder cancer local tumor control is virtually 100%.

Until now we treated 43 patients with T3-transitional cell carcinoma of the urinary bladder with integrated radio-chemotherapy. Fourty-one of these 43 are evaluable for the purpose of this analysis.

A complete remission was achieved in 75 and 80% of the patients respectively. This result is in accordance with the 84% which were reported by Shipley and coworkers (1984). That means that in about 20% of the patients we miss our aim to completely destruct the local tumor.

The patients with persistent tumor should certainly undergo radical cystectomy, but cystectomy was performed in 2 patients only. The other patients had at the time of the proposed cystectomy already locally far advanced tumors or were unfit to undergo major surgery.

A question which certainly arises in this respect is, how valid is the complete remission based on clinical evaluation. We looked through the charts of 29 patients who were followed for a minimum of 12 months and were staged post-therapeutically by CT scan, endoscopy and TUR of the tumor area. We obtained a 95% concordance in terms of complete tumor destruction or persistent tumor.

Acute, Chronic Morbidity and Mortality

The operative mortality in experienced hands in cystectomy series ranges from 1 to 7% (Hohenfellner and Jacobi, 1984; Skinner et al, 1980; Whitmore et al, 1977). Severe complications due to the operative intervention are reported in some 20% (Hohenfellner and Jacobi, 1984; Skinner et al, 1977). A second intervention is then necessary in about a third of these patients.

There is no acute death in our series of 43 patients with T3 tumors who were treated by combined radio-chemotherapy. If we consider a prolongation of the hospital stay, delay or stop of treatment and impairment of renal function as equivalent to the acute operative morbidity we observed a prolongation of the hospital stay in none of the patients, a stop of treatment was necessary in 4 due to uncontrolled urinary infection (n=1), gastro-intestinal symptoms (n=3) and renal impairment was observed in 1 respectively. The overall acute morbidity was 13%.

Skinner and coworkers (1980), Johnson and Lamy (1977), Whitmore and coworkers (1977) reported a late complication rate of about 33 to 41% of the patients who underwent cystectomy.

These late complications concern mostly the urinary diversion which results in impairment of renal function or even renal failure.

Late complications after radiotherapy are mainly reduced bladder capacity, shrunken bladder, severe radiocystitis, bowel stenosis and bowel fistula (Fish et al, 1976; Goffinet et al, 1975; Van der Werf-Messing, 1965). Secondary malignancies may also occur in a low percentage. If we consider our own group of patients and only those who were followed for at least 12 months we observed an overall late complication rate of 36%. But it has to be noted that proctitis (n=6) was always mild and these patients did not need medical treatment. We did not observe any bowel stenosis or fistula. Low bladder capacities were noted in 5 patients.
Two patients developed a bladder hemorrhage, in one of these it occurred 62 months after start of treatment and could not be controlled by conventional measures. This 78 year old patient died during the further course of the necessary interventions due to lung edema. On autopsy there was no evidence of local tumor or distant metastases.

Local Tumor Recurrence

Whitmore and others reported that after radical cystectomy pelvic tumors will develop in approximately 15% of the patients including those who undergo preoperative irradiation (Whitmore et al, 1977; Hohenfellner and Jacobi, 1984). The pelvic recurrence will occur in most of the patients within 2 years.

If we consider 33 patients in whom we achieved complete local tumor control and who were followed for a minimum of 12 months we observed 5 local recurrences, i.e. 15%. Topical chemotherapy (n=1) and cystectomy (n=1) were successful to control the local tumor in 2 patients. One patient could be controlled by TUR for his pT1 tumor but developed distant metastases. Two patients developed T4b tumors, in neither of these a TUR of the tumor area after completing treatment was performed. We feel that this post-therapeutic TUR is a necessity if we want to have optimal information about the treatment result. The interval between CR and tumor recurrence was 6 to 17 months.

There were no late recurrences until now, but the maximum follow-up of 79 months and the small group of patients do not allow to give any firm statement in this respect.

Distant Metastases

Distant metastases occur in some 20 to 40% of the patients who undergo cystectomy (Whitmore et al, 1977; Whitmore, 1983). Eight of 33 patients with CR in our series developed distant metastases within 2 to 28 months. One additional patient experienced a renal pelvic tumor with lung metastases. If we compare these figures with those reported by Blandy (1984) for definitive irradiation it is evident that the additional systemic chemotherapy is effective with regard to increasing local tumor control but not in the eradication of micrometastases.

Survival

The 5-year survival rates as correlated to the patho-histological stage in the cystectomy specimens vary from 30 to 58% (Bredael et al, 1980; Hohenfellner and Jacobi, 1984; Whitmore et al, 1977). This percentage considers cystectomy series with and without preoperative irradiation. The 5-year survival rate in our series of integrated radiochemotherapy is 46%. Patients in whom a complete remission was diagnosed after completing treatment had a 5-year survival rate of 66%. But we have to take into consideration that 1 out of 33 patients in whom a complete remission was achieved finally has lost his bladder because of local tumor recurrence.

CONCLUSIONS

Simultaneous radiotherapy and chemotherapy results in a 80% complete remission rate. In patients who undergo hyperfractionated, accelerated irradiation and chemotherapy the radiation dose can be reduced in 40% of them to 40 Gy. (The details are not given in this report). The acute and late morbidity is rather low compared to cystectomy series, especially considering the upper urinary tract. The local recurrence rate is higher in radio-chemotherapy patients than in patients who undergo cystectomy, but can be managed more successfully. That means we certainly can deal more effective-

ly with a superficial tumor recurrence in the bladder than
with a local recurrence in the true pelvis after cystectomy,
where an effective chemotherapy may salvage about 15% of the
patients.
The systemic chemotherapy applied in these two protocols
probably does not eradicate micrometastases. A 5-year survival rate is comparable to that obtained by radical cystectomy. We do not mean to advocate the integrated radiotherapy
and chemotherapy in patients with T3 bladder cancer as first
choice treatment, but it may be considered as a treatment
option in those patients who are unfit to undergo cystectomy
because of medical reasons or do not want to loose their
bladder as the initial step to the proposed cancer treatment.

REFERENCES

Blandy JP (1984). Salvage cystectomy in the treatment of in-
    vasive bladder cancer. Progress and Controversies in Onco-
    logical Urology. Alan R Liss Inc, New York, p 359.
Bredael JJ, Croker BP, Glenn JF (1980). The curability of in-
    vasive bladder cancer treated by radical cystectomy. Eur
    Urol 6:206.
Fish JC, Fayos JV (1976). Carcinoma of the urinary bladder.
    Radiology 118:179.
Goffinet DR, Schneider MJ, Glatstein EJ, Ludwig H, Ray GR,
    Dunnick NR, Bagshaw MA (1975). Bladder cancer results of
    radiation therapy in 384 patients. Radiology 117:149.
Hohenfellner R, Jacobi GH (1984). Radical cystectomy without
    preoperative radiotherapy for invasive bladder carcinoma -
    a justified approach. Progress and Controversies in Onco-
    logical Urology. Alan R Liss Inc, New York, p 313.
Hope-Stone HF, Blandy JP, Oliver RTD, England M (1981).
    Radical radiotherapy and salvage cystectomy in the treat-
    ment of invasive carcinoma of the bladder. In: Oliver RTC,
    Hendry WF, Bloom HGJ (eds) Bladder Cancer. Principles of
    Combination Therapy. Chap 15. Butterworths, London, Boston,
    Sydney, Wellington, p 127.
Jakse G, Frommhold H, zur Nedden D (1985). Combined radiation
    and chemotherapy for locally advanced transitional cell
    carcinoma of the urinary bladder. Cancer 55:1659.
Jakse G, Fritsch E, Frommhold H (1987). Hyperfractionated,
    accelerated irradiation and chemotherapy in locally ad-
    vanced bladder cancer. Eur Urol, in press.

Johnson DE, Lamy SM (1977). Complications of a single stage radical cystectomy and ileal conduit diversion: review of 214 cases. J Urol 117:171.

Lundbeck F, Christophersen IS (1979). Phase II study of adriamycin, 5-Fu, levamisole and irradiation in carcinoma of the bladder. Cancer Treat Rep 63:183.

Rhagavan D, Pearson B, Duval P, Rogers J, Meagher M, Wines R, Mameghon H, Boulas J, Green D (1985). Initial intravenous cisplatinum therapy: improved management for invasive high risk bladder cancer? J Urol 133:399.

Richards B, Bastable JR, Freedman L, Glashan RW, Harris G, Newling DWW, Robinson MRG, Smith PH (1983). Adjuvant chemotherapy with doxorubicin and 5-Fu in T_3, N_x, M_0 bladder cancer treated by radiotherapy. Brit J Urol 55:386.

Shipley WU, Coombs LJ, Einstein AB, Soloway MS, Wajsman Z, Prout GR (1984). Cisplatin and full irradiation for patients with invasive bladder carcinoma. J Urol 132:899.

Skinner DG, Crawford ED, Kaufman JJ (1980). Complications of radical cystectomy for carcinoma of the bladder. J Urol 123:640.

Skinner DG, Tift JP, Kaufman JJ (1982). High dose, short course preoperative radiation therapy and immediate single stage radical cystectomy with pelvic node dissection in the management of bladder cancer. J Urol 127:671.

Soloway MS, Morris CR, Sudderth B (1979). Radiation therapy and cis-diamminedichloroplatinum (II) in transplantable and primary murine bladder cancer. Int J Radiat Oncol Biol Phys 5:1355.

Teicher BA, Lazo JS, Sartorelli AC (1981). Classification of antineoplastic agents by their selective toxicities toward oxygenated and hypoxic tumor cells. Cancer Rep 41:73.

Wallace DM, Bloom HJG (1976). The management of deeply infiltrating (T_3) bladder carcinoma: controlled trial of radical radiotherapy versus preoperative radiotherapy and radical cystectomy. Brit J Urol 48:587.

Werf-Messing B van der (1965). Telecobalt treatment of carcinoma of the bladder. Clin Radiol 16:165.

Whitmore WF, Batata MA, Hilaris BS, Reddy GN, Unal A, Ghoneim MA, Grabstald H, Chu F (1977). A comparative study of two preoperative radiation regimes with bladder cancer. Cancer 40:1077.

Whitmore WF (1983). Management of invasive bladder neoplasms. Semin Urol 1:34.

EORTC Genitourinary Group Monograph 5: Progress
and Controversies in Oncological Urology II, pages 599–600
© 1988 Alan R. Liss, Inc.

Discussion: Combined Radiotherapy, Chemotherapy and
Surgery in the Management of Invasive Bladder Cancer

Gerrit Stoter, Rotterdam, The Netherlands

Zingg: Dr. Jakse, in your patient group can you compare the
late toxicity of Cisplatin chemotherapy and radiotherapy to
the standard approach of radical cystectomy and ureter
deviation? We tend to see complications 5 to 10 years later
usually due to upper urinary tract complications. Your
follow-up is only 12 months.

Jakse: The follow-up in our patient series is 12 to 79
months. The mean observation period of the complete
responders is 27 months. When I looked at the papers of
Whitmore, Skinner, Johnson and Lamey, I observed that they
had similar patients. These late complications in the upper
urinary tract as you mentioned will never occur in
radiotherapy treated patients, which has been confirmed by
others, but shrinkage of the bladder can occur, usually
within one year. Afterwards you do not see further reduction
of bladder capacity. However, what concerns me most is the
one patient I lost due to major hemorrhage from radiation
cystitis.

Debruyne: You mentioned that the local recurrence rate is
somewhat higher with your approach than with conventional
methods, but that the treatment of recurrence with surgery
is more successful. What do you mean by that?

Jakse: I only meant that salvage cystectomy or radical TUR
of local recurrence is more effective than systemic or
intra-arterial chemotherapy.

N.N.: You seem to be unfair towards cystectomy in the
comparison with other local therapy such as radiotherapy in
combination with systemic control by chemotherapy. Would you
please comment on that?

Jakse: A real comparison would require a randomized controlled study. However, the data I showed were realistic and

form a basis for such a randomized study.

Schröder: Would you prefer your study treatment regimen even if you were not performing a trial? Your study shows the same results with regard to local tumor control to the expense of 36% long term toxicity.

Jakse: Yes, I believe that a patient with a T3 lesion should be offered the chance of preserving his bladder by radio-chemotherapy. In case of failure one can still offer salvage cystectomy.

Zingg: Dr. Jakse, were your patients fit for cystectomy?

Jakse: We are very conservative with surgery in our department. All the patients who came to our department with a solitary muscle invasive bladder cancer were offered radio-chemotherapy. I think at least 60% of these patients were fit for cystectomy.

EORTC Genitourinary Group Monograph 5: Progress
and Controversies in Oncological Urology II, pages 601–610
© 1988 Alan R. Liss, Inc.

ROUND TABLE DISCUSSION: WHAT IS THE BEST MANAGEMENT OF
T2-3M0 CARCINOMA OF THE BLADDER? (Chairmen: E.J. Zingg and
A.W.S. Ritchie)

J.H.M. Blom

Department of Urology, Erasmus University
Hospital, Rotterdam, The Netherlands

ZINGG

In this round table discussion we have to give an
answer to the question: "What is the best management of
T2-3M0 carcinoma of the bladder?"

When we are dealing with an invasive tumor, the correlation between clinical and surgical-pathological staging is
about 50-60%, and most of the tumors are understaged. When
there is an invasive carcinoma of the bladder there is a
high probability of lymph node metastases, and when there
are lymph node metastases, there is a high probability of
disseminated disease. With all the loco-regional therapy
whatsoever we reach a survival rate of about 50%. Most of
the patients do not die from their local recurrence, but
because of the dissemination of the metastases. There is, at
least, some hypothesis that we could reach a better survival
rate by systemic chemotherapy for the micrometastases. I
would like to ask the panelists first: as you can see in the
program, ".... the best management of T2-3 tumors", so these
categories are considered as an entity: T2-3. When I heard
the figures of Mr. Hall and Dr. Jakse I heard them speaking
about the T3 tumors. So, I would first ask Prof. Denis: "Are
you happy about this?"

DENIS

I am not happy with the term T2-3, because to me it
means nothing. During the consensus meeting in Antwerp last
year we decided that with biopsy or TUR only it is

impossible to make the differentiation. When I am talking
about invasive disease, I would like to feel a mass of
tumor, I would like to confirm it by CT-scan or intravesical
ultrasound.

HALL

If we insist on only taking a biopsy before embarking
upon treatment then clearly we have to include all muscle
invasive tumors according to our TNM criteria. But a urologist does possess a resectoscope and if you use the resectoscope thoroughly and you follow the TNM criteria it is
possible to distinguish T2 tumors from T3. We accept them
within the TNM categorization and I think this distinction
can be made clinically in many patients. If you have G1T2
tumor no more treatment than a TUR is needed in by far the
majority. If you have a G2 or a G3T2 tumor then they tend to
behave like deeply invasive tumors.

JAKSE

I agree with Mr. Hall, but I would make it more precise. The patients with T2 solitary lesions without concomitant carcinoma in situ are the patients who can be cured by
TUR alone. If you have a patient who has multiple T2 tumors
with or without carcinoma in situ I think that is the patient who should undergo cystectomy.

ZINGG

Next point: It was already mentioned that adjuvant
chemotherapy is not worth while. On the other hand, at least
in my department, we see quite a few patients with invasive
tumor who have chemotherapy after a total cystectomy. The
surgeon wants to have a good conscience, as he is not sure
to have eradicated all the tumor. I would like to ask Dr.
Stoter the question: "Is there any rationale for adjuvant
chemotherapy after radical cystectomy?"

STOTER

I am not a urologist, but a medical oncologist. For me
it is a simple matter of methodology. The question to be
asked for adjuvant chemotherapy is whether that treatment is
effective in prolonging the disease-free and the overall

survival of the patients. That question can only be answered in a randomized controlled study with a standard treatment in the control arm. I still have to see data to prove that the existing treatment strategies that have been investigated, like for instance Cisplatin in protocol 7 of the NBCP, will be of benefit for the patients. In that protocol 7 there was a shift of the survival to the right side in the curves, but the results in terms of overall survival were the same. I am also doubtful about the promise which is held by the present chemotherapy that we have, i.e. Cisplatin, Methotrexate plus or minus Vinblastin and Adriamycin. It worries me. Those investigators who claim the best results in advanced disease with M-VAC therapy have only presented their initial results as promising and these are only data on a selected group of patients, who have achieved a clinical complete response, then were still fit enough to undergo a cystectomy and then were proven to have a pathological complete response or were rendered a pathological complete response. I think the survival data of over 26 months, as mentioned by Mr. Hall, are derived from that subset of patients and that worries me.

ZINGG

Is there any panelist here who is giving adjuvant chemotherapy?

RITCHIE

From the U.S. there has been no good study reported on adjuvant chemotherapy. Can we then take it that there is a consensus among us to exclude T2 lesions from further discussion and perhaps concentrate the discussion on T3 lesions? I think the point is that in trials of such treatment we should concentrate on patients who have a palpable residual lump of tumor, so that there is some measurable disease against which to test the effect of treatment.

ZINGG

About adjuvant chemotherapy: Do you have any experience?

RITCHIE

No, but we have a lot of patients referred to us, who have had chemotherapy out of the context of clinical trials. Patients with superficial disease, who failed to respond to intravesical chemotherapy, given M-VAC, then referred to us for subsequent treatment. And I think that it barely needs to be said in the context of a meeting such as this that I think that there ought to be a consensus that such treatment should not be given unless in a controlled clinical trial.

JAKSE

Dr. Stoter, considering the results of Sternberg and recently Dr. Scher from the Memorial Sloan-Kettering Cancer Center (MSKCC) who reported on 93 patients who were treated by M-VAC and the complete remission rate was about 37%. I think this is a rather important argument for considering adjuvant chemotherapy. May I have your comment on this?

STOTER

That is certainly a good reason to start a randomized trial of adjuvant or neo-adjuvant chemotherapy. I do not object to that. What I object to is to go bluntly into standard treatment in an adjuvant or neo-adjuvant setting. It is a pity that there are so many studies on their way which will not give an answer to the real question.

May I also come back to the MSKCC study? The median duration of the complete response in that study on the whole is 12+ months, and the median survival of the complete response is 16 months in the whole patient population. We have compared the duration of response and the duration of survival in our subsequent phase II studies of disseminated bladder cancer in the EORTC. We have shown no benefit at all for partial responders or stable disease in terms of survival or response duration, and there is only a marginal benefit in terms of survival advantage for complete responders. So, I would be very careful and hesitant to advocate this kind of treatment on a routine basis. I would strongly plead for randomized studies.

RITCHIE

In neo-adjuvant chemotherapy: which regime and what drugs should we use? Our experience is: we are using the full M-VAC regime. We use it specifically on patients with T3b and T4 lesions. Our philosophy is that the first thing we have to establish is that there is some measurable response and we are clearly selecting patients who have palpable disease. The way we give the treatment is: two courses of full M-VAC treatment followed by a reassessment and then the patient is given another one course according to a partial or complete response before having a cystectomy.

KATO

When we analysed our data for the T2 and the T3 tumors, which were improved by preoperative adjuvant chemotherapy, the difference came only from the grade 2 groups. In the grade 3 tumors we did not get beneficial results from the neo-adjuvant systemic chemotherapy.

ZINGG

Prof. Denis, what is your treatment modality?

DENIS

I work in the large context of the EORTC and we follow the advice of our Chemotherapy Committee as closely as possible. As soon as they enlarge the potential for our studies, and if my department is able to manage that, I will enlarge it, but for the time being we stick to what we have done in phase II studies: Cisplatin and Methotrexate. We can ask Dr. Stoter, but I think he will probably take the most cautious approach.

STOTER

The usual way is to determine in metastatic disease what is the most effective regimen. Now we have basically four regimens: Cisplatin alone, Cisplatin plus Methotrexate; Cisplatin, Methotrexate plus Vinblastine and the M-VAC regimen including Adriamycin. I think the current study, comparing Cisplatin alone versus M-VAC in disseminated disease is very valuable, because it will show how much extra you get by the combination therapy, if any. Suppose the outcome will be that M-VAC is more effective in terms of response and survival, then the next step will have to be: do a comparison between M-VAC and MVC without Adriamycin, because Adriamycin is a toxic drug and you want to get rid of it. In the meantime you could launch an adjuvant study with a control arm, either with Cisplatin alone (but that has been done in protocol 7 of the NBCP, and we know that that is not very effective) or with Cisplatin-Methotrexate, but even the two drugs are rather toxic. If I may give you some figures: the EORTC study, the Stanford study, the MSKCC study and the Australian study have toxic death rates from 2, 3, 5 and 2% respectively in disseminated disease. Fourty to fifty per cent of the patients have some degree of renal function disturbance. Twenty to fourty per cent (and in the EORTC study even 70%) have grade 3 and 4 mucositis, and also bone marrow toxicity from time to time is quite a problem. So, we have to be very careful and go step by step by implementing these strategies into our treatments.

DEBRUYNE

What is the influence of these very toxic regimens on the selection of patients? Is it a regimen that is just available to a very limited number of patients in a good condition, or do you have another scheme for patients with a poor prognosis or in poor condition?

STOTER

Generally you will have to make a patient selection because of the toxicity of the regimens. It is impossible to give more than four cycles of chemotherapy. That is probably good enough in an adjuvant situation.

I want to stress the fact that the concept of neo-adjuvant chemotherapy in bladder cancer was not based on theoretical advantages on the basis of the knowledge of tumor biology, but on the fact that adjuvant chemotherapy after local treatment in protocol 7 of the NBCP appeared to be inhuman. It could not be performed safely and adequately, and the toxicity was such that the message was: "Never perform systemic treatment after local treatment anymore." That was the reason that we are today talking about the concept of neo-adjuvant chemotherapy.

ZINGG

Dr. Splinter, did you have in your patient group cases who were not fit anymore for surgery after chemotherapy?

SPLINTER

As a matter of fact, of the 20 patients that I have shown, 18 have undergone a cystectomy, one patient had not undergone a cystectomy because the surgeon chose to do so, and the other patient had a second primary in the lung and therefore did not get his cystectomy. But there were no patients who could not undergo surgery and there was no more postsurgical morbidity than we see normally.

ZINGG

What about the implements on surgery? Have you not seen any complications in the bowel surgery, for instance in creating pouches after cystectomy?

SPLINTER

No, neither in our hospital, nor in the trial forms in this EORTC study. But I think that Prof. Denis can answer the question, because he has a series of 26 patients I think.

DENIS

Of 36 patients who I thought were going to die by standard treatment 13 were omitted from the study because we wanted to give them four cycles of chemotherapy before they would undergo cystectomy. We used the tumor as a local marker for chemotherapy. Seventeen of the patients were untreated. Over 60% of them, I think 9, were free of disease and they seem to do very well, but one of them developed a carcinoma in situ. And not to my agreement, but after discussing everything with these patients, five of them opted for partial cystectomy after we agreed that this would carry a risk for them, and after we were sure that the rest of the bladder was negative. So, I would say, this is still an investigative treatment, and the only excuse to do it is if you are absolutely sure that the patient will die by being treated in the usual way.

RITCHIE

Can I ask Mr. Hall how we would manage a patient who had concomitant carcinoma in situ, perhaps recognized for the first time at his first look after one of his extensive TUR's?

HALL

We have had a relatively low incidence of concurrent carcinoma in situ, but we have had some patients who had carcinoma in situ at subsequent cystoscopy. If it was localized they had a TUR, but if it was diffuse they had intravesical chemotherapy with success. We have not had to remove a bladder because of subsequent carcinoma in situ. It might be relevant, but in our series, using TUR and Methotrexate alone, 3 out of 63 patients subsequently got a new T4a tumor or more years later. They might have had carcinoma in situ in the prostatic ducts that was missed on diagnosis.

RITCHIE

I think before we leave the question of cystectomy for all it should be said that on the other side of the Atlantic there is a very strong feeling that the assessment of such treatment should include a cystectomy and you cannot really make a statement about response without performing a cystectomy. I appreciate that this afternoon there have been a lot of statements against that general policy. Dr. Splinter would you care to comment on that?

SPLINTER

Yes, I support that idea. First of all we should not give up the treatment therapy that offers the best chance for cure for the patients without being absolutely certain that we can properly replace its effect. And we must add neo-adjuvant chemotherapy to it and then do exactly the same as we used to do and find out what the results are. I prefer the radical cystectomy, because, as I showed you, the patient who had a pT0 and still had positive lymph nodes, will teach us in the future what to do with such a patient. I think we should first maintain the potentially curative kind of treatment we have and add chemotherapy to it. We should study its effect first before jumping to the next conclusion. And we need histology for that.

I must say that I am very impressed and very afraid of the fact that everyone is taking it a little bit for granted that the primary tumor is your parameter, and if the primary tumor disappears, all tumor disappears. I am afraid that that has been proven by no one.

RITCHIE

Certainly! We have had complete pathological response in the bladder and six months, nine months later patients are relapsed with lymph node or bone metastases.

CHODAK

We are designing these studies including cystectomy without very good evidence that we are really helping the patients in getting the information we are going to derive. And that is in the following way: the people who are dying are dying of metastases. And those metastases are more than likely present when we first see those patients. It is not very likely that they develop metastases because they happen to have bladder tumor that remains and then goes on to metastasize. Therefore, I am not sure that we are doing much in saying: "You have got to have your bladder out". We are learning from them whether or not the tumor is disappearing in the bladder, but we have already seen that patients may go on to metastasize later. The bottom line is whether or not they live longer and whether or not they do live with what time they have in a minimum amount of morbidity. So, I just suggest that maybe we need to ask the patients how they want the study designed. The thing is: how can we make them live longer and how can we minimize the morbidity of the length of time. I am concerned that we are going to design our studies with surgery in mind, because we are surgeons, but not so much because the patients will be better off.

ZINGG

Summarizing we can say that with the new prospect of adjuvant therapy there is a lot of evidence that there is no sense in a trial for adjuvant chemotherapy after radical cystectomy. There are a lot of trials going on. We have to wait, but at least we should not fiddle around with chemotherapeutic agents after total cystectomy.

For neo-adjuvant chemotherapy we have to rely on and to go into prospective randomized controlled studies. And I think that that is the most important point. Otherwise we have no figures and in 1, 2 or 3 years we will have the same questions raised as just now. We have to go into these studies. And we have to operate on the patient after neo-adjuvant chemotherapy for a palpable invasive tumor, because we got to have histological proof of the results and the achievement by the therapy and because we have to offer the patient maximal therapeutic benefit as long as he is potentially curable.

Index

611